cpt® changes 2006

An Insider's View

AMA
AMERICAN
MEDICAL
ASSOCIATION

CPT® 2006 Changes: An Insider's View

www.ama-assn.org

For information regarding the reprinting or licensing of *CPT® 2006 Changes: An Insider's View*, please contact:

CPT Intellectual Property Services
American Medical Association
515 N. State St.
Chicago, IL 60610
312 464-5022

Additional copies of this book may be ordered by calling: 800 621-8335 or from the secure AMA Web site at www.amabookstore.com. Refer to product number OP512906.

ISBN: 1-57947-706-2
AC34:05-P-004:11/05

Table of Contents

Foreword

The American Medical Association is pleased to offer *CPT® Changes 2006: An Insider's View*. Since this publication was first published in 2000 it has served as the definitive text on additions, revisions, and deletions to the CPT code set.

In developing this book, it was our intention to provide CPT users with a glimpse of the logic, rationale, and proposed function of CPT changes that resulted from the decisions of the CPT Editorial Panel and the yearly update process. AMA staff members have the unique perspective of being both participants in the CPT editorial process, and users of the CPT code set. *CPT Changes* is intended to bridge understanding between clinical decisions made at the CPT Editorial Panel regarding appropriate service/procedure descriptions, with functional interpretations of coding guidelines, code intent, and code combinations necessary for users of the CPT code set. A new edition of the book is published annually.

To assist CPT users in applying new and revised CPT codes, this book includes clinical examples that describe the typical patient who might receive the procedure and detailed descriptions of the procedure. Both of these are required as a part of the CPT code change proposal process and are used by the CPT Editorial Panel in crafting language, guidelines, and parenthetical notes associated with the new or revised codes. In addition, many of the clinical examples and descriptions of the procedures are used in the AMA/Specialty Society RVS Update process for conducting surveys on physician work and in developing work relative value recommendations to the Centers for Medicare and Medicaid Services (CMS) as part of the Medicare Physician Fee Schedule (MPFS).

We are confident that the information contained in *CPT Changes* each year will prove to be a valuable resource to CPT users not only as they apply changes for the year of publication but also as a resource for frequent reference as they continue their education in CPT coding. The American Medical Association makes every effort to be a voice of clarity and consistency in an otherwise confusing system of health care claims and payment and *CPT Changes 2006: An Insider's View* demonstrates our continued commitment to assist users of the CPT code set.

Acknowledgments

Thank you to these members of the AMA:

Anthony J. Frankos, Vice President, Business Products

Mike Desposito, Publisher

Jean Roberts, Director, Production and Manufacturing

Dan Reyes, Director, CPT Product Development

Erin Kalitowski, Marketing Manager

Carol Brockman, Developmental Editor

Rosalyn Carlton, Senior Production Coordinator

Ronnie Summers, Senior Print Coordinator

Boon Ai Tan, Senior Production Coordinator

Patrick Gallagher, Director of Physician Payment Policy and Systems

Todd Klemp, Senior Policy Associate

Using This Book

This book is designed to serve as a reference guide to understanding the changes contained in *Current Procedural Terminology (CPT®) 2006* and is not intended to replace the CPT codebook. Every effort is made to ensure accuracy; however, if differences exist, you should always defer to the information contained in the CPT codebook for 2006.

The Symbols

This book uses the same coding conventions that appear in the CPT nomenclature.

- ● Indicates that a new procedure number was added to the CPT nomenclature
- ▲ Indicates that a code revision has resulted in a substantially altered procedure descriptor
- ✚ Indicates a CPT add-on code
- ⊘ Indicates a codes that is exempt from the use of modifier 51 but is not designated as a CPT add-on procedure/service
- ▶◀ Indicate revised guidelines, cross-references, and/or explanatory text
- ⊙ Indicates a code that typically includes conscious sedation
- ✔ Indicates a code for a vaccine that is pending FDA approval

The FDA approval pending symbol (✔) has been added to the list of CPT code symbols for *CPT 2006*. Some vaccine products have been assigned a CPT Category I code in anticipation of future approval from the Food and Drug Administration (FDA). Upon revision of the approval status by the FDA, notation of this revision will be provided via the AMA CPT "Category I Vaccine Codes" Internet listing (www.ama-assn.org/ama/pub/category/10902.html) and in subsequent publications of the CPT codebook. A complete list of all procedures carrying this symbol can be found in Appendix K.

Whenever possible, complete segments of text from the CPT codebook are provided; however, in some cases, the text has been abbreviated.

The Rationale

After each change or series of changes is a rationale. The rationale is intended to provide a brief explanation as to why the change(s) occurred but may not answer every question that may arise as a result of the change(s).

Reading the Clinical Examples

The clinical examples and their procedural descriptions included in this text with many of the codes give practical situations for which the new and/or revised codes in the *CPT 2006* codebook would be appropriately reported. It is important to note that these examples do not suggest limiting the use of a code but only represent the typical patient and service/procedure. They do not describe the universe of patients for whom the service/procedure would be appropriate. In addition, third-party payer reporting policies may differ.

The Tabular Review of the Changes

The table beginning on page 359 allows you to see all of the code changes at a glance. By reviewing the table you can easily determine the level to which your particular field of interest has been affected by the changes in *CPT 2006*.

CPT Codebook Text and Guidelines

Guideline and revised CPT codebook text appears in green indented type. Any revised text, guidelines, and/or headings are indicated with the ▶◀ symbols. This convention in *CPT Changes 2006* differs slightly from the CPT codebook. Within the codebook, symbols are placed at the beginning and end of a paragraph that contains a revision or revisions. *CPT Changes 2006* offers readers a more detailed view of the changes to the codes and guidelines. In this book, the revision symbols (▶◀) are placed around each specific change.

Evaluation and Management

Most notable of the revisions of the Evaluation and Management section are the deletion of the Confirmatory Consult and Follow-up Inpatient Consult subsections and the deletion of the existing Nursing Facility, Subsequent Nursing Facility Care, and Domiciliary Care codes with the addition of new codes to describe these services.

Evaluation and Management

Office or Other Outpatient Services

The following codes are used to . . .

To report services provided to a patient who is admitted to a hospital or nursing facility in the course of an encounter in the office or other ambulatory facility, see the notes for initial hospital inpatient care (page 12) or ▶initial◀ nursing facility ▶care◀ (page ▶22)◀.

For services provided by physicians in . . .

Consultations

A "consultation" initiated by a patient and/or family, and not requested by a physician, is not reported using the consultation codes but may be reported using the office visit ▶codes◀, as appropriate.

If a consultation is ▶mandated◀, eg, by a third-party payer, modifier 32 should also be reported.

If subsequent to the completion of a consultation, the consultant assumes responsibility for management of a portion or all of the patient's condition(s), the ▶appropriate **Evaluation and Management** services code for the site of service should be reported.◀ In the hospital setting, the consulting physician should use the appropriate inpatient hospital consultation code for the initial encounter and then subsequent hospital care codes. In the office setting, the appropriate established patient code should be used.

For definitions of key components and . . .

Initial Inpatient Consultations

NEW OR ESTABLISHED PATIENT

▶(99261-99263 have been deleted)◀

▶(For follow-up inpatient consultation, see 99231-99233, 99307-99310)◀

Rationale

The follow-up inpatient consultation codes 99261-99263 have been deleted with instructions to report the subsequent hospital care codes (99231-99233) or the subsequent nursing facility care codes (99307-99310) depending on the site of service. In consideration of the typical use of these codes, it was found that these codes were redundant, and that other more specific E/M codes would be more appropriately reported (eg, Subsequent Hospital Care or Subsequent Nursing Facility codes). The initial inpatient consultation codes (99251-99255), which have been retained, are to be used only once by the reporting physician for an individual hospital or nursing facility patient for a particular episode of care. For example, a subsequent consultation that may be rendered in response to a change in patient's status or availability of new information (eg, test results) provided after the initial consultation during the same inpatient admission should be reported using the subsequent hospital care codes (99231-99233) and not as an initial inpatient consultation. Follow-up consultations that are performed in order to complete the initial consultation (eg, certain tests results previously not available are now ready) should also be reported using the subsequent hospital care codes (99231-99233). If the subsequent or follow-up consultation is provided in the nursing facility setting, the subsequent nursing facility care codes (99307-99310) should be reported.

►(99271-99275 have been deleted. For confirmatory consultation, see the appropriate E/M service code for the setting and type of service (eg, consultation))◄

Rationale

The confirmatory consultation codes (99271-99275) have been deleted with instructions to report the appropriate E/M service code for the setting and type of service (eg, consultation). The confirmatory consultation codes were believed to be redundant, as other more specific E/M consultation codes are available (99241-99245, 99251-99255) to report these services. For example, when a confirmatory consultation is provided in the outpatient setting, the office consultation codes (99241-99245) should be reported. Confirmatory consultations may be requested by any number of appropriate individuals or sources including the patient. When a consultation is mandated by a third-party payer, modifier 32 should be appended to the level of consultation code reported.

Inpatient Neonatal and Pediatric Critical Care Services

The following codes (99293-99296) are used . . .

The initial day neonatal critical care . . .

►Codes 99295, 99296 are used to report services provided by a physician directing the inpatient care of a critically ill neonate through the first 28 days of life. They represent care starting with the date of admission (99295) and subsequent day(s) (99296) and may be reported only once per day, per patient.◄

►Codes 99293, 99294 are used to report services provided by a physician directing the inpatient care of a critically ill infant or young child from 29 days of postnatal age through 24 months of age. They represent care starting with the date of admission (99293) and subsequent day(s) (99294) and may be reported by a single physician only once per day, per patient in a given setting. The critically ill or critically injured child older than 24 months of age would be reported with hourly critical care service codes (99291, 99292).◄

►When a neonate or infant is not critically ill, but requires intensive observation, frequent interventions and other intensive care services, the Continuing Intensive Care Services codes (99298, 99299, 99300) should be used to report services for those neonates/infants with present body weight of 5000 grams or less. When the present body weight of those neonates/infants exceeds 5000 grams, the Subsequent Hospital Care Services codes (99231-99233) should be used.◄

▶To report critical care services provided in the outpatient setting (eg, emergency department or office) for neonates and pediatric patients up through 24 months of age, see the hourly Critical Care codes 99291, 99292. If the same physician provides critical care services for a neonatal or pediatric patient in both the outpatient and inpatient settings on the same day, report only the appropriate Neonatal or Pediatric Critical Care code (99295-99296) for all critical care services provided on that day.◀

Care rendered under 99293-99296 includes management, . . .

The pediatric and neonatal critical care codes include those procedures listed above for the hourly critical care codes (99291, 99292). In addition, the following procedures are also included in the bundled (global) pediatric and neonatal critical care service codes (99293-99296): umbilical venous (36510) and umbilical arterial catheters (36660), ▶other arterial catheters (36140, 36620),◀ central (36555) or peripheral vessel catheterization (36000), ▶vascular access procedures (36400, 36405, 36406), vascular punctures (36420, 36600),◀ oral or nasogastric tube placement (43752), endotracheal intubation (31500), lumbar puncture (62270), suprapubic bladder aspiration (51000), bladder catheterization (51701, 51702), initiation and management of mechanical ventilation (94656, 94657) or continuous positive airway pressure (CPAP) (94660), surfactant administration, intravascular fluid administration (90760-90761), transfusion of blood components (36430, 36440), invasive or non-invasive electronic monitoring of vital signs, bedside pulmonary function testing (94375), and/or monitoring or interpretation of blood gases or oxygen saturation (94760-94762). Any services performed which are not listed above should be reported separately.

For additional instructions, see descriptions listed for 99293-99296

Rationale

The Pediatric and Neonatal Intensive Care guidelines have been revised by including codes 36400, 36405, and 36406 in the list of bundled services for neonatal and pediatric critical care codes in order to provide consistency among the critical care reporting guidelines.

Inpatient Pediatric Critical Care

99293 **Initial inpatient pediatric critical care,** per day, for the evaluation and management of a critically ill infant or young child, 29 days through 24 months of age

▸Continuing◂ Intensive ▸Care◂ Services

Codes 99298, 99299▶, 99300◀ are used to report services subsequent to the day of admission provided by a physician directing the continuing intensive care of the low birth weight (LBW▶, 1500-2500 grams present body weight◀) ▶infant, ◀very low birth weight (VLBW▶, less than 1500 grams present body weight◀) infant▶, or normal weight (2501-5000 grams present body weight) newborn◀ who ▶do not ◀meet the definition of critically ill▶ but continue to require intensive observation, frequent interventions, and other intensive services◀. Codes 99298, 99299▶, 99300 represent subsequent day(s) of care and may be reported only once per calendar day, per patient and ◀are global codes with the same services bundled as outlined under codes 99293-99296.

For additional instructions, see descriptions listed for 99298, 99299▶, 99300◀.

▲99298 **Subsequent intensive care,** per day, for the evaluation and management of the recovering very low birth weight infant (present body weight less than 1500 grams)

Infants with present body weight less than 1500 grams who are ▶not◀ critically ill ▶but◀ continue to require intensive cardiac and respiratory monitoring, continuous and/or frequent vital sign monitoring, heat maintenance, enteral and/or parenteral nutritional adjustments, laboratory and oxygen monitoring and constant observation by the health care team under direct physician supervision.

▲99299 **Subsequent intensive care,** per day, for the evaluation and management of the recovering low birth weight infant (present body weight of 1500-2500 grams)

Infants with present body weight of 1500-2500 grams who are ▶not◀ critically ill ▶but◀ continue to require intensive cardiac and respiratory monitoring, continuous and/or frequent vital sign monitoring, heat maintenance, enteral and/or parenteral nutritional adjustments, laboratory and oxygen monitoring, and constant observation by the health care team under direct physician supervision.

●99300 Subsequent intensive care, per day, for the evaluation and management of the recovering infant (present body weight of 2501-5000 grams)

▶Infants with present body weight of 2501-5000 grams who are not critically ill but continue to require intensive cardiac and respiratory monitoring, continuous and/or frequent vital sign monitoring, heat maintenance, enteral and/or parenteral nutritional adjustments, laboratory and oxygen monitoring, and constant observation by the health care team under direct physician supervision.◀

Rationale

The Continuing Intensive Care Services codes are noncritical care codes for low birth weight infants (99298 and 99299) who require intensive observation, frequent interventions, or other intensive management services. Examples of such care include continuous cardiac and/or respiratory monitoring; continuous and/or frequent vital signs; temperature maintenance; enteral and/or parenteral nutritional adjustments; and laboratory and oxygen monitoring. The addition of a new code, 99300, will now allow extension of these codes to infants weighing 2501 g or more. Neonatal intensive care units (NICUs) do not limit care to low birth weight premature infants. NICUs also care for term and normal birth weight infants who are not critically ill but whose level of illness require intensive care. New code 99300 has been added for these patients whose present body weight is 2501-5000 g. Intensive care services provided to a noncritically ill infant or child weighing more than 5000 g (approximately 11 lbs) would be reported using the Subsequent Hospital Care (99231-99233) codes.

Clinical Example **(99300)**

A 3500-g neonate is recovering from bacteremia and pneumonia following intrapartum acquisition of Group B strep organisms from his mother. He had severe pneumonia, pulmonary hypertension, neutropenia, thrombocytopenia, and septic shock requiring prolonged mechanical ventilation including nitric oxide, oscillatory ventilation, surfactant, and large pressor doses to maintain perfusion and blood pressure. He is now on low flow nasal cannula oxygen; his umbilical lines have been removed and a peripherally inserted central catheter (PICC) line is being placed to complete antibiotic therapy and for use in providing bridging parenteral nutrition until he is tolerating all enteral feeds.

Description of Procedure (99300)

The patient is examined with particular attention to overall cardiovascular stability, neurological function, pulmonary status post extubation, and gastrointestinal function. Comprehensive evaluations of these organ systems are completed. The PICC line site is carefully evaluated for any signs of cellulitis. The lungs are carefully evaluated for any evidence of post extubation atelectasis. The gastrointestinal tract is evaluated for any sign of mucosal or transmural injury leading to feeding intolerance, malabsorption, or perforation. The patient is evaluated neurologically to determine if physical therapy or occupational therapy would be indicated. The patient is visited throughout the day and evening to ensure that he continues to tolerate feedings and that there has been no change in his pulmonary, cardiovascular, or neurologic function.

Nursing Facility Services

The following codes are used to . . .

These codes should also be used . . .

Nursing facilities that provide convalescent, rehabilitative, . . .

Physicians have a central role in assuring that all residents receive thorough assessments and that medical plans of care are instituted or revised to enhance or maintain the residents' physical and psychosocial functioning. ►This role includes providing input in the development of the MDS and a multi-disciplinary plan of care, as required by regulations pertaining to the care of nursing facility residents.◄

Two ►major◄ subcategories of nursing facility services are recognized: ►Initial◄ Nursing Facility ►Care◄ and Subsequent Nursing Facility Care. Both subcategories apply to new or established patients.

For definitions of key components and . . .

►Initial◄ Nursing Facility ►Care◄

NEW OR ESTABLISHED PATIENT

When the patient is admitted to . . .

Hospital discharge or observation discharge services . . .

(For nursing facility care discharge, see 99315, 99316)

►Typical unit times have not been established for 99304-99306.◄

►(99301-99303 have been deleted)◄

●99304 Initial nursing facility care, per day, for the evaluation and management of a patient which requires these three key components:

- **a detailed or comprehensive history;**
- **a detailed or comprehensive examination; and**
- **medical decision making that is straightforward or of low complexity.**

Counseling and/or coordination of care with other providers or agencies are provided consistent with the nature of the problem(s) and the patient's and/or family's needs.

Usually, the problem(s) requiring admission are of low severity.

●99305 Initial nursing facility care, per day, for the evaluation and management of a patient which requires these three key components:

- **a comprehensive history;**
- **a comprehensive examination; and**
- **medical decision making of moderate complexity.**

Counseling and/or coordination of care with other providers or agencies are provided consistent with the nature of the problem(s) and the patient's and/or family's needs.

Usually, the problem(s) requiring admission are of moderate severity.

●99306 Initial nursing facility care, per day, for the evaluation and management of a patient, which requires these three key components:

- **a comprehensive history;**
- **a comprehensive examination; and**
- **medical decision making of high complexity.**

Counseling and/or coordination of care with other providers or agencies are provided consistent with the nature of the problem(s) and the patient's and/or family's needs.

Usually, the problem(s) requiring admission are of high severity.

Subsequent Nursing Facility Care

►All levels of subsequent nursing facility care include reviewing the medical record and reviewing the results of diagnostic studies and changes in the patient's status (ie, changes in history, physical condition, and response to management) since the last assessment by the physician.◄

●99307 Subsequent nursing facility care, per day, for the evaluation and management of a patient, which requires at least two of these three key components:

- **a problem focused interval history;**
- **a problem focused examination;**
- **straightforward medical decision making.**

Counseling and/or coordination of care with other providers or agencies are provided consistent with the nature of the problem(s) and the patient's and/or family's needs.

Usually, the patient is stable, recovering, or improving.

●**99308** Subsequent nursing facility care, per day, for the evaluation and management of a patient, which requires at least two of these three key components:

- **an expanded problem focused interval history;**
- **an expanded problem focused examination;**
- **medical decision making of low complexity.**

Counseling and/or coordination of care with other providers or agencies are provided consistent with the nature of the problem(s) and the patient's and/or family's needs.

Usually, the patient is responding inadequately to therapy or has developed a minor complication.

●**99309** Subsequent nursing facility care, per day, for the evaluation and management of a patient, which requires at least two of these three key components:

- **a detailed interval history;**
- **a detailed examination;**
- **medical decision making of moderate complexity.**

Counseling and/or coordination of care with other providers or agencies are provided consistent with the nature of the problem(s) and the patient's and/or family's needs.

Usually, the patient has developed a significant complication or a significant new problem.

●**99310** Subsequent nursing facility care, per day, for the evaluation and management of a patient, which requires at least two of these three key components:

- **a comprehensive interval history;**
- **a comprehensive examination;**
- **medical decision making of high complexity.**

Counseling and/or coordination of care with other providers or agencies are provided consistent with the nature of the problem(s) and the patient's and/or family's needs.

The patient may be unstable or may have developed a significant new problem requiring immediate physician attention.

(99311-99313 have been deleted)

Nursing Facility Discharge Services

The nursing facility discharge day management . . .

99315 Nursing facility discharge day management; 30 minutes or less

99316 more than 30 minutes

▶Other Nursing Facility Services◀

●99318 Evaluation and management of a patient involving an annual nursing facility assessment, which requires these three key components:

- **a detailed interval history;**
- **a comprehensive examination; and**
- **medical decision making that is of low to moderate complexity.**

Counseling and/or coordination of care with other providers or agencies are provided consistent with the nature of the problem(s) and the patient's and/or family's needs.

Usually, the patient is stable, recovering, or improving.

(Do not report 99318 on the same date of service as nursing facility services codes 99304-99316)

Rationale

The nursing facility services section has undergone comprehensive revisions to better reflect current practices which are driven by various regulations mandated for the care of patients receiving convalescent, rehabilitative, long-term care, or psychiatric care in nursing or residential facilities. These revisions also provide consistency in format with other codes in the CPT codebook. The existing codes 99301-99303, 99311-99313 have been deleted, and replaced with new codes. The time component has been excluded from the new codes to allow new corresponding typical times to be established. The primary changes to the nursing facility services section include creation of three levels of service for admissions (initial nursing facility care 99304-99306) consistent with the structure of the three levels of service for admission in the Initial Hospital Care section of the CPT codebook; replacement of subsequent care codes with codes 99307-99309, including creation of a fourth level of service (99310) to allow the reporting of a comprehensive level of care (comprehensive interval history, comprehensive exam, high complexity decision making); and, creation of a new code (99318) in a new subsection (Other Nursing Facility Care) to allow the reporting of a comprehensive annual assessment.

Clinical Example (99304)

An 80-year-old Alzheimer's patient with associated bowel and bladder incontinence plus controlled glaucoma, hypertension, and moderate osteoarthritis arrives for an admission visit because he is no longer able to be maintained at an assisted living facility and requires nursing facility placement. He is presently on a topical eye medication, a mild analgesic, and a cholinesterase inhibitor but no psychotropics.

Description of Procedure (99304)

The admission visit includes a detailed history of dietary and fluid intake, a review of the patient's chronic but stable vision, mild hearing loss, general arthritis, chronic constipation, a medication review, and a gathering of health history from his wife, the previous assisted living staff, and his previous medical care providers. A detailed physical exam is performed. Vital signs are noted. The skin is carefully inspected for ulceration or pre-ulceration. Oral hygiene is noted. Cardiovascular, pulmonary, abdominal, and genitourinary exams are performed with special attention to any evidence of obstructive urinary retention and fecal impaction. The patient's ability to communicate and gait safety is assessed.

Clinical Example (99305)

An 88-year-old, cognitively intact patient who suffered a hip fracture from a mechanical fall while living at home presents for a skilled nursing facility (SNF) admission. While in the hospital for treatment of the fracture, he developed a urinary tract infection and a stage II heel pressure ulcer. Prior to the fracture, he was known to have multiple health problems including controlled chronic heart failure and hypertension, chronic constipation, benign prostatic hyperplasia, osteoarthritis, old cerebrovascular accident, and depression. He was also known to have peripheral perfusion compromise.

Description of Procedure (99305)

The SNF admission includes a review of the patient's intake and hydration status; the postoperative course and initial rehabilitation results; the recent urosepsis and the development of the pressure ulcer; plus an evaluation of the status of the patient's multiple chronic health problems. A comprehensive physical exam is performed to assess the recent surgical site, the potential return of function, the need for the continued indwelling catheter, and the status of the pressure sore. Additionally, an examination of the patient's vision and hearing (especially in relation to rehabilitation potential), overall cardiovascular status in regard to stamina, plus a general abdominal, genitourinary, mental status, and neurological examination is performed and documented. A multidisciplinary plan of care is developed that includes physical therapy and occupational therapy services, initiation of a pressure wound care program, adjustments in diet, weaning off of the catheter, re-titration of medications, evaluation of dietary and fluid intake, and monitoring for mental status changes due to changes in environment.

Clinical Example (99306)

A 72-year-old diabetic patient who previously lived at the same skilled nursing facility (SNF) is now being admitted post hospitalization to the SNF for aspiration pneumonitis, blood sugars running in the 300+ range, chronic heart failure, and delirium associated with an ongoing history of dementia. She also suffers from chronic atrial fibrillation, constipation, stress incontinence, and a recent vertebral compression fracture associated with osteoporosis. She returns on IV hydration, antibiotics, O_2, and new psychotropics. She also requires continued titration of her diabetes and diuretic regimen, control of her pain (which is reducing her inspiratory effort), rehabilitation of swallowing and respiratory function, and stabilization of her cardiovascular and mental status.

Description of Procedure (99306)

The admission includes a comprehensive history including a review of the hospital records, labs and diagnostic findings, the patient's intake and hydration status, plus a review of the sliding scale insulin and psychotropic regimen. Additionally, there is a discussion with the patient's formal and informal care providers regarding a symptom review of the patient's multiple, still unstable, health problems. The comprehensive physical exam involved assessment of the current status of cardiopulmonary function, swallowing and mobility function, and cognitive function. Lab review includes assessing oxygenation, hydration, white count, cardiac rhythm, and glucose level trends. Orders are initiated for oxygen, IV fluids, antibiotics, pain control, and rehabilitation and diagnostic testing to assess status. Also, included in the multidisciplinary plan of care is physical therapy, repiratory therapy, and speech services; titration off of the insulin sliding scale; adjustments in diet and hydration; re-titration of psychotropic and analgesic medications; and monitoring for mental status changes.

Clinical Example (99307)

An 88-year-old demented, nondiabetic patient with a previously evaluated stage IV sacral pressure sore with peripheral, localized inflammation is seen in follow-up to evaluate the wound's response to the present plan of care.

Description of Procedure (99307)

The visit includes an interval history that reveals ongoing poor dietary intake and urinary incontinence in a patient who cannot cooperate in pressure relief activities because of cognitive impairment. It also includes a focused physical exam that reveals an improving lesion with no peripheral inflammation and no evidence of systemic involvement. The topical regimen is altered, a new nutritional program is ordered, and a support surface is authorized.

Clinical Example (99308)

During a nursing facility visit for evaluation and management of an acute urinary tract infection (UTI) in a 35-year-old male with multiple sclerosis with indwelling catheter, the patient presents with a new intermittent hematuria and fever.

Description of Procedure (99308)

The visit includes an expanded history review including intake and hydration information, discussion of the suprapubic-localizing discomfort and muscle spasm, and a psychosocial review of the patient's coping with his underlying disease. An expanded physical examination notes no evidence of dehydration, further gross hematuria, or focal neurological findings, but increased depression is detected. After necessary labs are ordered, he is treated for the UTI and started on an antidepressant.

Clinical Example (99309)

A 72-year-old patient with chronic obstructive pulmonary disease (COPD), hypertension, peripheral vascular disease, gastroesophageal reflux disease (GERD), chronic constipation, bladder stress incontinence, osteoarthritis, osteoporosis, dementia, and hypothyroidism on more than nine medications is seen for interval disease management of her chronic health issues and also to evaluate the status of a recent URI, increased constipation, new behavioral changes, and a skin tear that has occurred since the last medical visit.

Description of Procedure (99309)

The visit includes a detailed interval history review of each involved organ system that has an acute or active medical problem. This includes the status of the recent URI complicating her underlying COPD, any associated cardiovascular complication or decline, the status of the GERD, bowel and bladder function, and the recent change in mental status associated with the patient's dementia. Also included in the history is (a) a review of the patient's multiple medications for indication and efficacy; (b) recent lab and diagnostic data ordered to evaluate her recent respiratory compromise; and (c) the updated nursing plan of care. A detailed physical exam reveals a "frailer" more confused patient with normal vitals, resting comfortably in bed with a dry oral mucosa, "clear" lung fields, regular rhythm with no change in her AS murmur, no pedal edema, a vaguely tender abdomen, no lateralizing neurological signs, and a noninflamed skin tear.

Clinical Example (99310)

A 69-year-old, long-time resident of a nursing facility with a long history of multi-infarct dementia, non-insulin dependent diabetes mellitus, hypertension, and chronic renal insufficiency develops an acute decline in mental status with decreased intake and vague right-sided weakness. The family requests that she not be transferred to the hospital but receive treatment at the facility. Her blood pressure is 188/102, pulse 92/regular, and respirations are 20/min off O_2. Physical examination reveals a dry mucosa and decreased skin turgor, no cyanosis, reduced lung sounds, no pedal or sacral edema, a soft, nondistended abdomen, and a slight right hemiparesis. Lab values drawn just prior to visit reveal blood glucose 352, Na 152, BUN 78, creatinine 2.8, Hct 32, Hb10.1, a WBC of 18.0, O_2 sat of 87% on room air, and a portable chest X ray that "cannot rule out" an left lower lobe pneumonia.

Description of Procedure (99310)

The visit includes a comprehensive history including evaluation of hydration and intake, ability to swallow, cardiopulmonary status, abdominal bowel and bladder function, mental status, and sensori-motor function. The multifactorial etiologies and their effect on multiple, additional comorbidities require a comprehensive physical examination involving virtually every organ system. The resultant multidisciplinary care planning includes IV hydration and antibiotic therapy; nursing instructions regarding the monitoring of respiratory, mental, functional, and diabetic status; a respiratory therapy and physical therapy assessment with treatment as indicated; and further lab monitoring to track the effectiveness of the treatment.

Clinical Example (99318)

An annual nursing facility history, physical, and minimum data set/resident assessment instrument evaluation is undertaken for a 2-year nursing facility resident who is an 84-year-old female with multiple chronic health problems, including stable controlled hypertension, chronic constipation, osteoarthritis, and moderated stable dementia.

Description of Procedure **(99318)**

The visit includes a detailed review of the interval history for the occurrence and resolution of intercurrent episodes of illness or injury and for signs and symptoms of progression of the chronic conditions that justify continued nursing facility services. A review of systems may include an assessment of dietary and fluid intake with note of any dental concerns or changes in appetite; a review of worsening sensory impairments, such as vision or hearing loss; changes in functional level, especially related to mobility or continence, that might be amenable to therapy; a medication review with attention to the accumulation of therapies no longer needed and that screening tests for toxicity, side effects, and efficacy have been performed; and a review of any noted changes in behavior or affect. Also included is a review of compliance with routine specialty follow-up care and that health maintenance measures have been provided. Social history includes the relationship of the family with the patient, the staff, and the facility. A comprehensive physical exam is performed. Vital signs are noted, including a review of the patient's weight throughout the previous year. The skin is carefully inspected for ulceration. Evidence of sensory impairments and the status of oral hygiene is noted. Cardiovascular, pulmonary, abdominal, and genitourinary exams are performed with special attention to evidence of urinary retention and fecal impaction. The patient's ability to communicate and gait safety is assessed. Short form evaluations of interval changes in cognitive functioning and a screen for affective changes may be performed, as indicated. Assessment is made of the patient's and family's goals for care and their preferences for medical interventions, in light of the prognosis derived from the review of the chart, the interval history, and the physical examination.

Domiciliary, Rest Home (eg, Boarding Home), or Custodial Care Services

The following codes are used to report evaluation and management services in a facility which provides room, board and other personal assistance services, generally on a long-term basis. ►They also are used to report evaluation and management services in an assisted living facility.◄

►The facility's services do not include a medical component.◄

For definitions of key components and . . .

►(For care plan oversight services provided to a patient in a domiciliary facility under the individual supervision of a physician, see 99339, 99340)◄

►(99321-99323 have been deleted)◄

NEW PATIENT

●**99324** Domiciliary or rest home visit for the evaluation and management of a new patient, which requires these three key components:

- **a problem focused history;**
- **a problem focused examination; and**
- **straightforward medical decision making.**

Counseling and/or coordination of care with other providers or agencies are provided consistent with the nature of the problem(s) and the patient's and/or family's needs.

Usually, the presenting problem(s) are of low severity. Physicians typically spend 20 minutes with the patient and/or family or caregiver.

●**99325** Domiciliary or rest home visit for the evaluation and management of a new patient, which requires these three key components:

- **an expanded problem focused history;**
- **an expanded problem focused examination; and**
- **medical decision making of low complexity.**

Counseling and/or coordination of care with other providers or agencies are provided consistent with the nature of the problem(s) and the patient's and/or family's needs.

Usually, the presenting problem(s) are of moderate severity. Physicians typically spend 30 minutes with the patient and/or family or caregiver.

●**99326** Domiciliary or rest home visit for the evaluation and management of a new patient, which requires these three key components:

- **a detailed history;**
- **a detailed examination; and**
- **medical decision making of moderate complexity.**

Counseling and/or coordination of care with other providers or agencies are provided consistent with the nature of the problem(s) and the patient's and/or family's needs.

Usually, the presenting problem(s) are of moderate to high severity. Physicians typically spend 45 minutes with the patient and/or family or caregiver.

●**99327** Domiciliary or rest home visit for the evaluation and management of a new patient, which requires these three key components:

- **a comprehensive history;**
- **a comprehensive examination; and**
- **medical decision making of moderate complexity.**

Counseling and/or coordination of care with other providers or agencies are provided consistent with the nature of the problem(s) and the patient's and/or family's needs.

Usually, the presenting problem(s) are of high severity. Physicians typically spend 60 minutes with the patient and/or family or caregiver.

●99328 Domiciliary or rest home visit for the evaluation and management of a new patient, which requires these three key components:

- **a comprehensive history;**
- **a comprehensive examination; and**
- **medical decision making of high complexity.**

Counseling and/or coordination of care with other providers or agencies are provided consistent with the nature of the problem(s) and the patient's and/or family's needs.

Usually, the patient is unstable or has developed a significant new problem requiring immediate physician attention. Physicians typically spend 75 minutes with the patient and/or family or caregiver.

ESTABLISHED PATIENT

▶(99331-99333 have been deleted)◀

●99334 Domiciliary or rest home visit for the evaluation and management of an established patient, which requires at least two of these three key components:

- **a problem focused interval history;**
- **a problem focused examination;**
- **straightforward medical decision making.**

Counseling and/or coordination of care with other providers or agencies are provided consistent with the nature of the problem(s) and the patient's and/or family's needs.

Usually, the presenting problem(s) are self-limited or minor. Physicians typically spend 15 minutes with the patient and/or family or caregiver.

●99335 Domiciliary or rest home visit for the evaluation and management of an established patient, which requires at least two of these three key components:

- **an expanded problem focused interval history;**
- **an expanded problem focused examination;**
- **medical decision making of low complexity.**

Counseling and/or coordination of care with other providers or agencies are provided consistent with the nature of the problem(s) and the patient's and/or family's needs.

Usually, the presenting problem(s) are of low to moderate severity. Physicians typically spend 25 minutes with the patient and/or family or caregiver.

●99336 Domiciliary or rest home visit for the evaluation and management of an established patient, which requires at least two of these three key components:

- **a detailed interval history;**
- **a detailed examination;**
- **medical decision making of moderate complexity.**

⊘=Modifier 51 Exempt ⊙=Conscious Sedation ✚=Add-on Code ⁄⁄=FDA approval pending

Counseling and/or coordination of care with other providers or agencies are provided consistent with the nature of the problem(s) and the patient's and/or family's needs.

Usually, the presenting problem(s) are of moderate to high severity. Physicians typically spend 40 minutes with the patient and/or family or caregiver.

●**99337** Domiciliary or rest home visit for the evaluation and management of an established patient, which requires at least two of these three key components:

- **a comprehensive interval history;**
- **a comprehensive examination; and**
- **medical decision making of moderate to high complexity.**

Counseling and/or coordination of care with other providers or agencies are provided consistent with the nature of the problem(s) and the patient's and/or family's needs.

Usually, the presenting problem(s) are of moderate to high severity. The patient may be unstable or may have developed a significant new problem requiring immediate physician attention. Physicians typically spend 60 minutes with the patient and/or family or caregiver.

Rationale

The domiciliary, rest home, or custodial care services section has undergone comprehensive revisions to better capture the level of care provided in these settings consistent with the increase of patients with complex diseases who are eligible for this type of care (eg, Alzheimer patients) who remain in non-medical facilities to receive care made possible through advances in diagnostic and therapeutic technologies. The previous codes (99321-99323, 99331-99333) have been deleted and replaced with new codes (99324-99328, 99334-99337) that allow reporting higher levels of services provided to both new and established domiciliary and rest home patients with increasing medical complexity and frailty, due to mandates for movement of these patients from the hospital setting. Additionally, these new codes are applicable to evaluation and management services in assisted living facilities.

Clinical Example 1 (99324)

An 84-year-old male with advanced osteoarthritis, which has rendered him wheelchair bound and left him with persistent pain, is controlled on his current regimen.

Clinical Example 2 (99324)

An 84-year-old male with advanced osteoarthritis, which has rendered him wheelchair bound, complains of a rash and itching involving the plantar surface of the foot.

Description of Procedure (99324)

The intraservice period includes the services provided while the physician is with the patient and/or family. This includes the time in which the physician obtains the history, performs an evaluation, and counsels the patient.

Clinical Example 1 (99325)

An 85-year-old woman with non-insulin dependent diabetes, peripheral neuropathy with loss of sensory perception, hypertension, and heart failure was hospitalized 2 months ago with hypoglycemia. The patient has not kept appointments at the outpatient clinic due to dyspnea and fear of falling. Other related problems include very poor vision.

Clinical Example 2 (99325)

An 84-year-old male with advanced osteoarthritis and peripheral vascular disease, which has rendered him wheelchair bound, is followed for vascular insufficiency ulcers that have healed after treatment with custom shoes and topical wound care.

Description of Procedure (99325)

The intraservice period includes the services provided while the physician is with the patient and/or family. This includes the time in which the physician obtains the history, performs an evaluation, and counsels the patient.

Clinical Example (99326)

A 77-year-old woman with aortic valve replacement is maintained on Coumadin. Her past medical history includes atrial fibrillation and insulin dependent diabetes. She has had several falls recently. Anti-coagulation and diabetic management have been in good control through close monitoring by the nurse in the assisted living facility.

Preservice work includes record review of her previous primary care and assisted living facility records and communication with other professionals as appropriate. A detailed history includes an evaluation of antecedent symptoms to the falls, as well as adherence to diet, compliance with medications, glucose and anti-coagulation monitoring schedule, and the level of family support. A detailed examination includes vital signs in various positions; assessment of her cognitive status and stability of gait; and a detailed examination of the cardiac, musculoskeletal, and neurologic systems. A plan of care is developed that includes initiation of in-home physical therapy and adjustments, as appropriate, in diet, glucose monitoring, and medications. Postservice work includes telephone calls with the patient or family, plus all coordination of care, documentation, and interaction with other health professionals associated with delivery of care to this patient until the next face-to-face encounter.

Description of Procedure (99326)

The intraservice period includes the services provided while the physician is with the patient and/or family. This includes the time in which the physician obtains the history, performs an evaluation, and counsels the patient.

Clinical Example (99327)

A family refers a 73-year-old female patient for evaluation and management. Despite having been moved to an assisted living facility, she has had progressive weight loss, social withdrawal, and intermittent agitation over the past 2 months. She refuses to leave her room for visits to her physicians. Her meals are brought to her, but she eats sparingly. The patient has been followed through telephonic conversations between the nurse and the primary care physician, who has been ordering psychotropic medications to control behavior, and a cardiologist for management of her ischemic heart disease for which she takes four medications. She has seen neither physician for more than a year.

Preservice work includes a record review and communication with other professionals as appropriate. A comprehensive history includes signs and symptoms of depression and delirium, past medical history, review of systems, functional status, diet, medications, social interactions, and level of family support. An examination includes a comprehensive physical, functional assessment, and mental status testing. The patient is interviewed for depression and suicidal ideation. A new plan of care is developed, which includes adjustments in medications and diet, and the patient is referred to a visiting mental health counselor. Laboratory tests are drawn. Postservice work includes telephone calls with the patient or family and facility, plus all coordination of care, documentation, and interaction with other health professionals associated with delivery of care to this patient until the next face-to-face physician encounter.

Description of Procedure (99327)

The intraservice period includes the services provided while the physician is with the patient and/or family. This includes the time in which the physician obtains the history, performs an evaluation, and counsels the patient.

Clinical Example (99328)

An 83-year-old male presents with a history of schizophrenia, progressive neurologic degeneration with dementia, emphysema from smoking, osteoporosis with vertebral fractures and kyphosis, non-insulin dependent diabetes mellitus, and osteoarthritis of the back, hips, and knees. He now has a fever of 101.5°, productive cough, tachypnea, and delirium. Oral intake has dropped sharply for the past 2 days. His family does not want him to be hospitalized, accepts that this may be a terminal event, but wants to take all available measures to help him recover at the group home. The resident counselor is willing to participate in providing intravenous therapies.

Preservice work includes record review and communication with other professionals as appropriate. A comprehensive history includes the present illness, review of medications, glucose monitoring records, level of functional and mental status, and an assessment of the family's intentions. An examination includes vital signs; a comprehensive examination of the pulmonary, cardiac, musculoskeletal, and neuropsychiatric systems; and an assessment of the level of decisional capacity. Orders are initiated for IV fluids; antibiotics and oxygen with an infusion service; and daily nursing visits through a home care agency. Blood is drawn for laboratory testing and a portable radiography is ordered to verify the pneumonia. Postservice work includes review of the test results, telephone calls with the patient or family, instruction of the counselor, plus all coordination of care, documentation, and interaction with other health professionals associated with delivery of care to this patient until the next face-to-face physician encounter.

Description of Procedure (99328)

The intraservice period includes the services provided while the physician is with the patient and/or family. This includes the time in which the physician obtains the history, performs an evaluation, and counsels the patient.

Clinical Example (99334)

A 74-year-old man with hypertension and peripheral vascular disease has lived in a board and care home for 2 years following a stroke that resulted in right-sided hemiparesis. The patient is seen routinely for hypertension monitoring, medication refills, and preventive care.

Preservice work includes record review and communication with other professionals, as appropriate. Interval history includes stability of neurologic deficits, medication compliance with assessment for side-effects or toxicity, and adherence to diet; a review of systems includes a history of falls, incontinence, constipation, and cognitive status. An examination includes vital signs and a focused evaluation of the cardiovascular or neurologic systems. Medications are refilled, as appropriate. Postservice work includes telephone calls with the patient or his family plus all coordination of care, documentation, and interaction with other health professionals associated with delivery of care to this patient until the next face-to-face encounter.

Description of Procedure (99334)

The intraservice period includes the services provided while the physician is with the patient and/or family. This includes the time in which the physician obtains the history, performs an evaluation, and counsels the patient.

Clinical Example (99335)

A 78-year-old man with Alzheimer's disease had been agitated due to hallucinations and difficult to control for 2 weeks. Psychotropic medications were initiated with partial resolution of the agitation. The aides at the assisted living facility ensure his safety but are worried that he might fall.

Preservice work includes record review and communication with other professionals, as appropriate. A history includes a review of changes in behavior during the interval since the medications were begun and of any new neurologic symptoms. An expanded interval exam includes an assessment for change in behavior and neurologic assessment for medication side effects. Behavioral modifications are suggested for the staff and medications are adjusted as indicated. Postservice work includes follow-up of the laboratory tests, telephone calls with the family and facility staff plus all coordination of care, documentation, and interaction with other health professionals associated with delivery of care to this patient until the next face-to-face physician encounter.

Description of Procedure (99335)

The intraservice period includes the services provided while the physician is with the patient and/or family. This includes the time in which the physician obtains the history, performs an evaluation, and counsels the patient.

Clinical Example (99336)

A 78-year-old male patient with insulin dependent diabetes mellitus and chronic obstructive pulmonary disease, requiring continuous home oxygen, complains of worsening symptoms of peripheral vascular disease. He is becoming progressively more dependent for assistance with transfers and bathing. He complains of increasing left leg pain at night due to nocturnal ischemic claudication.

Preservice work includes record review and communication with other professionals, as appropriate. A history at the assisted living facility includes a detailed assessment of the changes in pain, functional status, and skin integrity; recent changes in caregiver support needs; and review of glucose monitoring and nutritional intake. A detailed examination includes the cardiovascular system and inspection of the skin with Doppler-assisted ankle-branchial index assessment; focused examination includes the patient's pulmonary status and bedside pulse oximetry. Blood is drawn to evaluate diabetic control. Postservice work includes a follow-up of the test results, telephone calls with the patient or his family, plus all coordination of care, documentation, and interaction with other health professionals associated with delivery of care to this patient until the next face-to-face physician encounter.

Description of Procedure (99336)

The intraservice period includes the services provided while the physician is with the patient and/or family. This includes the time in which the physician obtains the history, performs an evaluation, and counsels the patient.

Clinical Example (99337)

An 89-year-old female with a history of multi-infarct dementia, due to hypertension and insulin dependent diabetes mellitus, and chronic renal insufficiency has worsened with difficult to control hypertension and progressively more fatigue; but the nephrologist is reluctant to offer dialysis. Approximately 1 year ago, the patient became wheelchair bound and nonverbal. For 4 months, she has been unable to feed herself. Last month, she began to "pocket" her medications and solid foods in her cheek and was found to spit them out later. She has lost weight within the past 3 months, which has been associated with several episodes of hypoglycemia, and she recently developed a stage 3 pressure ulcer at her coccyx. Her family has been undecided as to resuscitation status.

Preservice work includes record review and communication with other professionals as appropriate. Comprehensive history includes a review of the interval changes in functional status, medications, glucose, blood pressure, and weight monitoring; cognitive and affective status; and an assessment of patient behavior. Comprehensive examination includes the cardiac, pulmonary, gastrointestinal, genitourinary, and neuro-psychiatric systems. She is also evaluated for anasarca and nutritional status. Decision making includes a review of the medication regimen in light of the progressive renal failure, delivery of instructions to the staff regarding monitoring parameters and updating the family, and emphasis on end-of-life care counseling. Postservice work includes telephone calls with the family and facility staff, coordination of all care, documentation, and interaction with other health professionals associated with delivery of care to this patient until the next face-to-face physician encounter.

Description of Procedure (99337)

The intraservice period includes the services provided while the physician is with the patient and/or family. This includes the time in which the physician obtains the history, performs an evaluation, and counsels the patient.

▸Domiciliary, Rest Home (eg, Assisted Living Facility), or Home Care Plan Oversight Services◂

▶(For instructions on the use of 99339, 99340, see introductory notes for 99374-99380)◀

▶(For care plan oversight services for patients under the care of a home health agency, hospice, or nursing facility, see 99374-99380)◀

●**99339** Individual physician supervision of a patient (patient not present) in home, domiciliary or rest home (eg, assisted living facility) requiring complex and multidisciplinary care modalities involving regular physician development and/or revision of care plans, review of subsequent reports of patient status, review of related laboratory and other studies, communication (including telephone calls) for purposes of assessment or care decisions with health care professional(s), family member(s), surrogate decision maker(s) (eg, legal guardian) and/or key caregiver(s) involved in patient's care, integration of new information into the medical treatment plan and/or adjustment of medical therapy, within a calendar month; 15-29 minutes

●**99340** 30 minutes or more

▶(Do not report 99339, 99340 for patients under the care of a home health agency, enrolled in a hospice program, or for nursing facility residents)◀

Home Services

▶(For care plan oversight services provided to a patient in the home under the individual supervision of a physician, see 99339, 99340)◀

Care Plan Oversight Services

Care Plan Oversight Services are reported . . .

The work involved in providing very . . .

▶(For care plan oversight services of patients in the home, domiciliary, or rest home (eg, assisted living facility) under the individual supervision of a physician, see 99339, 99340)◀

Rationale

The limitation imposed by the nursing facility setting designation of codes 99379 and 99380 prompted creation of two new codes 99339 and 99340, to describe care plan oversight services for patients receiving care in their home, domiciliary, or rest home (eg, assisted living facility) not provided under the auspices of a home health agency or hospice program.

Codes 99339, 99340 have been established to report the same services already described in existing codes 99379 and 99380 for care plan oversight services of patients residing in a nursing facility (eg, development and/or revision of care plans; review of subsequent reports of patient status; review of related laboratory and other studies; communication (including telephone calls) for purposes of assessment or care decisions with health care professional(s), family member(s), surrogate decision maker(s) (eg, legal guardian), and/or key caregiver(s) involved in patient's care; integration of new information into the medical treatment plan; and/or adjustment of medical therapy). All of the care plan oversight codes are time based, and are intended to be used only once within any given calendar month.

Codes 99339 and 99340 are intended to report care plan oversight services of children and adults with special health care needs and chronic medical conditions provided by primary care physicians who coordinate the medical care management with other medical and nonmedical service providers and family. These codes may encompass oversight of work or school programs the patient may be attending where therapy is provided.

A parenthetical note was added to exclude use of codes 99339, 99340 for nursing facility residents, patients enrolled in a hospice program, or patients under the care of a home health agency.

Clinical Example 1 (99339)

A 21-year-old with Down's syndrome is transitioning from home care and public special education to a sheltered work program operated by the community service agency. He is moderately mentally retarded and ongoing medical problems include hypothyroidism and sensorineural hearing loss. Over the past 2 months, his behavior has become progressively disruptive. His previously developed care plan includes the active medical and educational or vocational problems with ongoing adjustments being made based on feedback from the family and other health care professionals and service providers. The primary care physician (internal medicine, family physician, pediatrician) delivers primary care services and manages and coordinates care plan activities. Typical ongoing care plan oversight activities include:

- Review of reports including a new audiology assessment and endocrine consultation report
- Telephone call to the audiologist about results of the most recent hearing assessment and recommendations to provide hearing amplification to the patient

- Completion of medical forms for the vocational program listing medical problems, general cognitive and physical abilities, and recommendations for behavior management
- Discussion by phone with the family of recent appetite and weight gain noted by the family after beginning a new behavior medication and a subsequent call to the psychiatric nurse practitioner at the mental health center who recommends a dose change and a dietary consultation
- Review of endocrine recommendations to increase the thyroid dosage, with an ensuing telephone call to the family and pharmacy to prescribe a different dose form of Synthroid

The physician documents the relevant information in the record that summarizes these activities.

Clinical Example 2 (99339)

The patient is an 84-year-old female who lives with her daughter. She has advanced Alzheimer's disease and is dependent in all instrumental activities of daily living and most activities of daily living. She has begun to become increasingly agitated. She could not cooperate sufficiently to be brought to the office for evaluation so a home visit was made (reported separately). Over the next month, the physician will need to review the care of the patient, assessing progress and the effects of the interventions. This requires contact with the caregiver to review effects and to support the caregiver to avoid hospitalization and the likely cycle of delirium and nursing home placement that would result. Between 15 and 29 minutes are spent and documented in these activities.

Description of Procedure (99339)

Communication is provided for the purposes of assessment or care decisions with health care professional(s), family member(s), and/or key caregivers(s). A care plan is developed or revised.

Clinical Example 1 (99340)

A 21-year-old with Down's syndrome is transitioning from home care and public special education to a sheltered work program operated by the community service agency. He is moderately mentally retarded and ongoing medical problems include hypothyroidism and sensorineural hearing loss. Within the past 2 months, his behavior has become progressively disruptive. His previously developed care plan includes the active medical and educational or vocational problems with ongoing adjustments being made based on feedback from the family and other health care professionals and service providers. The primary care physician (internal medicine, family physician, pediatrician) delivers primary care services and manages and coordinates care plan activities. Typical ongoing care plan oversight activities include:

- Review of reports including a new audiology assessment and endocrine consultation report

- Telephone call to the audiologist about results of the most recent hearing assessment and recommendations to provide hearing amplification to the patient
- Completion of medical forms for the vocational program listing medical problems, general cognitive and physical abilities, and recommendations for behavior management
- Discussion by telephone with the family of recent appetite and weight gain noted by the family after beginning a new behavior medication and a subsequent call to the psychiatric nurse practitioner at the mental health center who recommends a dose change and a dietary consultation
- Review of endocrine recommendations to increase the thyroid dosage with an ensuing telephone call to the family and pharmacy to prescribe a different dose form of Synthroid

The physician documents the relevant information in the record that summarizes these activities.

Clinical Example 2 (99340)

The patient is an 84-year-old female who lives with her daughter. She has advanced Alzheimer's disease and is dependent in all instrumental activities of daily living and most activities of daily living. She has begun to become increasingly agitated. She could not cooperate sufficiently to be brought to the office for evaluation so a home visit was made (reported separately). Over the next month, the physician will need to review the care of the patient, assessing progress and the effects of the interventions. This requires contact with the caregiver to review effects and to support the caregiver to avoid hospitalization and the likely cycle of delirium and nursing home placement that would result. Thirty minutes or more are spent and documented in these activities.

Description of Procedure (99340)

Communication is provided for the purposes of assessment or care decisions with health care professional(s), family member(s), and or key caregivers(s). A care plan is developed or revised.

Anesthesia

Excluding minor editorial modifications, the revision of the Anesthesia section consists solely of the addition of two new codes to differentiate anesthesia services for incomplete or missed abortions and induced abortions and the revision of the Anesthesia guidelines to reflect the addition of new codes to report moderate sedation.

Anesthesia

Guidelines

Services involving administration of anesthesia are reported by the use of the anesthesia five-digit procedure code (00100-01999) plus modifier codes (defined under "Anesthesia Modifiers" later in these Guidelines).

The reporting of anesthesia services is . . .

Items used by all physicians in reporting their services are presented in the **Introduction.** Some of the commonalities are repeated in this section for the convenience of those physicians referring to this section on **Anesthesia.** Other definitions and items unique to anesthesia are also listed.

To report ▶moderate (conscious)◀ sedation provided by a physician also performing the service for which conscious sedation is being provided, see codes ▶99143-99145◀.

▶For the procedures listed in Appendix G, when a second physician other than the health care professional performing the diagnostic or therapeutic services provides moderate (conscious) sedation in the facility setting (eg, hospital, outpatient hospital/ambulatory surgery center, skilled nursing facility), the second physician reports the associated moderate sedation procedure/service 99148-99150; when these services are performed by the second physician in the nonfacility setting (eg, physician office, freestanding imaging center), codes 99148-99150 would not be reported. Moderate sedation does not include minimal sedation (anxiolysis), deep sedation, or monitored anesthesia care (00100-01999).◀

Rationale

The Anesthesia guidelines have been revised to instruct the circumstances for which codes 99148-99150 would be appropriately reported. Codes 99148-99150 were established to report moderate sedation services requiring the services of a second physician who is not performing the diagnostic or therapeutic procedure. Codes 99148-99150 are only reported by the second physician with the procedures listed in Appendix G when performed in the facility setting. When performed in the nonfacility setting, the efforts of the second physician are not reported with the codes in Appendix G because moderate sedation is included in these codes.

Obstetric

▶(01964 has been deleted. To report, see 01965, 01966)◀

●**01965** Anesthesia for incomplete or missed abortion procedures

●**01966** Anesthesia for induced abortion procedures

Rationale

Codes 01965 and 01966 have been added to *CPT 2006* to differentiate anesthesia for two different types of abortion procedures: spontaneous (incomplete or missed)

and induced abortions. Previously, code 01964 was used to identify anesthesia for either type of procedure and did not distinguish between the two types of anesthesia because the services were similar in performance. Codes 01965 and 01966 have been established to differentiate the varied types of abortions thus allowing physicians to specify the type of service for which the anesthesia service is being provided.

Spontaneous abortions are abortions that have not been artificially induced. This includes incomplete abortions (abortions in which part of the products of conception such as the placenta remain in the uterus) and missed abortion (abortions in which the fetus dies in utero but is retained within the mother's body for 2 months or longer). Induced abortions are abortions brought about by chemical or mechanical means. Because payment implications may be tied to each service, the anesthesia services have been differentiated to identify the specific type of anesthesia provided.

To accommodate the addition of codes 01965 and 01966, code 01964 has been deleted. A cross-reference has been included after code 01964 to identify the specific codes to use (01965, 01966) when identifying the type of anesthesia service provided.

Clinical Example (01965)

A 24-year-old female presents with a positive pregnancy test and heavy vaginal bleeding that started 1 day prior. By the last menstrual period, she should be 10-weeks pregnant. She denies passing tissue but has had large clots. On exam, she has a dilated cervical os with tissue at the os. The patient undergoes surgical treatment of an incomplete abortion.

Description of Procedure (01965)

An 18-gauge intravenous (IV) catheter was inserted in the patient's left forearm. After receiving a fluid bolus of crystalloid fluid, to correct her tachycardia, she received 2 mg of midazolam and 10 mg of metoclopramide and was taken to the operating room (OR). After moving to the OR table, EKG, non-invasive blood pressure, and pulse oximetry monitors were attached. Oxygen was administered by mask, and anesthesia was induced. Desflurane was added to the inspired oxygen, and she was ventilated by hand. After approximately 60 seconds, a laryngeal mask airway (LMA) was inserted. Proper positioning was ensured by chest movement and a satisfactory wave form and numerical value on the end-tidal CO_2 monitor. The patient was gently ventilated by hand for an additional 4 to 5 minutes before spontaneous respirations resumed. The patient was put in the lithotomy position, and after a vaginal prep, the procedure commenced.

At the request of the surgeon, 20 units of pitocin were added to the Ringer's Lactate solution that was infusing via the IV. Also, as prophylaxis against nausea, 4 mg of ondansetron was given by IV. The procedure lasted 20 minutes. Estimated blood loss was 150 cc.

At the conclusion of the procedure, the patient was taken out of the lithotomy position. The desflurane had been discontinued as the surgeon announced that she was finished; the patient was still breathing spontaneously and the LMA was removed 1 or 2 minutes later. The patient was moved to a recovery stretcher and taken to the post anesthesia care unit (PACU). Report was given to the PACU nurse as the monitors were being applied. After ensuring that the patient's condition was satisfactory, the anesthesiologist transferred care to the PACU nurse. A hemoglobin was obtained, demonstrating a slight additional drop to 9.5. After discussion with the surgeon, the decision was made to manage the patient's anemia conservatively.

Clinical Example (01966)

A 30-year-old female is pregnant. At 13-weeks gestation, an ultrasound reveals that her fetus has anencephaly. She consults her obstetrician about a termination of pregnancy. Except for some seasonal reactive airway disease, she is in otherwise good health.

Description of Procedure (01966)

An 18-gauge intravenous (IV) catheter was inserted in the patient's left forearm; she was given 2 mg of midazolam and 10 mg of metoclopramide and taken to the operating room (OR). After moving to the OR table, EKG, non-invasive blood pressure, and pulse oximetry monitors were attached. Oxygen was administered by mask, and anesthesia was induced with 100 mcg of fentanyl and 150 mg of propofol. Desflurane was added to the inspired oxygen, and she was ventilated by hand. After approximately 60 seconds, a laryngeal mask airway (LMA) was inserted. Proper positioning was ensured by chest movement and a satisfactory wave form and numerical value on the end-tidal CO_2 monitor. The patient was gently ventilated by hand for an additional 4 to 5 minutes before spontaneous respirations resumed. The patient was put in the lithotomy position, and after a vaginal prep, the procedure commenced.

At the request of the surgeon, 20 units of pitocin were added to the Ringer's Lactate solution that was infusing via the IV. Also, as prophylaxis against nausea, 4 mg of ondansetron was given by IV. The procedure lasted 20 minutes; at the conclusion of the procedure, the patient was taken out of the lithotomy position.

The desflurane had been discontinued as the surgeon announced that she was finished; the patient was still breathing spontaneously and the LMA was removed 1 or 2 minutes later, when the patient began to respond to verbal stimuli. The patient was moved to a recovery stretcher and taken to the post anesthesia care unit (PACU). The report was given to the PACU nurse as the monitors were being applied. After ensuring that the patient's condition was satisfactory, the anesthesiologist transferred care to the PACU nurse.

Other Procedures

(For intra-arterial or intravenous therapy for pain management, see ▶90774, 90775◀)

Surgery

For the 2006 CPT codebook, extensive revisions to the Integumentary subsection include substantial revision of the existing guidelines, the addition of 37 codes, and the deletion and revision of many other codes in the Free Skin Graft and Burns, Local Treatment subsections. Other significant changes are the revisions of the Respiratory and Digestive System subsections. In the Digestive System subsection, nine gastric restrictive procedure codes and 11 laparoscopic intestinal procedure codes have been added. Also noteworthy is the conversion of the descending thoracic aortic aneurysm Category III series of codes 0033T-0040T to Category I, with the addition of seven codes.

Also, significant is the addition of several other series of codes, including those to describe mechanical thrombectomy, percutaneous renal pelvis catheter, intracranial balloon angioplasty, and percutaneous vertebral augmentation procedures. Several guidelines have been revised to clarify reporting, including the guidelines to clarify reporting biopsies, bone grafts, and adjacent tissue transfer procedures. Code revisions include turbinate and operating telescope codes in the Respiratory subsection, and the lung resection and venous ligation procedures.

Surgery

Integumentary System

Skin, Subcutaneous and Accessory Structures

EXCISION—DEBRIDEMENT

+11008 Removal of prosthetic material or mesh, abdominal wall for necrotizing soft tissue infection (List separately in addition to code for primary procedure)

(Report skin grafts or flaps separately when performed for closure at the same session as 11004-11008)

►(When insertion of mesh is used for closure, use 49568)◄

(If testicular transplantation is performed, use 54680)

Rationale

A parenthetical note has been included to identify the approriate code to report when insertion of mesh is used for closure. Although code 49568 includes language that specifies use "*for incisional or ventral hernia repair*," this code may also be used to identify insertion of mesh for closure of this nature, as the effort to perform mesh insertion for repair associated with necrotizing soft tissue infection is the same as that provided for the implantation of mesh for incisional or ventral hernia repair.

Repair (Closure)

►SKIN REPLACEMENT SURGERY AND SKIN SUBSTITUTES◄

Identify by size and location of the defect (recipient area) and the type of graft ►or skin substitute◄; includes simple debridement of granulation ►tissue◄ or recent avulsion.

When a primary procedure such as orbitectomy, radical mastectomy, or deep tumor removal requires skin graft for definitive closure, see appropriate anatomical subsection for primary procedure and this section for skin graft ►or skin substitute◄.

Use 15000►, 15001◄ for initial wound ►recipient site◄ preparation.

Use 15100-15261 for ►autologous◄ skin grafts. For ►autologous◄ tissue-cultured ►epidermal◄ grafts, use ►15150-15157◄. ►For harvesting of autologous keratinocytes and dermal tissue for tissue-cultured skin grafts, use 15040.◄ Procedures are coded by recipient site. Use ►15170-15176 for acellular dermal replacement◄. Use modifier 58 for staged application procedure(s).

Repair of donor site requiring skin . . .

Codes 15000 ►and◄ 15001 describe burn and wound preparation ►or incisional or excisional release of scar contracture resulting in an open wound requiring a skin graft. Codes 15100-15431 describe the application of skin replacements and skin substitutes◄. The following definition should be applied to those codes that reference "100 sq cm or one percent of body area of infants and children" when determining the involvement of body size ▶:◀ The measurement of 100 sq cm is applicable to adults and children age 10 and older, percentages ▶of body surface area◀ apply to infants and children under the age of 10.

▶These codes are not intended to be reported for simple graft application alone or application stabilized with dressings (eg, by simple gauze wrap) without surgical fixation of the skin substitute/graft. The skin substitute/graft is anchored using the surgeon's choice of fixation. When services are performed in the office, the supply of the skin substitute/graft should be reported separately. Routine dressing supplies are not reported separately.◀

(For microvascular flaps, see 15756-15758)

▶*Surgical Preparation*◀

▲15000 Surgical preparation or creation of recipient site by excision of open wounds, burn eschar, or scar (including subcutaneous tissues), or incisional release of scar contracture; first 100 sq cm or one percent of body area of infants and children

(For appropriate skin grafts ▶or replacements◀, see 15050-15261▶, 15330-15336◀▶.◀ ▶L◀ist the graft ▶or replacement◀ separately by its procedure number when the graft, immediate or delayed, is applied)

+15001 each additional 100 sq cm or each additional one percent of body area of infants and children (List separately in addition to code for primary procedure)

(Use 15001 in conjunction with 15000)

(For excision of benign lesions, see 11400-11471)

(For excision of malignant lesions, see 11600-11646)

(For excision ▶to prepare or create recipient site◀ with dressing▶s or materials not listed in 15040-15431◀, use 15000▶-15001◀ only)

(For excision with immediate skin grafting use 15000, 15001 in conjunction with 15050-15261)

(For excision with immediate allograft ▶skin◀ placement, use ▶15000, 15001 in conjunction with 15300-15366◀)

(For excision with immediate ▶xenogeneic dermis◀ placement use ▶15000, 15001 in conjunction with◀ 15400▶-15431◀)

▶*Grafts*◀

▶Autograft/Tissue Cultured Autograft◀

●15040 Harvest of skin for tissue cultured skin autograft, 100 sq cm or less

15050 Pinch graft, single or multiple, to cover small ulcer, tip of digit, or other minimal open area (except on face), up to defect size 2 cm diameter

▲15100 Split-thickness autograft, trunk, arms, legs; first 100 sq cm or less, or one percent of body area of infants and children (except 15050)

+15101 each additional 100 sq cm, or each additional one percent of body area of infants and children, or part thereof (List separately in addition to code for primary procedure)

(Use 15101 in conjunction with 15100)

●15110 Epidermal autograft, trunk, arms, legs; first 100 sq cm or less, or one percent of body area of infants and children

+●15111 each additional 100 sq cm, or each additional one percent of body area of infants and children, or part thereof (List separately in addition to code for primary procedure)

►(Use 15111 in conjunction with 15110)◄

●15115 Epidermal autograft, face, scalp, eyelids, mouth, neck, ears, orbits, genitalia, hands, feet, and/or multiple digits; first 100 sq cm or less, or one percent of body area of infants and children

+●15116 each additional 100 sq cm, or each additional one percent of body area of infants and children, or part thereof (List separately in addition to code for primary procedure)

►(Use 15116 in conjunction with 15115)◄

▲15120 Split-thickness autograft, face, scalp, eyelids, mouth, neck, ears, orbits, genitalia, hands, feet, and/or multiple digits; first 100 sq cm or less, or one percent of body area of infants and children (except 15050)

+15121 each additional 100 sq cm, or each additional one percent of body area of infants and children, or part thereof (List separately in addition to code for primary procedure)

(Use 15121 in conjunction with 15120)

(For eyelids, see also 67961 et seq)

●15130 Dermal autograft, trunk, arms, legs; first 100 sq cm or less, or one percent of body area of infants and children

+●15131 each additional 100 sq cm, or each additional one percent of body area of infants and children, or part thereof (List separately in addition to code for primary procedure)

►(Use 15131 in conjunction with 15130)◄

●15135 Dermal autograft, face, scalp, eyelids, mouth, neck, ears, orbits, genitalia, hands, feet, and/or multiple digits; first 100 sq cm or less, or one percent of body area of infants and children

+●15136 each additional 100 sq cm, or each additional one percent of body area of infants and children, or part thereof (List separately in addition to code for primary procedure)

►(Use 15136 in conjunction with 15135)◄

●15150 Tissue cultured epidermal autograft, trunk, arms, legs; first 25 sq cm or less

+●15151 additional 1 sq cm to 75 sq cm (List separately in addition to code for primary procedure)

►(Do not report 15151 more than once per session)◄

►(Use 15151 in conjunction with 15150)◄

+●15152 each additional 100 sq cm, or each additional one percent of body area of infants and children, or part thereof (List separately in addition to code for primary procedure)

▶(Use 15152 in conjunction with 15151)◀

●15155 Tissue cultured epidermal autograft, face, scalp, eyelids, mouth, neck, ears, orbits, genitalia, hands, feet, and/or multiple digits; first 25 sq cm or less

+●15156 additional 1 sq cm to 75 sq cm (List separately in addition to code for primary procedure)

▶(Do not report 15156 more than once per session)◀

▶(Use 15156 in conjunction with 15155)◀

+●15157 each additional 100 sq cm, or each additional one percent of body area of infants and children, or part thereof (List separately in addition to code for primary procedure)

▶(Use 15157 in conjunction with 15156)◀

▶Acellular Dermal Replacement◀

●15170 Acellular dermal replacement, trunk, arms, legs; first 100 sq cm or less, or one percent of body area of infants and children

+●15171 each additional 100 sq cm, or each additional one percent of body area of infants and children, or part thereof (List separately in addition to code for primary procedure)

▶(Use 15171 in conjunction with 15170)◀

●15175 Acellular dermal replacement, face, scalp, eyelids, mouth, neck, ears, orbits, genitalia, hands, feet, and/or multiple digits; first 100 sq cm or less, or one percent of body area of infants and children

+●15176 each additional 100 sq cm, or each additional one percent of body area of infants and children, or part thereof (List separately in addition to code for primary procedure)

▶(Use 15176 in conjunction with 15175)◀

▶Allograft/Tissue Cultured Allogeneic Skin Substitute◀

▶Application of a non-autologous human skin graft (ie, homograft) from a donor to a part of the recipient's body to resurface an area damaged by burns, traumatic injury, soft tissue infection and/or tissue necrosis or surgery.◀

●15300 Allograft skin for temporary wound closure, trunk, arms, legs; first 100 sq cm or less, or one percent of body area of infants and children

+●15301 each additional 100 sq cm, or each additional one percent of body area of infants and children, or part thereof (List separately in addition to code for primary procedure)

▶(Use 15301 in conjunction with 15300)◀

●15320 Allograft skin for temporary wound closure, face, scalp, eyelids, mouth, neck, ears, orbits, genitalia, hands, feet, and/or multiple digits; first 100 sq cm or less, or one percent of body area of infants and children

+●15321 each additional 100 sq cm, or each additional one percent of body area of infants and children, or part thereof (List separately in addition to code for primary procedure)

▶(Use 15321 in conjunction with 15320)◀

⊘=Modifier 51 Exempt ⊙=Conscious Sedation ✚=Add-on Code ✓=FDA approval pending

●15330 Acellular dermal allograft, trunk, arms, legs; first 100 sq cm or less, or one percent of body area of infants and children

+●15331 each additional 100 sq cm, or each additional one percent of body area of infants and children, or part thereof (List separately in addition to code for primary procedure)

▶(Use 15331 in conjunction with 15330)◀

●15335 Acellular dermal allograft, face, scalp, eyelids, mouth, neck, ears, orbits, genitalia, hands, feet, and/or multiple digits; first 100 sq cm or less, or one percent of body area of infants and children

+●15336 each additional 100 sq cm, or each additional one percent of body area of infants and children, or part thereof (List separately in addition to code for primary procedure)

▶(Use 15336 in conjunction with 15335)◀

●15340 Tissue cultured allogeneic skin substitute; first 25 sq cm or less

+●15341 each additional 25 sq cm

▶(Use 15341 in conjunction with 15340)◀

▶(Do not report 15340, 15341 in conjunction with 11040-11042, 15000)◀

▶(15342 has been deleted. To report, see 15170, 15175, 15340, 15360, 15365)◀

▶(15343 has been deleted. To report, see 15171, 15176, 15341, 15361, 15366)◀

▶(15350 has been deleted. To report, see 15300, 15320, 15330, 15335)◀

▶(15351 has been deleted. To report, see 15301, 15321, 15331, 15336)◀

●15360 Tissue cultured allogeneic dermal substitute; trunk, arms, legs; first 100 sq cm or less, or one percent of body area of infants and children

+●15361 each additional 100 sq cm, or each additional one percent of body area of infants and children, or part thereof (List separately in addition to code for primary procedure)

▶(Use 15361 in conjunction with 15360)◀

●15365 Tissue cultured allogeneic dermal substitute, face, scalp, eyelids, mouth, neck, ears, orbits, genitalia, hands, feet, and/or multiple digits; first 100 sq cm or less, or one percent of body area of infants and children

+●15366 each additional 100 sq cm, or each additional one percent of body area of infants and children, or part thereof (List separately in addition to code for primary procedure)

▶(Use 15366 in conjunction with 15365)◀

▶Xenograft◀

▶Application of a non-human skin graft or biologic wound dressing (eg, porcine tissue or pigskin) to a part of the recipient's body following debridement of the burn wound or area of traumatic injury, soft tissue infection and/or tissue necrosis, or surgery.◀

▲15400 Xenograft, skin (dermal), for temporary wound closure; trunk, arms, legs; first 100 sq cm or less, or one percent of body area of infants and children

+▲15401 each additional 100 sq cm, or each additional one percent of body area of infants and children, or part thereof (List separately in addition to code for primary procedure)

(Use 15401 in conjunction with 15400)

●15420 Xenograft skin (dermal), for temporary wound closure, face, scalp, eyelids, mouth, neck, ears, orbits, genitalia, hands, feet, and/or multiple digits; first 100 sq cm or less, or one percent of body area of infants and children

+●15421 each additional 100 sq cm, or each additional one percent of body area of infants and children, or part thereof (List separately in addition to code for primary procedure)

▶(Use 15421 in conjunction with 15420)◀

●15430 Acellular xenograft implant; first 100 sq cm or less, or one percent of body area of infants and children

+●15431 each additional 100 sq cm, or each additional one percent of body area of infants and children, or part thereof (List separately in addition to code for primary procedure)

▶(Use 15431 in conjunction with 15430)◀

▶(Do not report 15430, 15431 in conjunction with 11040-11042, 15000)◀

Rationale

Comprehensive changes (ie, additions, deletions, and revisions of codes accompanied by new and revised introductory language, parenthetical notes, subheadings, and cross-references) have been made to the Integumentary, Repair (Closure) subsection of Surgery to accommodate reporting of skin grafts, skin replacements, skin substitutes, and local burn wound care.

The Free Skin Grafts subheading under the Repair (Closure) heading was deleted and replaced with a new subheading titled Skin Replacement Surgery and Skin Substitutes. Revisions have been made to the introductory language to clarify the appropriate reporting of the new and revised codes. An additional paragraph was added at the end of the introductory language to specify that reporting of the codes in this section must involve surgical fixation of the skin substitute or graft, which is anchored by the surgeon's choice of fixation to clarify the level of effort required to report these codes. Additional language clarifies that supply of the skin substitute or graft should be reported separately, whereas routine dressing supplies should not be reported separately.

Code 15000 was revised to include "incisional release of scar contracture" and the parenthetical note following this code was revised to include "replacements" and the new code range 15330-15336 for acelluar autograft procedures.

The fourth cross-reference following 15001, previously referencing alloplastic dressing, has been revised to specify that only 15000-15001 should be used for excision to prepare or create a recipient site with dressings or materials not listed in the subsequent cross-references. The sixth and seventh cross-references have also been revised to reference the new range of codes applicable to allograft skin and xenogeneic dermis placements.

Following the new subheading titled Autograft/Tissue Cultured Autograft, code 15040 has been added to describe harvest of skin for tissue cultured skin autograft.

Codes 15100 and 15120 have been editorially revised to describe split-thickness autograft.

Codes 15110 and 15115 have been added to describe epidermal autografts for the first 100 sq cm or less, or 1% of body area of infants and children. Add-on codes 15111 and 15116 have been established to report epidermal autografts for each additional 100 sq cm, or each additional 1% of body area of infants and children, or part thereof.

Codes 15130 and 15135 have been added to describe dermal autografts for the first 100 sq cm or less, or 1% of body area of infants and children. Add-on codes 15131 and 15136 have been established to report dermal autografts for each additional 100 sq cm, or each additional 1% of body area of infants and children, or part thereof.

Codes 15150 and 15155 have been added to describe tissue cultured epidermal autograft for the first 25 sq cm or less. Add-on codes 15151, 15152, 15156, and 15157 have been established to report each additional 1 sq cm to 75 sq cm, and each additional 100 sq cm, or each additional 1% of body area of infants and children, or part thereof. Instructional parenthetical notes following 15151 and 15156 have been added to preclude the reporting of 15151 and 15156 more than once per session.

Codes 15170 and 15175 have been added to describe acellular dermal replacement for the first 100 sq cm or less, or 1% of body area of infants and children. Add-on codes 15171 and 15176 have been established to report each additional 100 sq cm, or each additional 1% of body area of infants and children, or part thereof.

Following the new subheading titled Allograft/Tissue Cultured and the accompanying introductory language; codes 15300 and 15320 have been added to describe allograft skin for temporary wound closure for the first 100 sq cm or less, or 1% of body area of infants and children. Add-on codes 15301 and 15321 have been established to report each additional 100 sq cm, or each additional 1% of body area of infants and children, or part thereof.

Codes 15330 and 15335 have been added to describe acellular dermal allograft for the first 100 sq cm or less, or 1% of body area of infants and children. Add-on codes 15331 and 15336 have been established to report each additional 100 sq cm, or each additional 1% of body area of infants and children, or part thereof.

Code 15340 has been added to describe tissue cultured allogeneic skin substitute for the first 25 sq cm or less. Add-on code 15341 has been established to report each additional 25 sq cm. As the site preparation for these procedures is typically minimal, an exclusionary parenthetical note has been added to preclude reporting 15340 and 15341 with the site preparation code 15000 and the debridement codes 11040-11042.

Codes 15342 and 15343 have been deleted and replaced with codes 15170-15176, 15340-15341, and 15360-15366. Additionally, 15350 and 15351 have been deleted and replaced with 15300-15321.

Codes 15360 and 15365 have been added to describe tissue cultured allogeneic dermal substitute for the first 100 sq cm or less, or 1% of body area of infants and children. Add-on codes 15361 and 15366 have been established to report each additional 100 sq cm, or each additional 1% of body area of infants and children, or part thereof.

Following the new subheading titled Xenograft and the accompanying introductory language, 15400 has been revised to include "(dermal)" and "or one percent of body area of infants and children." Additionally, add-on code 15401 has been revised to include "or each additional one percent of body area of infants and children or part thereof."

Code 15420 has been added to describe xenograft skin (dermal) for temporary wound closure for the first 100 sq cm or less, or 1% of body area of infants and children. Add-on code 15421 has been established to report each additional 100 sq cm, or each additional 1% of body area of infants and children, or part thereof.

Code 15430 has been added to describe acellular xenograft implant for the first 100 sq cm or less, or 1% of body area of infants and children. Add-on code 15431 has been established to report each additional 100 sq cm, or each additional 1% of body area of infants and children, or part thereof. As the site preparation required for these procedures is minimal, an exclusionary parenthetical note has been added to preclude reporting 15430 and 15431 with the site preparation code 15000 and the debridement codes 11040-11042.

Clinical Example (15000)

A 27-year-old cook was admitted to the burn center with grease scald burns involving the left neck, shoulder, chest, arm, and hand. A total of 25% body surface area was burned full thickness. Under general anesthesia, the left arm and hand burns were excised down to viable subcutaneous tissue; a total of 500 sq cm was excised. Vigorous bleeding was controlled by electrocautery, selective suture ligation, and topical thrombin application. Blood loss was estimated at 500 ml.

Description of Procedure (15000)

After the induction of anesthesia, the subcutaneous tissue beneath the full-thickness burn is infiltrated with crystalloid solution containing epinephrine in order to minimize blood loss. The eschar is excised down to viable subcutaneous tissue. Hemostasis is obtained with electrocautery, epinephrine-soaked laparotomy pads, and/or topical thrombin. A total of 100 sq cm is excised in preparation for immediate or staged skin grafting and/or application of a skin substitute/replacement.

Clinical Example (15040)

A 10-year-old boy was rescued from a burning building. Due to altered mental status and suspicion of inhalation injury, he was intubated at the scene. He was transported to the nearby emergency department where he was assessed to have 80% total body surface area burns. Intravenous fluid resuscitation was initiated and ventilatory support maintained. He was transferred to the regional burn center for definitive management. Once hemodynamically stable, he was taken to the operating room for excision of his extensive full-thickness burns (the excision is separately reported); however, due to the extent of the burn and lack of sufficient donor sites, his remaining excised wounds were covered with cadaveric allograft and/or other skin substitute or replacement. Because inadequate skin graft donor sites were available for immediate, permanent wound coverage, a split-thickness skin biopsy was harvested for the preparation of cultured autologous skin grafts to be applied in 3 to 4 weeks, when available.

Description of Procedure (15040)

After the induction of anesthesia, the subcutaneous tissue beneath the donor site is infiltrated with crystalloid solution containing epinephrine in order to minimize blood loss and facilitate donor skin harvesting. A split-thickness skin graft 0.010 to 0.015 inches in depth is harvested using a dermatome. A total of 100 sq cm is recovered. Hemostasis is obtained with epinephrine-soaked laparotomy pads and/or topical thrombin. A dressing is applied to the donor site and covered with dry gauze.

Clinical Example (15110)

A 10-year-old boy was rescued from a burning building. Due to altered mental status and suspicion of inhalation injury, he was intubated at the scene. He was transported to the nearby emergency department where he was assessed to have 80% total body surface area burns. Intravenous fluid resuscitation was initiated and ventilatory support maintained. He was transferred to the regional burn center for definitive management. Once hemodynamically stable, he was taken to the operating room for excision of his extensive full-thickness burns; however, due to the extent of the burn and lack of sufficient donor sites available for immediate, permanent wound coverage, his wounds were covered with an acellular dermal replacement (ie, Integra®). He is returned to the operating room for harvesting of "ultrathin" epidermal skin autografts to be placed on the now vascularized acellular dermal replacement covering his torso, arms, and legs.

Description of Procedure (15110)

After the induction of anesthesia, the subcutaneous tissue beneath the donor site is infiltrated with crystalloid solution containing epinephrine in order to minimize blood loss and facilitate donor skin harvesting. An epidermal skin graft 0.004 to 0.006 inches in depth is harvested using a dermatome. The dermatome is adjusted as necessary during donor skin harvesting to ensure that almost no dermal tissue is harvested. A total of 100 sq cm is recovered and is meshed for expansion prior to placement on the excised wound. Hemostasis of the graft site is obtained with epinephrine-soaked laparotomy pads and/or topical thrombin. The epidermal skin graft is applied to the trunk and secured to the excised wound with interrupted sutures, surgical staples, and/or fibrin sealant. A dressing is applied to the graft site and secured to prevent mechanical shear. A dressing is applied to the donor site and covered with dry gauze.

Clinical Example (15111)

A 10-year-old boy was rescued from a burning building. Due to altered mental status and suspicion of inhalation injury, he was intubated at the scene. He was transported to the nearby emergency department where he was assessed to have 80% total body surface area burns. Intravenous fluid resuscitation was initiated and ventilatory support maintained. He was transferred to the regional burn center for definitive management. Once hemodynamically stable, he was taken to the operating room for excision of his extensive full-thickness burns; however, due to the extent of the burn and lack of sufficient donor sites available for immediate, permanent wound coverage, his wounds were covered with an acellular dermal replacement (ie, Integra®). He is returned to the operating room for harvesting of "ultrathin" epidermal skin autografts to be placed on the now vascularized acellular dermal replacement covering his torso, arms, and legs.

Description of Procedure (15111)

After the induction of anesthesia, the subcutaneous tissue beneath the donor site is infiltrated with crystalloid solution containing epinephrine in order to minimize blood loss and facilitate donor skin harvesting. An epidermal skin graft 0.004 to 0.006 inches in depth is harvested using a dermatome. The dermatome is adjusted as necessary during donor skin harvesting to ensure that almost no dermal tissue is harvested. An additional 400 sq cm is recovered and is meshed for expansion prior to placement on the excised wound. Hemostasis of the graft site is obtained with epinephrine-soaked laparotomy pads and/or topical thrombin. The epidermal skin graft is applied to the trunk and arm and secured to the excised wound with interrupted sutures, surgical staples, and/or fibrin sealant. A dressing is applied to the graft site and secured to prevent mechanical shear. A dressing is applied to the donor site and covered with dry gauze.

Clinical Example (15115)

A 10-year-old boy was rescued from a burning building. Due to altered mental status and suspicion of inhalation injury, he was intubated at the scene. He was transported to the nearby emergency department where he was assessed to have 80% total body surface area burns. Intravenous fluid resuscitation was initiated and ventilatory support maintained. He was transferred to the regional burn center for definitive management. Once hemodynamically stable, he was taken to the operating room for excision of his extensive full-thickness burns; however, due to the extent of the burn and lack of sufficient donor sites available for immediate, permanent wound coverage, his wounds were covered with an acellular dermal replacement (ie, Integra®). He is returned to the operating room for harvesting of "ultrathin" epidermal skin autografts to be placed on the now vascularized acellular dermal replacement covering his hands.

Description of Procedure (15115)

After the induction of anesthesia, the subcutaneous tissue beneath the donor site is infiltrated with crystalloid solution containing epinephrine in order to minimize blood loss and facilitate donor skin harvesting. An epidermal skin graft 0.004 to 0.006 inches in depth is harvested using a dermatome. The dermatome is adjusted as necessary during donor skin harvesting to ensure that almost no dermal tissue is harvested. A total of 100 sq cm is recovered and is meshed for expansion prior to placement on the excised wound. Hemostasis of the graft site is obtained with epinephrine-soaked laparotomy pads and/or topical thrombin. The epidermal skin graft is applied to the hands and secured to the excised wound with interrupted sutures, surgical staples, and/or fibrin sealant. A dressing is applied to the graft site and secured to prevent mechanical shear. A dressing is applied to the donor site and covered with dry gauze.

Clinical Example (15116)

A 10-year-old boy was rescued from a burning building. Due to altered mental status and suspicion of inhalation injury, he was intubated at the scene. He was transported to the nearby emergency department where he was assessed to have 80% total body surface area burns. Intravenous fluid resuscitation was initiated and ventilatory support maintained. He was transferred to the regional burn center for definitive management. Once hemodynamically stable, he was taken to the operating room for excision of his extensive full-thickness burns; however, due to the extent of the burn and lack of sufficient donor sites available for immediate, permanent wound coverage, his wounds were covered with an acellular dermal replacement (ie, Integra®). He is returned to the operating room for harvesting of "ultrathin" epidermal skin autografts to be placed on the now vascularized acellular dermal replacement covering both of his hands. The first 100 sq cm will be coded separately.

Description of Procedure (15116)

After the induction of anesthesia, the subcutaneous tissue beneath the donor site is infiltrated with crystalloid solution containing epinephrine in order to minimize blood loss and facilitate donor skin harvesting. An epidermal skin graft 0.004 to 0.006 inches in depth is harvested using a dermatome. The dermatome is adjusted as necessary during donor skin harvesting to ensure that almost no dermal tissue is harvested. Two hundred square centimeters is recovered and is meshed for expansion prior to placement on the excised wound. Hemostasis of the graft site is obtained with epinephrine-soaked laparotomy pads and/or topical thrombin. The epidermal skin graft is applied to the hands and secured to the excised wound with interrupted sutures, surgical staples, and/or fibrin sealant. A dressing is applied to the graft site and secured to prevent mechanical shear. A dressing is applied to the donor site and covered with dry gauze.

Clinical Example (15130)

A 62-year-old male has recurrent metastatic cancer to his left popliteal fossa. He has previously had radiation therapy to this area and undergoes surgical exploration. The popliteal artery is exposed and has evidence of radiation injury.

Description of Procedure (15130)

After the induction of anesthesia, the subcutaneous tissue beneath the donor site is infiltrated with crystalloid solution containing epinephrine in order to minimize blood loss and facilitate donor skin harvesting. A split-thickness skin graft 0.010 to 0.015 inches in depth is raised but not removed from the underlying dermal bed using a dermatome. The dermatome is adjusted to facilitate removal of the graft from the device. A second pass of the dermatome is made over the freshly created donor site at a depth of 0.010 inches for the recovery of the dermal graft. A total of 100 sq cm of dermal autograft tissue is recovered. Hemostasis of the donor site is obtained with epinephrine-soaked laparotomy pads and/or topical thrombin. The split-thickness skin graft that was originally raised is applied to the donor site and secured with interrupted sutures, surgical staples, and/or fibrin sealant. The dermal graft is secured to the surgically prepared wound in the popliteal fossa. Dressings are applied to both the grafted donor site and the surgically prepared wound in the popliteal fossa and both are secured to prevent mechanical shear.

Clinical Example (15131)

A 62-year-old male has recurrent metastatic cancer to his left popliteal fossa. He has previously had radiation therapy to this area and undergoes surgical exploration. The popliteal artery is exposed and has evidence of radiation injury.

Description of Procedure (15131)

After the induction of anesthesia, the subcutaneous tissue beneath the donor site is infiltrated with crystalloid solution containing epinephrine in order to minimize blood loss and facilitate donor skin harvesting. A split-thickness skin graft 0.010 to 0.015 inches in depth is raised but not removed from the underlying dermal bed using a dermatome. The dermatome is adjusted to facilitate removal of the graft from the device. A second pass of the dermatome is made over the freshly created donor site at a depth of 0.010 inches for the recovery of the dermal graft. Two hundred square centimeters of dermal autograft tissue is recovered. Hemostasis of the donor site is obtained with epinephrine-soaked laparotomy pads and/or topical thrombin. The split-thickness skin graft that was originally raised is applied to the donor site and secured with interrupted sutures, surgical staples, and/or fibrin sealant. The dermal graft is secured to the surgically prepared wound in the popliteal fossa. The first 100 sq cm is separately reported. Dressings are applied to both the grafted donor site and the surgically prepared wound in the popliteal fossa and both are secured to prevent mechanical shear.

Clinical Example (15135)

A 62-year-old male has recurrent metastatic cancer to his left neck. He has previously had radiation therapy to this area and undergoes surgical exploration with radical neck dissection. The carotid artery is exposed and has evidence of radiation injury.

Description of Procedure (15135)

After the induction of anesthesia, the subcutaneous tissue beneath the donor site is infiltrated with crystalloid solution containing epinephrine in order to minimize blood loss and facilitate donor skin harvesting. A split-thickness skin graft 0.010 to 0.015 inches in depth is raised but not removed from the underlying dermal bed using a dermatome. The dermatome is adjusted to facilitate removal of the graft from the device. A second pass of the dermatome is made over the freshly created donor site at a depth of 0.010 inches for the recovery of the dermal graft.

A total of 100 sq cm of dermal autograft tissue is recovered. Hemostasis of the donor site is obtained with epinephrine-soaked laparotomy pads and/or topical thrombin. The split-thickness skin graft that was originally raised is applied to the donor site and secured with interrupted sutures, surgical staples, and/or fibrin sealant. The dermal graft is secured to the surgically prepared wound in the neck. Dressings are applied to both the grafted donor site and the surgically prepared wound on the trunk and both are secured to prevent mechanical shear.

Clinical Example (15136)

A 62-year-old male has recurrent metastatic cancer to his left neck. He has previously had radiation therapy to this area and undergoes surgical exploration with radical neck dissection. The carotid artery is exposed and has evidence of radiation injury.

Description of Procedure (15136)

After the induction of anesthesia, the subcutaneous tissue beneath the donor site is infiltrated with crystalloid solution containing epinephrine in order to minimize blood loss and facilitate donor skin harvesting. A split-thickness skin graft 0.010 to 0.015 inches in depth is raised but not removed from the underlying dermal bed using a dermatome. The dermatome is adjusted to facilitate removal of the graft from the device. A second pass of the dermatome is made over the freshly created donor site at a depth of 0.010 inches for the recovery of the dermal graft. Two hundred square centimeters of dermal autograft tissue is recovered. The first 100 sq cm is coded separately. Hemostasis of the donor site is obtained with epinephrine-soaked laparotomy pads and/or topical thrombin. The split-thickness skin graft that was originally raised is applied to the donor site and secured with interrupted sutures, surgical staples, and/or fibrin sealant. The dermal graft is secured to the surgically prepared wound in the neck. Dressings are applied to both the grafted donor site and the surgically prepared wound on the trunk and both are secured to prevent mechanical shear.

Clinical Example (15150)

A 10-year-old boy was rescued from a burning building. Due to altered mental status and suspicion of inhalation injury, he was intubated at the scene. He was transported to the nearby emergency department where he was assessed to have 80% total body surface area burns. Intravenous fluid resuscitation was initiated and ventilatory support maintained. He was transferred to the regional burn center for definitive management. Once hemodynamically stable, he was taken to the operating room for excision of his extensive full-thickness burns; however, due to the extent of the burn and lack of sufficient donor sites, his remaining excised wounds were covered with cadaveric allograft and/or other skin substitute or replacement. Because inadequate skin graft donor sites were available for immediate, permanent wound coverage, a small split-thickness skin graft was harvested for the preparation of cultured autologous skin grafts 3 to 4 weeks previously. He is now returned to the operating room for the application of cultured autologous epidermal autografts to his torso and lower extremities.

Description of Procedure (15150)
After the induction of anesthesia, hemostasis of the graft site is obtained with epinephrine-soaked laparotomy pads and/or topical thrombin. The tissue-cultured epidermal autografts are removed from the transport medium and a total of 25 sq cm is applied to the trunk and secured to the excised wound with interrupted sutures, surgical staples, and/or fibrin sealant. A dressing is applied to the graft site and secured to prevent mechanical shear.

Clinical Example (15151)
A 10-year-old boy was rescued from a burning building. Due to altered mental status and suspicion of inhalation injury, he was intubated at the scene. He was transported to the nearby emergency department where he was assessed to have 80% total body surface area burns. Intravenous fluid resuscitation was initiated and ventilatory support maintained. He was transferred to the regional burn center for definitive management. Once hemodynamically stable, he was taken to the operating room for excision of his extensive full-thickness burns; however, due to the extent of the burn and lack of sufficient donor sites, his remaining excised wounds were covered with cadaveric allograft and/or other skin substitute/skin replacement. Because inadequate skin graft donor sites were available for immediate, permanent wound coverage, a small split-thickness skin graft was harvested for the preparation of cultured autologous skin grafts 3 to 4 weeks previously. He is now returned to the operating room for the application of cultured autologous epidermal autografts to his torso and lower extremities.

Description of Procedure (15151)
After the induction of anesthesia, hemostasis of the graft site is obtained with epinephrine-soaked laparotomy pads and/or topical thrombin. The tissue-cultured epidermal autografts are removed from the transport medium. Additional grafts measuring 100 sq cm (the first 25 sq cm will be coded separately) are applied to the trunk and secured to the excised wound with interrupted sutures, surgical staples, and/or fibrin sealant. A dressing is applied to the graft site and secured to prevent mechanical shear.

Clinical Example (15152)
A 10-year-old boy was rescued from a burning building. Due to altered mental status and suspicion of inhalation injury, he was intubated at the scene. He was transported to the nearby emergency department where he was assessed to have 80% total body surface area burns. Intravenous fluid resuscitation was initiated and ventilatory support maintained. He was transferred to the regional burn center for definitive management. Once hemodynamically stable, he was taken to the operating room for excision of his extensive full-thickness burns; however, due to the extent of burn and lack of sufficient donor sites, his remaining excised wounds were covered with cadaveric allograft and/or other skin substitute or replacement. Because inadequate skin graft donor sites were available for immediate, permanent wound coverage, a small split-thickness skin graft was harvested for the preparation of cultured autologous skin grafts 3 to 4 weeks previously. He is now returned to the operating room for the application of cultured autologous epidermal autografts to his torso, lower extremities, and hands.

Description of Procedure (15152)

After the induction of anesthesia, hemostasis of the graft site is obtained with epinephrine-soaked laparotomy pads and/or topical thrombin. The tissue-cultured epidermal autografts are removed from the transport medium. Two hundred square centimeters (the first 100 sq cm will be coded separately) of grafts are applied to the trunk and secured to the excised wound with interrupted sutures, surgical staples, and/or fibrin sealant. A dressing is applied to the graft site and secured to prevent mechanical shear.

Clinical Example (15155)

A 10-year-old boy was rescued from a burning building. Due to altered mental status and suspicion of inhalation injury, he was intubated at the scene. He was transported to the nearby emergency department where he was assessed to have 80% total body surface area burns. Intravenous fluid resuscitation was initiated and ventilatory support maintained. He was transferred to the regional burn center for definitive management. Once hemodynamically stable, he was taken to the operating room for excision of his extensive full-thickness burns; however, due to the extent of the burn and lack of sufficient donor sites, his remaining excised wounds were covered with cadaveric allograft and/or other skin substitute or replacement. Because inadequate skin graft donor sites were available for immediate, permanent wound coverage, a small split-thickness skin graft was harvested for the preparation of cultured autologous skin grafts 3 to 4 weeks previously. He is now returned to the operating room for the application of cultured autologous epidermal autografts to hands.

Description of Procedure (15155)

After the induction of anesthesia, hemostasis of the graft site is obtained with epinephrine-soaked laparotomy pads and/or topical thrombin. The tissue-cultured epidermal autografts are removed from the transport medium and a total of 25 sq cm is applied to the hand and secured to the excised wound with interrupted sutures, surgical staples, and/or fibrin sealant. A dressing is applied to the graft site and secured to prevent mechanical shear.

Clinical Example (15156)

A 10-year-old boy was rescued from a burning building. Due to altered mental status and suspicion of inhalation injury, he was intubated at the scene. He was transported to the nearby emergency department where he was assessed to have 80% total body surface area burns. Intravenous fluid resuscitation was initiated and ventilatory support maintained. He was transferred to the regional burn center for definitive management. Once hemodynamically stable, he was taken to the operating room for excision of his extensive full-thickness burns; however, due to the extent of the burn and lack of sufficient donor sites, his remaining excised wounds were covered with cadaveric allograft and/or other skin substitute or replacement. Because inadequate skin graft donor sites were available for immediate, permanent wound coverage, a small split-thickness skin graft was harvested for the preparation of cultured autologous skin grafts 3 to 4 weeks previously. He is now returned to the operating room for the application of cultured autologous epidermal autografts to his hands.

Description of Procedure (15156)

After the induction of anesthesia, hemostasis of the graft site is obtained with epinephrine-soaked laparotomy pads and/or topical thrombin. The tissue-cultured epidermal autografts are removed from the transport medium. Grafts measuring 100 sq cm (the first 25 sq cm will be coded separately) are applied to the hand and secured to the excised wound with interrupted sutures, surgical staples, and/or fibrin sealant. A dressing is applied to the graft site and secured to prevent mechanical shear.

Clinical Example (15157)

A 10-year-old boy was rescued from a burning building. Due to altered mental status and suspicion of inhalation injury, he was intubated at the scene. He was transported to the nearby emergency department where he was assessed to have 80% total body surface area burns. Intravenous fluid resuscitation was initiated and ventilatory support maintained. He was transferred to the regional burn center for definitive management. Once hemodynamically stable, he was taken to the operating room for excision of his extensive full-thickness burns; however, due to the extent of burn and lack of sufficient donor sites, his remaining excised wounds were covered with cadaveric allograft and/or other skin substitute or replacement. Because inadequate skin graft donor sites were available for immediate, permanent wound coverage, a small split-thickness skin graft was harvested for the preparation of cultured autologous skin grafts 3 to 4 weeks previously. He is now returned to the operating room for the application of cultured autologous epidermal autografts to hands.

Description of Procedure (15157)

After the induction of anesthesia, hemostasis of the graft site is obtained with epinephrine-soaked laparotomy pads and/or topical thrombin. The tissue-cultured epidermal autografts are removed from the transport medium. Two hundred square centimeters of grafts (the first 100 sq cm will be coded separately) are applied to the hands and fingers and secured to the excised wound with interrupted sutures, surgical staples, and/or fibrin sealant. A dressing is applied to the graft site and secured to prevent mechanical shear.

Clinical Example (15170)

A 45-year-old man was rescued from a burning building. Due to altered mental status and suspicion of inhalation injury, the patient was intubated at the scene. He was transported to the nearby burn center where he was assessed to have 75% total body surface area burns. Intravenous fluid resuscitation was initiated and ventilatory support maintained. He underwent bilateral upper extremity escharotomies for circumferential full-thickness burns and his wounds were subsequently dressed with a topical antimicrobial agent and gauze. He required continuous ventilatory support, enteral nutrition, and continued intravenous fluid administration due to his inability to eat. Five days postburn, he underwent excision and split-thickness autografting for full-thickness burns of his hands and upper extremities with meshed skin grafts. He is now being returned to the operating room for excision of the full-thickness burns of his posterior trunk with simultaneous application of an acellular dermal replacement.

Description of Procedure (15170)

After the induction of anesthesia, hemostasis of the graft site is obtained with epinephrine-soaked laparotomy pads and/or topical thrombin. The acellular dermal replacement is removed from the rinsing solution and a total of 100 sq cm is applied to the trunk and secured to the excised wound with interrupted sutures or surgical staples. A net dressing is applied and expanded over the graft site and secured with staples to prevent mechanical shear. The wound is covered with gauze dressings and secured with a bulky dressing to further prevent mechanical shear.

Clinical Example (15171)

A 45-year-old man was rescued from a burning building. Due to altered mental status and suspicion of inhalation injury, the patient was intubated at the scene. He was transported to the nearby burn center where he was assessed to have 75% total body surface area burns. Intravenous fluid resuscitation was initiated and ventilatory support maintained. He underwent bilateral upper extremity escharotomies for circumferential full-thickness burns and his wounds were subsequently dressed with a topical antimicrobial agent and gauze. He required continuous ventilatory support, enteral nutrition, and continued intravenous fluid administration due to his inability to eat. Five days postburn, he underwent excision and split-thickness autografting for full-thickness burns of his hands and upper extremities with meshed skin grafts. He is now being returned to the operating room for excision of the full-thickness burns of his posterior trunk with simultaneous application of an acellular dermal replacement.

Description of Procedure (15171)

After the induction of anesthesia, hemostasis of the graft site is obtained with epinephrine-soaked laparotomy pads and/or topical thrombin. The acellular dermal replacement is removed from the rinsing solution. Two hundred square centimeters (the first 100 sq cm will be coded separately) is applied to the trunk and secured to the excised wound with interrupted sutures or surgical staples. A net dressing is applied and expanded over the graft site and secured with staples to prevent mechanical shear. The wound is covered with gauze dressings and secured with a bulky dressing to further prevent mechanical shear.

Clinical Example (15175)

A 45-year-old man was rescued from a burning building. Due to altered mental status and suspicion of inhalation injury, the patient was intubated at the scene. He was transported to the nearby burn center where he was assessed to have 75% total body surface area burns. Intravenous fluid resuscitation was initiated and ventilatory support maintained. He underwent bilateral upper extremity escharotomies for circumferential full-thickness burns and his wounds were subsequently dressed with a topical antimicrobial agent and gauze. He required continuous ventilatory support, enteral nutrition, and continued intravenous fluid administration due to his inability to eat. Five days postburn, he underwent excision and split-thickness autografting for full-thickness burns of his hands and upper extremities with meshed skin grafts. He is now being returned to the operating room for excision of the full-thickness burns of his hands with simultaneous application of an acellular dermal replacement.

Description of Procedure (15175)

After the induction of anesthesia, hemostasis of the graft site is obtained with epinephrine-soaked laparotomy pads and/or topical thrombin. The acellular dermal replacement is removed from the rinsing solution and a total of 100 sq cm is applied to the hands and secured to the excised wound with interrupted sutures or surgical staples. A net dressing is applied and expanded over the graft site and secured with staples to prevent mechanical shear. The wound is covered with gauze dressings and secured with a bulky dressing to further prevent mechanical shear.

Clinical Example (15176)

A 45-year-old man was rescued from a burning building. Due to altered mental status and suspicion of inhalation injury, the patient was intubated at the scene. He was transported to the nearby burn center where he was assessed to have 75% total body surface area burns. Intravenous fluid resuscitation was initiated and ventilatory support maintained. He underwent bilateral upper extremity escharotomies for circumferential full-thickness burns and his wounds were subsequently dressed with a topical antimicrobial agent and gauze. He required continuous ventilatory support, enteral nutrition, and continued intravenous fluid administration due to his inability to eat. Five days postburn, he underwent excision and split-thickness autografting for full-thickness burns of his hands and upper extremities with meshed skin grafts. He is now being returned to the operating room for excision of the full-thickness burns of his posterior hands with simultaneous application of an acellular dermal replacement.

Description of Procedure (15176)

After the induction of anesthesia, hemostasis of the graft site is obtained with epinephrine-soaked laparotomy pads and/or topical thrombin. The acellular dermal replacement is removed from the rinsing solution. Two hundred square centimeters (the first 100 sq cm is coded separately) is applied to the hands and fingers and secured to the excised wound with interrupted sutures or surgical staples. A net dressing is applied and expanded over the graft site and secured with staples to prevent mechanical shear. The wound is covered with gauze dressings and secured with a bulky dressing to further prevent mechanical shear.

Clinical Example (15300)

A 74-year-old mechanic was admitted to the burn center with burns of both legs, lower back, and abdomen after his gasoline-saturated clothing was ignited from a spark. The burns involved 40% body surface area. During the first operative session, the patient underwent surgical excision of the burn tissue from the left lower leg beginning at the ankle and extending to the popliteal area (reported separately). After excision and hemostasis, allografts were obtained from the skin bank. Approximately 100 sq cm of allograft skin was grafted to the excised surface on the left lower leg and secured with interrupted absorbable sutures. The graft was dressed with a low adherent dressing and reinforced with absorbent dressing and secured with net dressing.

Description of Procedure (15300)

After the induction of anesthesia, hemostasis of the graft site is obtained with epinephrine-soaked laparotomy pads and/or topical thrombin. Human allograft skin is obtained from the skin bank. A total of 100 sq cm is applied to the leg and secured to the excised wound with interrupted sutures or surgical staples. The wound is covered with gauze dressings and secured with a bulky dressing to prevent mechanical shear.

Clinical Example (15301)

A 74-year-old mechanic was admitted to the burn center with burns of both legs, lower back, and abdomen after his gasoline-saturated clothing was ignited from a spark. The burns involved 40% body surface area. During the first operative session, the patient underwent surgical excision of the burn tissue from the lower legs beginning at the ankle and extending to the popliteal area (reported separately). After excision and hemostasis, allografts were obtained from the skin bank. Approximately 200 sq cm of allograft skin was then grafted to the excised surface on the lower legs and secured with interrupted absorbable sutures and surgical staples (the first 100 sq cm is reported separately). The graft was dressed with a low adherent dressing and reinforced with absorbent dressing and secured with net dressing.

Description of Procedure (15301)

After the induction of anesthesia, hemostasis of the graft site is obtained with epinephrine-soaked laparotomy pads and/or topical thrombin. Human allograft skin is obtained from the skin bank. An additional 400 sq cm is applied to the legs and secured to the excised wound with interrupted sutures or surgical staples. The wound is covered with gauze dressings and secured with a bulky dressing to prevent mechanical shear.

Clinical Example (15320)

A 74-year-old mechanic was admitted to the burn center with burns of both hands and feet after his gasoline-saturated clothing was ignited from a spark. The burns involved 40% body surface area. During the first operative session, the patient underwent surgical excision of the burn tissue from the left hand beginning at the wrist (reported separately). After excision and hemostasis, allografts were obtained from the skin bank. Approximately 100 sq cm of allograft skin was grafted to the excised surface on the left hand and secured with interrupted absorbable sutures. The graft was dressed with a low adherent dressing and reinforced with absorbent dressing and secured with net dressing.

Description of Procedure (15320)

After the induction of anesthesia, hemostasis of the graft site is obtained with epinephrine-soaked laparotomy pads and/or topical thrombin. Human allograft skin is obtained from the skin bank. A total of 100 sq cm is applied to the hands and fingers and secured to the excised wound with interrupted sutures or surgical staples. The wound is covered with gauze dressings and secured with a bulky dressing to prevent mechanical shear.

Clinical Example (15321)

A 74-year-old mechanic was admitted to the burn center with burns of both hands and feet after his gasoline-saturated clothing was ignited from a spark. The burns involved 40% body surface area. During the first operative session, the patient underwent surgical excision of the burn tissue from the hands and feet beginning at the wrist and ankle (reported separately). After excision and hemostasis, allografts were obtained from the skin bank. Approximately 200 sq cm of allograft skin was grafted to the excised surfaces on the hands and secured with interrupted absorbable sutures and surgical staples (the first 100 sq cm is reported separately). The graft was dressed with a low adherent dressing, reinforced with absorbent dressing, and secured with net dressing.

Description of Procedure (15321)

After the induction of anesthesia, hemostasis of the graft site is obtained with epinephrine-soaked laparotomy pads and/or topical thrombin. Human allograft skin is obtained from the skin bank. An additional 200 sq cm (the first 100 sq cm is coded separately) is applied to the hands and fingers and secured to the excised wound with interrupted sutures or surgical staples. The wound is covered with gauze dressings and secured with a bulky dressing to prevent mechanical shear.

Clinical Example (15330)

A 20 year-old with a history of burns presents with scarring and contracture of the axilla. The patient underwent surgery 2 years prior with split-thickness skin grafts for burns over 80% of his body. He now has limited range of motion and limited function of his shoulder as a result of the burn. He has failed physical therapy intervention and continues with functional deficits as a result of this contracture.

Description of Procedure (15330)

After the induction of anesthesia, hemostasis of the graft site is obtained with epinephrine-soaked laparotomy pads and/or topical thrombin. Acellular dermal allograft is removed from the transport package. A total of 100 sq cm is applied to the trunk and secured to the wound with absorbable sutures. The dermal graft is covered with a local skin flap (separately coded). The wound is covered with gauze dressings and secured with a bulky dressing to prevent mechanical shear.

Clinical Example (15331)

A 20-year-old with history of burns presents with scarring and contracture of the axilla. The patient underwent surgery 2 years prior with split-thickness skin grafts for burns over 80% of his body. He now has limited range of motion and limited function of his shoulder as a result of the burn. He has failed physical therapy intervention and continues with functional deficits as a result of this contracture.

Description of Procedure (15331)

After the induction of anesthesia, hemostasis of the graft site is obtained with epinephrine-soaked laparotomy pads and/or topical thrombin. Acellular dermal allograft is removed from the transport package. Two hundred square centimeters (the first 100 sq cm is coded separately) is applied to the trunk and secured to the wound with absorbable sutures. The dermal graft is covered with a local skin flap (separately coded). The wound is covered with gauze dressings and secured with a bulky dressing to prevent mechanical shear.

Clinical Example (15335)

A 38-year-old female experienced second- and third-degree grease burns to the dorsum of her right hand extending to the palmar surface, covering 3% of her total body surface area.

Description of Procedure (15335)

After the induction of anesthesia, hemostasis of the graft site is obtained with epinephrine-soaked laparotomy pads and/or topical thrombin. Acellular dermal allograft is removed from the transport package. A total of 100 sq cm is applied to the hand and fingers and secured to the wound with absorbable sutures. The dermal graft is covered with a local skin flap (separately coded). The wound is covered with gauze dressings and secured with a bulky dressing to prevent mechanical shear.

Clinical Example (15336)

A 38-year-old female experienced second- and third-degree grease burns to the dorsum of her right hand and fingers extending to the palmar surface, covering 3% of her total body surface area.

Description of Procedure (15336)

After the induction of anesthesia, hemostasis of the graft site is obtained with epinephrine-soaked laparotomy pads and/or topical thrombin. Acellular dermal allograft is removed from the transport package. Two hundred square centimeters (the first 100 sq cm is coded separately) is applied to the hand and fingers and secured to the wound with absorbable sutures. The dermal graft is overgrafted with a split-thickness skin graft that is also secured with interrupted sutures or surgical staples (separately coded). The wound is covered with gauze dressings and secured with a bulky dressing to prevent mechanical shear.

Clinical Example (15340)

A 68-year-old male with type II diabetes presents with a 3 × 3-cm noninfected, full-thickness chronic ulceration of the plantar aspect of the right heel. The decision is made to debride the wound and proceed with application of a tissue-cultured allogeneic skin substitute.

Description of Procedure (15340)

The wound is debrided and, after adequate hemostasis has been achieved and administration of anesthesia has occurred, graft materials were obtained. The wound was measured. Approximately 25 sq cm of tissue-cultured allogeneic skin substitute was fenestrated, grafted to the excised surface, and secured with interrupted sutures.

Clinical Example (15341)

A 68-year-old male with type II diabetes presents with a 6 × 6-cm noninfected, full-thickness chronic ulceration of the plantar aspect of the right heel. The decision is made to debride the wound and proceed with application of a tissue-cultured allogeneic skin substitute.

Description of Procedure **(15341)**

The wound is debrided and, after adequate hemostasis has been achieved and administration of anesthesia has occurred, graft materials were obtained. The wound was measured. Approximately 50 sq cm of tissue-cultured allogeneic skin substitute was fenestrated, grafted to the excised surface, and secured with interrupted sutures.

Clinical Example **(15360)**

A 15-year-old child sustained 20% total body surface area second-degree burns. The wounds are superficial and of intermediate depth. In an effort to promote healing without the use of topical antibiotic dressings, the patient is taken to the operating room for debridement of the burn wounds and simultaneous application of a tissue-cultured allogeneic dermal substitute.

Description of Procedure **(15360)**

Hemostasis of the debrided or excised graft site is obtained. The tissue-cultured allogeneic dermal substitute is removed from the transport container and a total of 100 sq cm is applied to the trunk and secured to the excised wound with interrupted sutures, surgical staples, or sterile adhesive strips. The wound is covered with gauze dressings and secured with a bulky dressing to prevent mechanical shear.

Clinical Example **(15361)**

A 15-year-old child sustained 20% total body surface area second-degree burns. The wounds are superficial and of intermediate depth. In an effort to promote healing without the use of topical antibiotic dressings, the patient is taken to the operating room for debridement of the burn wounds and simultaneous application of a tissue-cultured allogeneic dermal substitute.

Description of Procedure **(15361)**

Hemostasis of the debrided or excised graft site is obtained. The tissue-cultured allogeneic dermal substitute is removed from the transport container. Two hundred square centimeters (the first 100 sq cm is coded separately) is applied to the trunk and secured to the excised wound with interrupted sutures, surgical staples, or sterile adhesive strips. The wound is covered with gauze dressings and secured with a bulky dressing to prevent mechanical shear.

Clinical Example **(15365)**

A 15-year-old child sustained 20% total body surface area second-degree burns. The wounds are superficial and of intermediate depth. In an effort to promote healing without the use of topical antibiotic dressings, the patient is taken to the operating room for debridement of the burn wounds and simultaneous application of a tissue-cultured allogeneic dermal substitute.

Description of Procedure **(15365)**

Hemostasis of the debrided or excised graft site is obtained. The tissue-cultured allogeneic dermal substitute is removed from the transport container and a total of 100 sq cm is applied to the hands and fingers and secured to the excised wound with interrupted sutures, surgical staples, or sterile adhesive strips. The wound is covered with gauze dressings and secured with a bulky dressing to prevent mechanical shear.

Clinical Example **(15366)**

A 15-year-old child sustained 20% total body surface area second-degree burns. The wounds are superficial and of intermediate depth. In an effort to promote healing without the use of topical antibiotic dressings, the patient is taken to the operating room for debridement of the burn wounds and simultaneous application of a tissue-cultured allogeneic dermal substitute.

Description of Procedure **(15366)**

Hemostasis of the debrided or excised graft site is obtained. The tissue-cultured allogeneic dermal substitute is removed from the transport container. Two hundred square centimeters (the first 100 sq cm is coded separately) is applied to the hands and fingers and secured to the excised wound with interrupted sutures, surgical staples, or sterile adhesive strips. The wound is covered with gauze dressings and secured with a bulky dressing to prevent mechanical shear.

Clinical Example **(15400)**

A 22-year-old mechanic suffered burns of the left neck, shoulder, and arm from a radiator scald injury. The burns involved 10% body surface and were deep partial thickness. During the first operative session, the patient underwent surgical preparation of the burn on the left shoulder and arm by excision down to viable dermis. After adequate hemostasis had been achieved in the excised surface, the xenograft was grafted to the excised surface and secured with 60 interrupted sutures. The graft was dressed with a low adherent dressing and reinforced with absorbent dressing and secured with net dressing.

Description of Procedure **(15400)**

After adquate hemostasis had been achieved in the excised surface, xenograft dressings were obtained from the skin bank and thawed. Approximately 500 sq cm of xenograft was grafted to the excised surface and secured with 60 interrupted sutures.

Clinical Example **(15401)**

A 22-year-old mechanic suffered burns of the left shoulder, arm, and forearm from a radiator scald injury. The burns involved 10% body surface. These burns were deep partial thickness. During the first operative session, the patient underwent surgical preparation of the burn on the left shoulder, arm, and forearm by excision down to viable dermis (reported separately). After adequate hemostasis had been achieved in the excised surface, xenograft skin was grafted to the excised surface and secured with interrupted sutures and surgical staples. The graft was dressed with a low adherent dressing and reinforced with net dressing. The initial 100 sq cm has already been applied (coded separately). A second 100 sq cm is now applied.

Description of Procedure (15401)

Hemostasis of the debrided or excised graft site is obtained. Xenograft skin (dermal) is obtained from the skin bank and thawed. Two hundred sq cm (the first 100 sq cm is coded separately) is applied to the left shoulder and arm and secured to the excised wound with interrupted sutures or surgical staples. The wound is covered with gauze dressings and secured with a bulky dressing to prevent mechanical shear.

Clinical Example (15420)

A 22-year-old mechanic suffered burns of the face and neck from a radiator scald injury. The burns involved 10% body surface. These burns were deep partial thickness. During the first operative session, the patient underwent surgical preparation of the burns of the face and neck by excision down to viable dermis (reported separately). After adequate hemostasis had been achieved in the excised surface, 100 sq cm of xenograft skin was grafted to the excised surface and secured with interrupted sutures and surgical staples. The graft was dressed with a low adherent dressing and reinforced with absorbent dressing and secured with net dressing.

Description of Procedure (15420)

Hemostasis of the debrided or excised graft site is obtained. Xenograft skin (dermal) is obtained from the tissue bank. A total of 100 sq cm is applied to the face and neck and secured to the excised wound with interrupted sutures or surgical staples. The wound is covered with gauze dressings and secured with a bulky dressing to prevent mechanical shear.

Clinical Example (15421)

A 22-year-old mechanic suffered burns of the face, neck, and hands from a radiator scald injury. The burns involved 10% body surface. These burns were deep partial thickness. During the first operative session, the patient underwent surgical preparation of the burns of the face, neck, and hands by excision down to viable dermis (reported separately). After adequate hemostasis had been achieved in the excised surface, 200 sq cm of xenograft skin was grafted to the excised surface and secured with interrupted sutures and surgical staples (the first 100 sq cm is reported separately). The graft was dressed with a low adherent dressing and reinforced with absorbent dressing and secured with net dressing.

Description of Procedure (15421)

Hemostasis of the debrided or excised graft site is obtained. Xenograft skin (dermal) is obtained from the tissue bank. Two hundred square centimeters (the first 100 sq cm is coded separately) is applied to the hand and fingers and secured to the excised wound with interrupted sutures or surgical staples. The wound is covered with gauze dressings and secured with a bulky dressing to prevent mechanical shear.

Clinical Example (15430)

A 72-year-old female presents with a 2 × 2-cm noninfected venous stasis ulceration in the area of the medial mallelous. The decision is made to debride the wound and proceed with application of an acellular xenogeneic implant.

Description of Procedure (15430)

The wound is debrided and after adequate hemostasis has been achieved in the excised surface, the acellular xenograft implant was obtained. The wound was measured and the acellular xenograft implant was cut to shape, grafted to the excised surface, and secured.

OTHER PROCEDURES

►(15810, 15811 have been deleted)◄

Rationale

Codes 15810 and 15811 have been deleted. Salabrasion is an outdated procedure and is currently performed by physicians on an infrequent basis.

BURNS, LOCAL TREATMENT

Procedures 16000-16036 refer to local treatment of burned surface only.► Codes 16020-16030 include the application of materials (eg, Biobrane®, other dressings) not described in 15100-15431.◄

List percentage of body surface involved . . .

For necessary related medical services (eg, . . .

►For the application of skin grafts or skin substitutes, see 15100-15650.◄

16000 Initial treatment, first degree burn, when no more than local treatment is required

►(16010, 16015 have been deleted. To report, see 16020-16030)◄

▲16020 Dressings and/or debridement of partial-thickness burns, initial or subsequent; small (less than 5% total body surface area)

▲16025 medium (eg, whole face or whole extremity, or 5% to 10% total body surface area)

▲16030 large (eg, more than one extremity, or greater than 10% total body surface area)

16035 Escharotomy; intial incision

+16036 each additional incision (List separately in addition to code for primary procedure)

(Use 16036 in conjunction with 16035)

(For debridement, curettement of burn wound, see 160►2◄0-16030)

Rationale

The introductory language in the Burns, Local Treatment subsection has been revised to include a sentence specifying that codes 16020-16030 include application of materials (eg, Biobrane®, other dressings) not described in 15100-15431. At the end of the introductory language, a cross-reference has been added to refer to the application of skin grafts or skin substitutes codes (15100-15650).

Codes 16010 and 16015 have been deleted. Codes 16020-16030 have been editorially revised by omitting "without anesthesia" and "office or hospital."

Description of Procedure (16020)
The burn wound is surgically debrided of blisters and nonadherent devitalized tissue. The extent of the debridement is small and involves less than 5% of the total body surface area. The wound is dressed with a gauze dressing or other skin substitute (separate procedure).

Description of Procedure (16025)
The burn wound is surgically debrided of blisters and nonadherent devitalized tissue. The debridement involves the entire upper extremity and 5% to 10% of the total body surface area. The wound is dressed with a gauze dressing or other skin substitute (separate procedure).

Description of Procedure (16030)
The burn wound is surgically debrided of blisters and nonadherent devitalized tissue. The debridement involves both upper extremities and more than 10% of the total body surface area. The wound is dressed with a gauze dressing or other skin substitute (separate procedure).

Breast

EXCISION

19260 Excision of chest wall tumor including ribs

19271 Excision of chest wall tumor involving ribs, with plastic reconstruction; without mediastinal lymphadenectomy

19272 with mediastinal lymphadenectomy

►(Do not report 19260, 19271, 19272 in conjunction with 32002, 32020, 32100, 32503, 32504)◄

Rationale

To reflect the addition of new codes to report apical lung tumor resection with chest wall and ribs resections, neurovascular dissection, and chest wall resection, a cross-reference was added following 19260, 19271, and 19272. This cross-reference directs users to 32002, 32020, 32100, 32503, and 32504 for removal of tumors in the upper apex of the lung and to differentiate these from other chest wall tumor resections.

FRACTURE AND/OR DISLOCATION

►(21493 and 21494 have been deleted. To report, use the applicable Evaluation and Management codes)◄

21495 Open treatment of hyoid fracture

►(For laryngoplasty with open reduction of fracture, use 31584)◄

►(To report treatment of closed fracture of larynx, use the applicable Evaluation and Management codes)◄

Rationale

Codes 21493 and 21494 have been deleted because these procedures are performed infrequently. A cross-reference has been added to indicate that closed treatment of a larynx fracture is reported with the appropriate evaluation and management code.

Neck (Soft Tissues) and Thorax

INCISION

21501 Incision and drainage, deep abscess or hematoma, soft tissues of neck or thorax;

►(For posterior spine subfascial incision and drainage, see 22010-22015)◄

Rationale

In tandem with the establishment of 22010 and 22015 to report incision and drainage of posterior deep spinal abscesses, a cross-reference has been added to direct users to these codes.

Spine (Vertebral Column)

(For injection procedure, chemonucleolysis, single or multiple levels, use 62292)

(For injection procedure for facet joints, see 64470-64476, 64622-64627)

(For needle or trocar biopsy, see 20220-20225)

►INCISION◄

●22010 Incision and drainage, open, of deep abscess (subfascial), posterior spine; cervical, thoracic, or cervicothoracic

●22015 lumbar, sacral, or lumbosacral

►(Do not report 22015 in conjunction with 22010)◄

►(Do not report 22015 in conjunction with instrumentation removal, 10180, 22850, 22852)◄

►(For incision and drainage of abscess or hematoma, superficial, see 10060, 10140)◄

Rationale

Codes 22010 and 22015 were established to report incision and drainage of posterior deep spinal abscesses. The codes are differentiated according to region: cervical, thoracic, or cervicothoracic (22010) and lumbar, sacral, or lumbosacral (22015). An exclusionary parenthetical note following these codes indicates the mutually exclusive nature of these procedures, precluding the ability to report both codes for the same session. An exclusionary parenthetical note was added to restrict the use of these codes in conjunction with the postoperative incision and drainage code 10180 and the spinal instrumentation codes 22850 and 22852. A cross-reference directs the users to 10060 and 10140 to report superficial incision and drainage of hematoma of unspecified locations. Incision and drainage at the thoracolumbar junction would be reported with the code describing the region where the majority of the work is performed.

Clinical Example (22010)

A 47-year-old man underwent C3-C7 posterior spinal fusion. Two months postoperatively, he presents febrile with erythema, drainage of the neck wound, and neck pain. He undergoes incision and drainage of a deep abscess of the cervical spine.

Description of Procedure (22010)

A posterior approach to the spine is performed using the prior midline incision, which may require extension. The deep fascia is incised. Cultures are obtained. The midline wound is widely opened, irrigated, and debrided. Hematoma, necrotic tissue, and/or purulent collections are carefully debrided and the entire field irrigated using copious amounts of fluid. Hemostasis is obtained and the wound is closed over drains that are packed open or closed over a wound vacuum device. A sterile dressing is applied.

Clinical Example (22015)

A 51-year-old woman underwent L4-S1 posterior spinal fusion. Seven weeks postoperatively, she presents febrile with erythema, drainage of the back wound, and back pain. She undergoes incision and drainage of a deep abscess of the lumbar spine.

Description of Procedure (22015)

A posterior approach to the spine is performed using the prior midline incision, which may require extension. The deep fascia is incised. Cultures are obtained. The midline wound is widely opened, irrigated, and debrided. Hematoma, necrotic tissue, and/or purulent collections are carefully debrided and the entire field irrigated using copious amounts of fluid. Hemostasis is obtained and the wound is closed over drains that are packed open or closed over a wound vacuum device. A sterile dressing is applied.

VERTEBRAL BODY, EMBOLIZATION OR INJECTION

22520 Percutaneous vertebroplasty, one vertebral body, unilateral or bilateral injection; thoracic

22521 lumbar

+22522 each additional thoracic or lumbar vertebral body (List separately in addition to code for primary procedure)

(Use 22522 in conjunction with 22520, 22521 as appropriate)

(For radiological supervision and interpretation, see 76012, 76013)

●22523 Percutaneous vertebral augmentation, including cavity creation (fracture reduction and bone biopsy included when performed) using mechanical device, one vertebral body, unilateral or bilateral cannulation (eg, kyphoplasty); thoracic

●22524 lumbar

+●22525 each additional thoracic or lumbar vertebral body (List separately in addition to code for primary procedure)

►(Do not report 22525 in conjunction with 20225 when performed at the same level as 22523-22525)◄

►(Use 22525 in conjunction with 22523, 22524)◄

►(For radiological supervision and interpretation, see 76012, 76013)◄

Rationale

Codes 22523 and 22524 were added to describe percutaneous vertebral augmentation, including cavity creation using a mechanical device at a single thoracic and lumbar vertebral body respectively. As indicated in the code descriptors, fracture reduction and bone biopsy are incidental to the procedure and not reported separately. An exclusionary parenthetical note was added following 22525 to preclude the use of the deep bone biopsy code 20225 with the vertebral augmentation codes 22523-22525.

Add-on code 22525 was established to describe each additional thoracic or lumbar vertebral body on which percutaneous vertebral augmentation is performed. A parenthetical note was added to delineate the reporting of 22525 in conjunction with 22523 and 22524, as appropriate.

Radiological Supervision and Interpretation (S&I) code 76012 should be reported separately for the fluoroscopic guidance performed in conjunction with codes 22523-22525. It would also be appropriate to separately report radiological S&I code 76013 performed under CT guidance in conjunction with codes 22523-22525.

The percutaneous vertebral augmentation, mechanical device procedure is designed to treat patients with vertebral body compression fractures commonly caused by primary osteoporosis, secondary osteoporosis, multiple myeloma, osteolytic metastatic disease, benign lesions, and traumatic fractures.

Vertebral compression fracture (VCF) repair procedures by open or percutaneous methods are performed for the treatment of progressive osteoporotic and osteolytic compression fractures. New mechanical devices (miniature expandable jacks, curved tamps, expandable balloon tamps, or otherwise) have been developed to provide surgeons with new tools and options to treat VCFs. Previous CPT codes reflected only traditional open and closed treatment or reduction of vertebral fractures (22305-22328) and were not intended to report the open or percutaneous creation of a cavity in a vertebral body or the restoration of spinal alignment achievable through kyphoplasty. The vertebroplasty codes (22520-22522) do not encompass the different steps involved with kyphoplasty or the restoration of vertebral body height.

The procedure described by codes 22523-22525 is performed under either local or general anesthesia and involves percutaneous access into the vertebral body by introduction of a working cannula. This is followed by the insertion of a mechanical device (expandable jack, curved tamp, expandable balloon, or otherwise) containing radiopaque dye to create a cavity or void, reduce the endplate fractures (ie, restore the height, elevate the collapsed endplates), and restore overall spinal alignment from within the vertebral body. The final step involves the vertebral body augmentation and internal stabilization by introducing or filling the resultant cavity with bone graft, enhanced bone graft slurries, allograft bone, polymethylmethacrylate, or bone graft substitute at the surgeon's discretion. The vertebral augmentation or cavity filling after cannulation, cavity creation, or fracture reduction steps during kyphoplasty are significantly different procedures than the high-pressure injection of cement as embodied in 22851.

Clinical Example (22523)

A 75-year-old woman presents with severe, persistent back pain and progressive spinal deformity, secondary to osteoporotic vertebral collapse. Radiographic imaging, including magnetic resonance imaging, confirms the recent compression fracture at T10. A bone biopsy is performed as well as a percutaneous vertebral augmentation with fracture reduction using a mechanical device to create a cavity.

Description of Procedure (22523)

A small skin incision is made at the appropriate position based on fluoroscopic visualization of the pertinent anatomy. Using anteroposterior and lateral plane fluoroscopy (separately reported), the following (in contrast to just using a small bone biopsy needle to inject bone cement into a vertebral body) are sequentially placed: a needle, guidewire, 4.2-mm cannula (working channel), and drill. These are followed by a mechanical cavity creation device that is placed via either a transpedicular or extrapedicular approach into the compressed vertebral body. The entire process is repeated on the contralateral side; hence, this is a bilateral procedure. The mechanical cavity creation fracture reduction device is gradually deployed to create a cavity. The device is removed, leaving behind the formed cavity. Bone cement is mixed and allowed 18 to 25 minutes for the mixed cement to have a consistency appropriate for injection. The cavities are filled with the bone substitute. Final intraoperative imaging is obtained to confirm alignment and fill. The working cannulae are removed and the incisions are closed with a single stitch. Sterile dressings are applied.

Clinical Example (22524)

A 75-year-old woman presents with severe, persistent back pain and progressive spinal deformity, secondary to osteoporotic vertebral collapse. Radiographic imaging, including magnetic resonance imaging, confirms the recent compression fracture at L3. A bone biopsy is performed as well as a percutaneous vertebral augmentation with fracture reduction using a mechanical device to create a cavity.

Description of Procedure (22524)

A small skin incision is made at the appropriate position based on fluoroscopic visualization of the pertinent anatomy. Using anteroposterior and lateral plane fluoroscopy (separately reported), the following (in contrast to just using a small bone biopsy needle to inject bone cement into a vertebral body) are sequentially placed: a needle, guidewire, 4.2-mm cannula (working channel), and drill. These are followed by a mechanical cavity creation device that is placed via either a transpedicular or extrapedicular approach into the compressed vertebral body. The entire process is repeated on the contralateral side; hence, this is a bilateral procedure. The mechanical cavity creation fracture reduction device is gradually deployed to create a cavity. The device is removed, leaving behind the formed cavity. Bone cement is mixed and allowed 18 to 25 minutes for the mixed cement to have a consistency appropriate for injection. The cavities are filled with the bone substitute. Final intraoperative imaging is obtained to confirm alignment and fill. The working cannulae are removed and the incisions are closed with a single stitch. Sterile dressings are applied.

Clinical Example (22525)

A 75-year-old woman presents with severe, persistent back pain and progressive spinal deformity, secondary to osteoporotic vertebral collapse. Radiographic imaging, including magnetic resonance imaging, confirms the recent compression fracture at T9 and T10. After undergoing vertebral augmentation of T10 (coded separately), the additional level at T9 is treated.

Note: When completing this survey, only "add-on" work for the additional vertebral body should be considered. The primary procedure would be billed separately.

Description of Procedure (22525)

After completion of the first vertebral level treated, the physician proceeds to the next level, repositioning the patient and draping as necessary to ensure a sterile field.

A small skin incision is made at the appropriate position based on fluoroscopic visualization of the pertinent anatomy. Using anteroposterior and lateral plane fluoroscopy (separately reported), the following (in contrast to just using a small bone biopsy needle to inject bone cement into a vertebral body) are sequentially placed: a needle, guidewire, 4.2-mm cannula (working channel), and drill. These are followed by a mechanical cavity creation device that is placed via either a transpedicular or extrapedicular approach into the compressed vertebral body. The entire process is repeated on the contralateral side; hence, this is a bilateral procedure. The mechanical cavity creation fracture reduction device is gradually deployed to create a cavity. The device is removed, leaving behind the formed cavity. Bone cement is mixed and allowed 18 to 25 minutes for the mixed cement to have a consistency appropriate for injection. The cavities are filled with the bone substitute. Final intraoperative imaging is obtained to confirm alignment and fill. The working cannulae are removed and the incisions are closed with a single stitch. Sterile dressings are applied.

Foot and Toes

OTHER PROCEDURES

●**28890** Extracorporeal shock wave, high energy, performed by a physician, requiring anesthesia other than local, including ultrasound guidance, involving the plantar fascia

(For extracorporeal shock wave therapy involving musculoskeletal system▶ not otherwise specified◀, see Category III codes 0019T, ▶0101T, 0102T◀)

Rationale

Code 28890 has been added to identify high-energy extracorporeal shock wave (ESW) treatment of the plantar fascia. A cross-reference has been added subsequent to 28890 to direct users to high-energy ESW procedures of other areas.

This code (previously included as part of the Category III listing) has been included as part of the Musculoskeletal listing to identify the additional effort necessary to perform this procedure vs other ESW treatments. The language included in the code descriptor helps to differentiate this procedure, indicating that (1) it is an ESW treatment that is high energy (usually involving pain), (2) it requires performance by a physician, and (3) it necessitates use of a non-local anesthetic. As is also indicated in the descriptor, it includes ultrasound guidance and is specific to treatment for plantar fasciitis. Parenthetical notes also guide the user, notating the appropriate codes to use for other ESW procedures (Category III codes 0019T, 0101T, 0102T). The language in these procedure codes does not include language regarding anesthesia, further notifying the user of the different intents for use of these codes.

Clinical Example (28890)

A 43-year-old female with chronic plantar fasciitis, who has undergone more than 6 months of conservative therapy without resolution of her symptoms, presents to the DPM, MD, or DO and the decision is made to proceed with high energy extracorporeal shock wave (ESW) of the plantar fascia requiring anesthesia other than local (separately reportable).

Description of Procedure (28890)

The point of maximal tenderness is identified and marked on the patient's heel. The foot is prepped and a local heel block is placed. Coupling gel is applied to the heel, and the shock wave generating device is positioned over the heel. Shock waves are then administered according to the manufacturers' protocol until the appropriate energy level is achieved. During shock wave administration, the position of the shock wave generating device is adjusted, and the power level and shock frequency is increased according to a standard protocol.

Application of Casts and Strapping

The listed procedures apply when the . . .

A physician who applies the initial cast, strap or splint and also assumes all of the subsequent fracture, dislocation, or injury care cannot use the application of casts and strapping codes as an initial service, since the first cast/splint or strap application is included in the treatment of fracture and/or dislocation codes. (See notes under Musculoskeletal System, page 71.) A temporary cast/splint/strap is not considered to be part of the preoperative care, and the use of the modifier 56 is not applicable. Additional evaluation and management services are reportable only if significant identifiable further services are provided at the time of the cast application or strapping.

If cast application or strapping is . . .

Listed procedures include removal of cast . . .

(For orthotics ►management◄ and training, ►see 97760-97762◄)

Endoscopy/Arthroscopy

29866 Arthroscopy, knee, surgical; osteochondral autograft(s) (eg, mosaicplasty) (includes harvesting of the autograft)

(Do not report 29866 in conjunction with 29870, 29871, 29875, 29884 when performed at the same session and/or ►29874, 29877,◄ 29879, 29885-29887 when performed in the same compartment)

29867 osteochondral allograft (eg, mosaicplasty)

(Do not report 29867 in conjunction with 27570, 29870, 29871, 29875, 29884 when performed at the same session and/or ►29874, 29877,◄ 29879, 29885-29887 when performed in the same compartment)

(Do not report 29867 in conjunction with 27415)

29868 meniscal transplantation (includes arthrotomy for meniscal insertion), medial or lateral

(Do not report 29868 in conjunction with 29870, 29871, 29875, 29880, 29883, 29884 when performed at the same session or ►29874, 29877,◄ 29881, 29882 when performed in the same compartment)

Rationale

The exclusionary notes following the arthroscopic osteochondral and meniscal graft codes 29866, 29867, and 29868 have been editorially revised to instruct that arthroscopic removal of foreign bodies (29874) and/or debridement of shaving of articular cartilage (29877) is appropriately reported when performed in a compartment other than the arthroscopic graft procedure.

Respiratory System

Nose

EXCISION

▲30130 Excision inferior turbinate, partial or complete, any method

▶(For excision of superior or middle turbinate, use 30999)◀

▲30140 Submucous resection inferior turbinate, partial or complete, any method

▶(Do not report 30130 or 30140 in conjunction with 30801, 30802, 30930)◀

▶(For submucous resection of superior or middle turbinate, use 30999)◀

▶(For endoscopic resection of concha bullosa of middle turbinate, use 31240)◀

(For submucous resection of nasal septum, use 30520)

(For reduction of turbinates, use 30140 with modifier 52)

DESTRUCTION

▲30801 Cautery and/or ablation, mucosa of inferior turbinates, unilateral or bilateral, any method; superficial

▶(For cautery and ablation of superior or middle turbinates, use 30999)◀

30802 intramural

▶(Do not report 30801, 30802, 30930 in conjunction with 30130 or 30140)◀

▶(For cautery performed for control of nasal hemorrhage, see 30901-30906)◀

OTHER PROCEDURES

▲30930 Fracture nasal inferior turbinate(s), therapeutic

▶(Do not report 30801, 30802, 30930 in conjunction with 30130 or 30140)◀

▶(For fracture of superior or middle turbinate(s), use 30999)◀

Rationale

Codes 30130, 30140, 30801, 30802, and 30930 have been revised to clarify their widespread usage specific to the inferior turbinates and primary reporting for procedures performed for the treatment of inferior turbinate hypertrophy causing nasal airway obstruction and to eliminate frequent confusion with middle and superior turbinates when other intra-nasal surgeries (eg, endoscopic sinus surgery) are performed.

Resection of the middle turbinate is generally performed for endoscopic treatment of enlargement with pneumatization and is reported using code 31240 (nasal endoscopy with concha bullosa resection). If this turbinate is removed in association with ethmoidectomy, it should be considered integral to that resection

⊘=Modifier 51 Exempt ⊙=Conscious Sedation ✚=Add-on Code ⁄⁄=FDA approval pending

and not reported separately. The middle and superior turbinates are rarely treated with cautery and/or ablation nor laterally fractured. For this reason, cross-references have been added to direct that fracture, cautery, and/or ablation of superior or middle turbinates is reported with the unlisted nose procedure code 30999. A cross-reference has also been added following code 30801 (cautery and ablation of inferior turbinates) to direct the user to the appropriate range of codes to report cautery for control of nasal hemorrhage (30901-30906).

The superior turbinate is usually resected only with ethmoidectomy and not separately reported.

Codes 30801, 30802, and 30930 were additionally revised with the removal of "separate procedure" from the descriptors. Cross-references were added in support of these revisions to indicate codes 30130 (partial or complete excision of turbinate bone) and 30140 (partial or complete submucous resection of turbinate bone), which report larger procedures for which removal of the inferior turbinates are inherent, would not be appropriately reported in conjunction with these codes.

When reporting 30130, 30140, 30801, 30802, and 30930, it should be noted that these codes are unilateral because there are three turbinates in each right and left nasal cavity. If the turbinate procedure was performed to gain access to the ethmoid bone, neither 30130, 30140, nor 31240 would typically be reported.

Larynx

ENDOSCOPY

For endoscopic procedures, code appropriate endoscopy of each anatomic site examined. ►If using operating microscope, telescope, or both, use the applicable code only once per operative session.◄

31515 Laryngoscopy direct, with or without tracheoscopy; for aspiration

▲31526 diagnostic, with operating microscope or telescope

31530 Laryngoscopy, direct, operative, with foreign body removal;

▲31531 with operating microscope or telescope

31535 Laryngoscopy, direct, operative, with biopsy;

▲31536 with operating microscope or telescope

31540 Laryngoscopy, direct, operative, with excision of tumor and/or stripping of vocal cords or epiglottis;

▲31541 with operating microscope or telescope

31560 Laryngoscopy, direct, operative, with arytenoidectomy;

▲31561 with operating microscope or telescope

31570 Laryngoscopy, direct, with injection into vocal cord(s), therapeutic;

▲31571 with operating microscope or telescope

(Do not report code 69990 in addition to code 31571)

Rationale

An editorial change was made for 31526, 31531, 31536, 31541, 31561, and 31571 to allow for reporting the use of telescopes during direct laryngoscopic surgery. In addition, the Larynx, Endoscopy guidelines have been revised to indicate that use of both an operating microscope and telescope during the same session should be reported only *once* per session.

Clinical Example (31541)

A patient presents with hoarseness, probable airway compromise that is more significant with exercise. Patients of all ages may present with lesions; however, the lesions will vary with age. Children most frequently have recurrent respiratory papilloma as the source of their lesions. Adult lesions will most frequently be secondary to vocal polyps or squamous cell carcinoma.

Description of Procedure (31541)

The patient may have the procedure performed under local or general anesthesia; both forms have their advantages and disadvantages. The local anesthesia is more difficult and the larynx more difficult to operate on. General anesthesia complicates visualization of the larynx with the endotracheal tube. The larynx is visualized through a specially designed laryngoscope. It must have a wide inlet to allow visualization of the larynx. A microscope with a long focal length lens is used to give good visualization of the larynx. With long and specialized instruments, the tumor can be removed and the vocal cord mucosa removed. This has to be performed delicately and atraumatically.

Clinical Example (31561)

Usually an adult patient will present with bilateral vocal cord paralysis and consequent laryngeal airway obstruction. The patient is tracheotomy dependent with the desire to be made independent of a tracheostomy.

Description of Procedure (31561)

General anesthesia is induced, followed by the placement of the endoscope and microscope, through which the surgical procedure is performed, in many cases with the use of laser. The patient is monitored as he/she awakens. The scope is placed and the microscope set up. Through the microscope the injection is performed with meticulous technique. The immediate result is assessed and may require additional injections and assessments. The equipment is disassembled.

Clinical Example (31571)

Usually an adult patient will present with vocal cord paralysis and chronic or life-threatening aspiration or with breathy or weakened voice. In some cases, the patient may present also with other forms of vocal dysfunction such as spastic dysphemia. The procedure is carried out commonly under general anesthesia.

Description of Procedure (31571)

The intraservice includes administering general anesthesia (if required) and topical or local anesthesia to the larynx and pharynx; placing the scope; setting up and working through the microscope; performing injection with meticulous technique; assessing the immediate result, which may require additional injections and assessments; and disassembling the equipment.

REPAIR

►(31585 and 31586 have been deleted. To report, use the appropriate Evaluation and Management codes)◄

Rationale

Codes 31585 and 31586 have been deleted because these procedures are performed infrequently. An instructional parenthetical note has been added to indicate that closed treatment of a larynx fracture without manipulation is reported with the appropriate evaluation and management code.

Lungs and Pleura

INCISION

⊘32002 Thoracentesis with insertion of tube with or without water seal (eg, for pneumothorax) (separate procedure)

►(Do not report 32002 in conjunction with 19260, 19271, 19272, 32503, 32504)◄

(If imaging guidance is performed, see 76003, 76360, 76942)

⊘ ⊙32020 Tube thoracostomy with or without water seal (eg, for abscess, hemothorax, empyema) (separate procedure)

►(Do not report 32020 in conjunction with 19260, 19271, 19272, 32503, 32504)◄

(If imaging guidance is performed, use 75989)

32100 Thoracotomy, major; with exploration and biopsy

►(Do not report 32100 in conjunction with 19260, 19271, 19272, 32503, 32504)◄

Rationale

The three parenthetical exclusionary notes following the thoracentesis, tube thoracostomy, and thoracotomy incision codes 32002, 32020, and 32100 have been added to instruct that these codes represent component procedures of the larger procedures and are, therefore, not appropriately reported separately in conjunction with the chest wall (19260, 19271, 19272) and apical lung tumor resection (32503, 32504) codes.

32160 with cardiac massage

(For segmental or other resections of lung, see 32480-►32504◄)

EXCISION

32440 Removal of lung, total pneumonectomy;

32442 with resection of segment of trachea followed by broncho-tracheal anastomosis (sleeve pneumonectomy)

32445 extrapleural

(For extrapleural pneumonectomy, with empyemectomy, use 32445 and 32540)

►(If lung resection is performed with chest wall tumor resection, report the appropriate chest wall tumor resection code, 19260-19272, in addition to lung resection code 32440-32445)◄

32480 Removal of lung, other than total pneumonectomy; single lobe (lobectomy)

32500 wedge resection, single or multiple

►(If lung resection is performed with chest wall tumor resection, report the appropriate chest wall tumor resection code, 19260-19272, in addition to lung resection code 32480-32500)◄

✍ Rationale

Two instructional parentheticals following the total pneumonectomy (32440-32445) and partial pneumonectomy (32480-32500) code series have been added to indicate that if a chest wall resection is performed at the same time as lung resection codes, these are considered to be distinct procedures and, as such, are separately reported.

✚32501 Resection and repair of portion of bronchus (bronchoplasty) when performed at time of lobectomy or segmentectomy (List separately in addition to code for primary procedure)

(Use 32501 in conjunction with 32480, 32482, 32484)

(32501 is to be used when a portion of the bronchus to preserved lung is removed and requires plastic closure to preserve function of that preserved lung. It is not to be used for closure for the proximal end of a resected bronchus)

●32503 Resection of apical lung tumor (eg, Pancoast tumor), including chest wall resection, rib(s) resection(s), neurovascular dissection, when performed; without chest wall reconstruction(s)

●32504 with chest wall reconstruction

►(Do not report 32503, 32504 in conjunction with 19260, 19271, 19272, 32002, 32020, 32100)◄

►(32520, 32522, and 32525 have been deleted)◄

►(For performance of lung resection in conjunction with chest wall resection, see 19260, 19271, 19272 and 32480-32500, 32503, 32504)◄

SURGICAL COLLAPSE THERAPY; THORACOPLASTY

(See also ►32503, 32504◄)

32900 Resection of ribs, extrapleural, all stages

⃠=Modifier 51 Exempt ⊙=Conscious Sedation ✚=Add-on Code ⁄⁄=FDA approval pending

Rationale

In order to address the need for flexibility in reporting the treatment of lung cancers, with wide variability in regard to the amount of both lung and chest wall involvement (pleura, ribs, sternum, cartilage, muscle, subcutaneous tissue, and skin), three codes have been deleted (32520, 32522, 32525), two codes added, and instructional cross-references added to direct appropriate reporting for those procedures that should be additionally reported to capture the surgical variations of lung resection procedures.

Codes 32503 and 32504 have been added to report apical lung resection tumors that typically include lobectomy with resection of the ribs in the thoracic inlet and dissection of the tumor away from the brachial plexus and the subclavian artery.

In conjunction with the deletion of codes 32520, 32522, and 32525, the instructional references that have been added direct the use of existing lung resection codes in conjunction with the chest wall resection codes 19260, 19271, and 19272 for selection of the appropriate code combinations. The cross-reference preceding 32900 has also been revised to reflect the deletion of these codes.

In tandem with the deletion of codes 32520 and 32525, the cross-reference preceding code 32900 has been revised to direct the user to the new lung resection codes.

Clinical Example **(32503)**

A 66-year-old female, overweight, heavy smoker presents with a 4-month history of right shoulder and/or arm pain. An apical lung biopsy confirms non-small cell lung cancer.

Description of Procedure **(32503)**

A high thoracotomy is performed with a planned entry into the fourth intercostal space, dividing extrathoracic muscles with electrocautery for hemostasis and resecting a 1-cm segment of the rib posteriorly to facilitate exposure and spreading of the ribs. (Care is taken to avoid injury to the intercostal neurovascular bundles.) The chest is explored, assessing for the presence of adhesions between the lung and the chest wall, which are carefully divided before inserting the rib spreader to prevent a tear of the lung. The superior sulcus lung tumor is carefully palpated and its specific relationship to the chest wall, vertebral column, thoracic inlet, great vessels, and brachial plexus as well as its specific pulmonary vasculature and bronchial tree anatomy, and its relationship to the right middle and right lower lobe is defined to determine that a resection of this superior sulcus tumor with right upper lobectomy and chest wall of ribs 1, 2, and 3 is required and feasible.

Single lung ventilation of the contralateral lung is instituted to facilitate exposure of the operative lung side, the chest wall, vasculature, and bronchus. The extent of the tumor is identified from within the thorax and its anterior-ventral and posterior-caudal extent is defined. The trapezius and rhomboid muscles are divided between the posterior medial border of the scapula and the spinous processes such that the scapula can be elevated. A retractor is placed to elevate the scapula superiorly and laterally and the fourth rib inferiorly. Exposure to the ribs of the thoracic inlet/superior sulcus is thus obtained. The third rib is divided anteriorly 5 cm beyond the closest tumor margin. An additional 1-cm piece of rib is resected to facilitate exposure of the second rib. The third rib is divided posteriorly at the level of the transverse process. If the tumor involves this area, the rib is resected from the transverse process by dividing the costo-transversus ligament and then the costo-vertebral ligament, thus freeing the rib from the vertebral body. The intercostal bundle is identified, ligated, and divided. The second rib is divided anteriorly 5 cm beyond the closest tumor margin. An additional 1-cm piece of rib is resected to facilitate exposure of the second rib. The second rib is divided posteriorly at the level of the transverse process. If the tumor involves this area, the rib is resected from the transverse process by dividing the costo-transversus ligament and then the costo-vertebral ligament, thus freeing the rib from the vertebral body. The intercostal bundle is identified, ligated, and divided. The sympathetic ganglion is resected with the specimen. The first rib is divided anteriorly at the junction of the first rib with the sternum and the clavicle. Care is taken in dissecting the tumor off the great vessels, especially the subclavian artery, the vena cava, and innominate vein as well as the phrenic nerve and the brachial plexus. The first rib is divided posteriorly at the level of the transverse process. If the tumor involves this area, the rib is resected from the transverse process by dividing the costo-transversus ligament and then the costo-vertebral ligament, thus freeing the rib from the vertebral body. The T1 nerve root (just inferior to the posterior aspect of the first rib) is divided where it is involved with the tumor. The C8 nerve root is inspected and, if involved, is resected en bloc. The tumor is freed from its fibrous adhesions to the brachial plexus. The en bloc resection is thus allowed to drop into the chest. The lung is retracted posteriorly and inferiorly and as appropriate for the mediastinal pleura to be incised, carefully avoiding injury to the phrenic nerve. The lobar arterial blood supply is carefully dissected, mobilized, and encircled with ties. The upper and lower lobes are carefully separated by dissecting within the major fissure until the appropriate lobar arteries are identified. The isolated lobar arteries to the right upper lobe are ligated, suture-ligated, and then divided, carefully inspecting for bleeding from the proximal end. Specifically, the major fissure is dissected to facilitate exposure and precise identification of the lobar branch to the posterior segment of the right upper lobe (posterior ascending branch of the pulmonary artery), care being taken to identify and protect the superior segmental artery to the right lower lobe, and the middle lobe artery. The lung is retracted appropriately to permit exposure of the pulmonary venous drainage returning to the heart. Two pulmonary veins are confirmed. The pulmonary vein to just the right upper lobe is carefully dissected, mobilized, and encircled with ties. Specifically, the venous drainage to the right middle lobe is identified, care being taken to identify and protect the venous drainage from the right middle and lower lobe. The veins (from the right upper lobe) are ligated proximally with heavy suture, its distal branches ligated, the proximal end suture-ligated, and the vein divided, carefully assessing for bleeding from the proximal end. The lobar bronchus to the right upper lobe is carefully dissected, mobilized, and encircled with a tape. Specifically, the bronchus to the right middle lobe is identified, care being taken to identify and protect this bronchus, as well as the superior segmental bronchus and the basilar bronchi to the right lower lobe. The right upper lobe bronchus is individually crossed with a surgical stapler as close as possible to its origin with the bronchus intermedius. After ascertaining that ventilation of the remaining lobe has not been compromised by clamping of the bronchus, the lobar bronchus is divided sharply and the stapler is removed. The lobe is removed from the field and submitted for frozen section confirmation of a "clear" bronchial margin of resection. The divided bronchial stump is oversewn distal to the staples suture line with interrupted sutures. The pleural cavity is filled with warm saline. The anesthetist is asked to inflate the airway with 20 cm to 40 cm of water pressure, and the bronchial stump is carefully inspected for an air leak. The saline is aspirated from the chest. Chest tubes are inserted through separate interspace incisions to provide optimal drainage of air from the apex of the chest and of fluid from the base. The chest tubes are secured to the skin with sutures. The ribs are reapproximated with heavy pericostal sutures, carefully avoiding injury to the intercostal neurovascular bundles. The extrathoracic chest wall musculature is closed in layers with running suture. Subcutaneous tissue and skin are approximated

Clinical Example (32504)

A 66-year-old female, overweight, heavy smoker presents with a 4-month history of right shoulder and/or arm pain. An apical lung biopsy confirms non-small cell lung cancer.

Description of Procedure (32504)

A high thoracotomy is performed with a planned entry into the fifth intercostal space, dividing extrathoracic muscles with electrocautery for hemostasis and resecting a 1-cm segment of the rib posteriorly to facilitate exposure and spreading of the ribs. (Care is taken to avoid injury to the intercostal neurovascular bundles.) The chest is explored, assessing for the presence of adhesions between the lung and the chest wall, which are carefully divided before inserting the rib spreader to prevent a tear of the lung. The superior sulcus lung tumor is carefully palpated and its specific relationship to the chest wall, vertebral column, thoracic inlet, great vessels, and brachial plexus as well as its specific pulmonary vasculature and bronchial tree anatomy, and its relationship to the right middle and right lower lobe, defined to determine that a resection of this superior sulcus tumor with right upper lobectomy and chest wall of ribs 1, 2, 3, and 4 is required and is feasible.

Single-lung ventilation of the contralateral lung is instituted to facilitate exposure of the operative lung side, the chest wall, vasculature, and bronchus. The extent of the tumor is identified from within the thorax, and its anterior-ventral and posterior-caudal extent is defined. The trapezius and rhomboid muscles are divided between the posterior medial border of the scapula and the spinous processes such that the scapula can be elevated. A retractor is placed to elevate the scapula superiorly and laterally and the fifth rib inferiorly. Exposure to the ribs of the thoracic inlet/superior sulcus is thus obtained. The fourth rib is divided anteriorly 5 cm beyond the closest tumor margin. An additional 1-cm piece of rib is resected to facilitate exposure of the third rib. The fourth rib is divided posteriorly at the level of the transverse process. If the tumor involves this area, the rib is resected from the transverse process by dividing the costo-transversus ligament and then the costo-vertebral ligament, thus freeing the rib from the vertebral body. The intercostal bundle is identified, ligated, and divided. The third rib is divided anteriorly 5 cm beyond the closest tumor margin. An additional 1-cm piece of rib is resected to facilitate exposure of the second rib. The third rib is divided posteriorly at the level of the transverse process. If the tumor involves this area, the rib is resected from the transverse process by dividing the costo-transversus ligament and then the costo-vertebral ligament, thus freeing the rib from the vertebral body. The intercostal bundle is identified, ligated, and divided. The second rib is divided anteriorly 5 cm beyond the closest tumor margin. An additional 1-cm piece of rib is resected to facilitate exposure of the second rib. The second rib is divided posteriorly at the level of the transverse process. If the tumor involves this area, the rib is resected from the transverse process by dividing the costo-transversus ligament and then the costo-vertebral ligament, thus freeing the rib from the vertebral body. The intercostal bundle is identified, ligated, and divided. The sympathetic ganglion is resected with the specimen. The first rib is divided anteriorly at the junction of the first rib with the sternum and the clavicle. Care is taken in dissecting the tumor off the great vessels, especially the subclavian artery, the vena cava, and innominate vein as well as the phrenic nerve and the brachial plexus. The first rib is divided posteriorly at the level of the transverse process. If the tumor involves this area, the rib is resected from the transverse process by dividing the costo-transversus ligament and then the costo-vertebral ligament, thus freeing the rib from the vertebral body. The T1 nerve root (just inferior to the posterior aspect of the first rib) is divided where it is involved with the tumor. The C8 nerve root is inspected and, if involved, is resected en bloc. The tumor is freed from its fibrous adhesions to the brachial plexus. The en bloc resection is thus allowed to drop into the chest. The lung is retracted posteriorly and inferiorly and as appropriate for the mediastinal pleura to be incised, carefully avoiding injury to the phrenic nerve. The lobar arterial blood supply is carefully dissected, mobilized, and encircled with ties. The upper and lower lobes are carefully separated by dissecting within the major fissure until the appropriate lobar arteries are identified. The isolated lobar arteries to the right upper lobe are ligated, suture-ligated, and divided, carefully inspecting for bleeding from the proximal end. Specifically, the major fissure is dissected to facilitate exposure and precise identification of the lobar branch to the posterior segment of the right upper lobe (posterior ascending branch of the pulmonary artery), care being taken to identify and protect the superior segmental artery to the right lower lobe, and the middle lobe artery. The lung is retracted appropriately to permit exposure of the pulmonary venous drainage returning to the heart. Two pulmonary veins are confirmed. The pulmonary vein to just the right upper lobe is carefully dissected, mobilized, and encircled with ties. Specifically, the venous drainage to the right middle lobe is identified, care being taken to identify and protect the venous drainage from the right middle and lower lobe. The veins (from the right upper lobe) are ligated proximally with heavy suture, its distal branches ligated, the proximal end suture-ligated, and the vein divided, carefully assessing for bleeding from the proximal end. The lobar bronchus to the right upper lobe is carefully dissected, mobilized, and encircled with a tape. Specifically, the bronchus to the right middle lobe is identified, care being taken to identify and protect this bronchus as well as the superior segmental bronchus and the basilar bronchi to the right lower lobe. The right upper lobe bronchus is individually crossed with a surgical stapler as close as possible to its origin with the bronchus intermedius. After ascertaining that ventilation of the remaining lobe has not been compromised by clamping of the bronchus, the lobar bronchus is divided sharply and the stapler is removed.

The lobe is removed from the field and submitted for frozen section confirmation of a "clear" bronchial margin of resection. The divided bronchial stump is oversewn distal to the staple suture line with interrupted sutures. The pleural cavity is filled with warm saline. The anesthetist is asked to inflate the airway with 20 cm to 40 cm of water pressure, and the bronchial stump is carefully inspected for an air leak. The saline is aspirated from the chest. The musculoskeletal defect is measured and a prolene mesh patch is cut to the appropriate size. Holes are drilled in the ribs anteriorly and the fifth rib posteriorly to faciltate anchoring the patch. The patch is sewn into the ribs anteriorly and inferiorly with interrupted 2-0 nonabsorbable, surgical sutures. The posterior aspect of the patch is fixed either to the transverse processes or the paraspinous musculature with 2-0 nonabsorbable, surgical sutures. The apex of the patch is bordered by the subclavian vessels and brachial plexus so no fixation sutures are placed in that site. Chest tubes are inserted through separate interspace incisions to provide optimal drainage of air from the apex of the chest and of fluid from the base. The chest tubes are secured to the skin with sutures. The ribs are reapproximated with heavy pericostal sutures, carefully avoiding injury to the intercostal neurovascular bundles. The extrathoracic chest wall musculature is closed in layers with running suture. Subcutaneous tissue and skin are approximated.

Cardiovascular System

Heart and Pericardium

CARDIAC VALVES

Pulmonary Valve

33478 Outflow tract augmentation (gusset), with or without commissurotomy or infundibular resection

►(Use 33478 in conjunction with 33768 when a cavopulmonary anastomosis to a second superior vena cava is performed)◄

Rationale

In support of the establishment of add-on code 33768 to report performance of cavopulmonary anastomosis for the repair of bilateral superior venae cavae, an instructional parenthetical note indicates the appropriate reporting of the add-on code with the outflow tract augmentation code 33478.

CORONARY ARTERY ANOMALIES

▲33502 Repair of anomalous coronary artery from pulmonary artery origin; by ligation

33506 by translocation from pulmonary artery to aorta

(Do not report modifier 63 in conjunction with 33505, 33506)

●33507 Repair of anomalous (eg, intramural) aortic origin of coronary artery by unroofing or translocation

Rationale

Code 33507 was established to report repair of a coronary artery from an anomalous origin on the aorta. Consistent with this revision, code 33502 was editorially revised with the addition of the phrase "from pulmonary artery origin" to the descriptor to differentiate and clarify the artery origins in these codes. Due to improved imaging capabilities, this condition has become easier to diagnose and is recognized increasingly as a cause of sudden death in young patients.

Clinical Example (33507)

A 3-month-old child presents with tachypnea and poor feeding and has marked cardiomegaly on his chest X ray. An electrocardiogram shows deep Q waves in the left precordial leads. Echocardiogram demonstrates a poorly contractile left ventricle and anomalous origin of the left coronary from the pulmonary artery. Catheterization demonstrates a left ventricular end diastolic pressure of 25 mm Hg and retrograde flow for the left coronary into the pulmonary artery.

Description of Procedure (33507)

Under general endotracheal anesthesia, in the supine position, the patient was prepped and draped in standard aseptic fashion. A skin incision was made via standard median sternotomy and the sternum was divided in the midline. A cardiac cannulas placed cardiopulmonary bypass was initiated. The aortic cross clamp was applied and cardioplegic arrest was obtained. Aortotomy and repair of the defect is accomplished via unroofing an intramural anomalous coronary artery or through translocation of the origin to the anatomically correct position. The aortotomy is closed. The heart and aorta are de-aired, the cross-clamp is removed, and the patient is rewarmed and separated from bypass. Chest tubes and temporary pacing wires are placed. The sternum is closed with wires; the abdominal fascia, skin, and subcutaneous tissue are closed in layers.

ARTERIAL GRAFTING FOR CORONARY ARTERY BYPASS

33545 Repair of postinfarction ventricular septal defect, with or without myocardial resection

●33548 Surgical ventricular restoration procedure, includes prosthetic patch, when performed (eg, ventricular remodeling, SVR, SAVER, DOR procedures)

▶(Do not report 33548 in conjunction with 32020, 33210, 33211, 33310, 33315)◀

▶(For Batista procedure or pachopexy, use 33999)◀

Rationale

Code 33548 was established to report ventricular restoration procedures. This procedure focuses on reshaping the geometry of the heart as a treatment for left ventricular failure and includes preoperative assessment and planning the most optimal geometry of the heart muscle. This procedure is performed as an alternative to cardiac transplantation for the patient with end-stage cardiac disease with advanced stages of heart failure. Bypass surgery is also frequently performed in addition to this procedure and would be separately reported. As indicated by the code descriptor, placement of a prosthetic patch of autologous or artificial material sutured at the level of the Fontan to close the defect is included in the procedure and not separately reported. Also included in this procedure is the ventricular remodeling when performed. A cross-reference has been added to refer the user to unlisted code 33999 to report the Batista or pachopexy procedures. The Batista procedure is performed for patients with nonischemic cardiomyopathy. Ventricular restoration is performed for patients with ischemic cardiomyopathy. An exclusionary parenthetical note has been added following 33548 to preclude reporting tube thoracostomy (32020); insertion of temporary transvenous single or dual chamber catheters (33210-33211); and cardiotomy procedures (33310-33315) because these procedures are also inherent. This procedure is frequently performed in conjunction with other cardiac repair codes (eg, mitral valve replacement, valvuloplasty, coronary artery bypass graft), which may be separately reported when performed.

Clinical Example (33548)

A 56-year-old man presents with class IV congestive heart failure symptoms that are refractory to medical management and have required four hospitalizations in the past 6 months. He has no angina pectoris but has a history of multiple myocardial infarctions and several percutaneous revascularizations. Cardiac catheterization reveals a totally occluded proximal LAD and a poor distal LAD supplied by right-to-left collaterals and a diminuitive circulflex coronary system. The right coronary is dominant and without significant in-stent restenosis. Left ventriculography shows anterior and anteroapical akinesis, trace mitral regurgitation, global left ventricular dilatation, and an overall ejection fraction of 15%. Left ventricular regional and global function is carefully assessed through echocardiography and viability studies. He is evaluated for cardiac transplantation and is found to have prohibitive preformed antibodies. He is considered unsuitable for transplantation due to this finding, his weight of 250 lbs, and an O blood type. A surgical ventricular restoration procedure is recommended and accepted by the patient.

Description of Procedure (33548)

A skin incision is made via standard median sternotomy. The sternum is divided in the midline. Cannulation is accomplished using the ascending aorta and two-stage right atrium venous return. A cardiopulmonary bypass is initiated. A left ventricular vent is inserted via the right superior pulmonary vein. The heart is carefully inspected to assess the anteroapical akinetic area for resectability; the left anterior descending (LAD) is confirmed to be inoperable and the supplied tissue is nonviable. The ascending aorta is clamped and cardioplegic arrest is instituted. An anterior ventriculotomy is performed to the left of the LAD, and extended to the apex of the heart. The junction between scarred abnormal myocardium and normal myocardium is determined by visual inspection and palpation. An encircling 0-prolene suture is placed at the junction and tied to reduce the orifice and restore the normal elliptical shape of the left ventricle (Fontan stitch). Available sizers and intraventricular balloons may be used to determine the final corrected left ventricular volume. A circular patch of autologous or artificial material is sutured at the level of the Fontan stitch to close the defect without reducing ventricular volume further. The left ventriculotomy is closed in layers. The patient is rewarmed and weaned from cardiopulmonary bypass using moderate doses of inotropic agents. Hemostasis is obtained and the surgical wound is repaired after placing appropriate drainage tubes.

SINGLE VENTRICLE AND OTHER COMPLEX CARDIAC ANOMALIES

33608 Repair of complex cardiac anomaly other than pulmonary atresia with ventricular septal defect by construction or replacement of conduit from right or left ventricle to pulmonary artery

(For repair of pulmonary ►artery arborization anomalies by unifocalization, see 33925-33926◄)

33617 Repair of complex cardiac anomalies (eg, single ventricle) by modified Fontan procedure

►(Use 33617 in conjunction with 33768 when a cavopulmonary anastomosis to a second superior vena cava is performed)◄

Rationale

In support of the establishment of add-on code 33768 to report performance of cavopulmonary anastomosis for the repair of bilateral superior venae cavae an instructional parenthetical note indicates appropriate reporting of the add-on code with Fontan procedure code 33617.

SHUNTING PROCEDURES

33750 Shunt; subclavian to pulmonary artery (Blalock-Taussig type operation)

33767 superior vena cava to pulmonary artery for flow to both lungs (bidirectional Glenn procedure)

+●33768 Anastomosis, cavopulmonary, second superior vena cava (List separately in addition to primary procedure)

►(Use 33768 in conjunction with 33478, 33617, 33767)◄

►(Do not report 33768 in conjunction with 32020, 33210, 33211)◄

Rationale

Add-on code 33768 was established to report performance of cavopulmonary anastomosis for treatment of bilateral superior venae cavae at the same session as the performance of the complex cardiac anomaly repair procedures: 33478 (outflow tract augmentation), 33617 (Fontan), or 33767 (bidirectional Glenn).

A parenthetical note instructs the appropriate reporting of the cavopulmonary anastomosis with these procedures.

An exclusionary parenthetical note has been added to instruct that component procedures of the larger procedure (33768) would not be separately reported. These component procedures include tube thoracostomy (32020) and insertion of temporary transvenous single- or dual-chamber pacing cardiac electrodes (33210, 33211).

Clinical Example (33768)

A child with single ventricle physiology presents with bilateral superior venae cavae with low pulmonary vascular resistance.

Description of Procedure (33768)

The additional superior vena cava is dissected out along with the adjacent branch pulmonary artery. The physician prepares the additional vena cava for insertion of bypass cannula, divides the azygos vein or hemi-azygos vein, and inserts the bypass cannula in the additional superior vena cava. The additional superior vena cava is divided and the cardiac end is oversewn. An incision is made in the superior aspect of the adjacent pulmonary artery and an end-to-side anastomosis of the additional superior vena cava to the adjacent pulmonary artery is performed. The second superior vena cava is de-cannulated and the cannulation site is repaired.

▶ENDOVASCULAR REPAIR OF DESCENDING THORACIC AORTA◀

▶Codes 33880-33891 represent a family of procedures to report placement of an endovascular graft for repair of the descending thoracic aorta. These codes include all device introduction, manipulation, positioning, and deployment. All balloon angioplasty and/or stent deployment within the target treatment zone for the endoprosthesis, either before or after endograft deployment, are not separately reportable. Open arterial exposure and associated closure of the arteriotomy sites (eg, 34812, 34820, 34833, 34834), introduction of guidewires and catheters (eg, 36140, 36200-36218), and extensive repair or replacement of an artery (eg, 35226, 35286) should be additionally reported. Transposition of subclavian artery to carotid, and carotid-carotid bypass performed in conjunction with endovascular repair of the descending thoracic aorta (eg, 33889, 33891) should be separately reported. The primary codes, 33880 and 33881, include placement of all distal extensions, if required, in the distal thoracic aorta, while proximal extensions, if needed, are reported separately.◀

▶For fluoroscopic guidance in conjunction with endovascular repair of the thoracic aorta, see codes 75956-75959 as appropriate. Codes 75956 and 75957 include all angiography of the thoracic aorta and its branches for diagnostic imaging prior to deployment of the primary endovascular devices (including all routine components of modular devices), fluoroscopic guidance in the delivery of the endovascular components, and intraprocedural arterial angiography (eg, confirm position, detect endoleak, evaluate runoff). Code 75958 includes the analogous services for placement of each proximal thoracic endovascular extension. Code 75959 includes the analogous services for placement of a distal thoracic endovascular extension(s) placed during a procedure after the primary repair.◀

▶Other interventional procedures performed at the time of endovascular repair of the descending thoracic aorta should be additionally reported (eg, innominate, carotid, subclavian, visceral, or iliac artery transluminal angioplasty or stenting, arterial embolization, intravascular ultrasound) when performed before or after deployment of the aortic prostheses.◀

●33880 Endovascular repair of descending thoracic aorta (eg, aneurysm, pseudoaneurysm, dissection, penetrating ulcer, intramural hematoma, or traumatic disruption); involving coverage of left subclavian artery origin, initial endoprosthesis plus descending thoracic aortic extension(s), if required, to level of celiac artery origin

►(For radiological supervision and interpretation, use 75956 in conjunction with 33880)◄

●33881 not involving coverage of left subclavian artery origin, initial endoprosthesis plus descending thoracic aortic extension(s), if required, to level of celiac artery origin

►(For radiological supervision and interpretation, use 75957 in conjunction with 33881)◄

●33883 Placement of proximal extension prosthesis for endovascular repair of descending thoracic aorta (eg, aneurysm, pseudoaneurysm, dissection, penetrating ulcer, intramural hematoma, or traumatic disruption); initial extension

►(For radiological supervision and interpretation, use 75958 in conjunction with 33883)◄

►(Do not report 33881, 33883 when extension placement converts repair to cover left subclavian origin. Use only 33880)◄

✚●33884 each additional proximal extension (List separately in addition to code for primary procedure)

►(Use 33884 in conjunction with 33883)◄

►(For radiological supervision and interpretation, use 75958 in conjunction with 33884)◄

●33886 Placement of distal extension prosthesis(s) delayed after endovascular repair of descending thoracic aorta

►(Do not report 33886 in conjunction with 33880, 33881)◄

►(Report 33886 once, regardless of number of modules deployed)◄

►(For radiological supervision and interpretation, use 75959 in conjunction with 33886)◄

●33889 Open subclavian to carotid artery transposition performed in conjunction with endovascular repair of descending thoracic aorta, by neck incision, unilateral

►(Do not report 33889 in conjunction with 35694)◄

●33891 Bypass graft, with other than vein, transcervical retropharyngeal carotid-carotid, performed in conjunction with endovascular repair of descending thoracic aorta, by neck incision

►(Do not report 33891 in conjunction with 35509, 35601)◄

Rationale

Consistent with the deletion and conversion of Category III codes 0033T-0040T, seven Category I codes, guidelines, and cross-references have been established to report placement of an endovascular graft for repair of the descending thoracic aorta. These codes include all device introduction, manipulation, positioning, and deployment. All balloon angioplasty and/or stent deployment within the target treatment zone for the endoprosthesis, before or after endograft deployment, is also included and, therefore, not separately reported. Conversely, balloon angioplasty and/or stent deployment outside of the target zone is separately reportable.

The primary codes of the series, 33880 and 33881, describe endovascular repair of the descending thoracic aorta and are differentiated by the coverage or noncoverage of the subclavian artery. Endovascular prostheses for the descending aorta are obtained in modules. The first component of the endovascular repair is deployed such that the leading edge lands in a nearly normal segment of proximal aorta, allowing firm fixation. Subsequent components are deployed through the diseased portion of aorta such that each partially overlaps the preceding one, thereby preventing any leaks between modules. Components are "tiled" in this way until the diseased portion of aorta is completely covered and the distal-most component lies in normal aorta. While some repairs require only one component, the typical patient requires two, three, or more modules to cover the diseased segment of descending thoracic aorta. The primary treatment code 33880 includes deployment of the initial module and the placement of all distal extensions required in the descending aorta up to the origin of the celiac artery. The celiac artery is generally felt to be the distinguishing landmark between the thoracic and abdominal portions of the aorta. As indicated in the guidelines for codes 33880 and 33881, all balloon angioplasties and/or stent deployments within the target treatment zone for the endoprosthesis, either before or after endograft deployment, are not separately reportable. Those balloon angioplasties outside of the target treatment zone are separately reportable. When thoracic aorta endovascular repair involves coverage of the subclavian artery, code 33880 is reported. When subclavian coverage is not involved, code 33881 is reported.

The open arterial exposure codes (34812, 34820, 34833, 34834) are separately reported for preparation of the arterial access for the endovascular graft, based upon the site of access. One of the first key steps in endovascular repair procedures is open arterial exposure of peripheral arteries (femoral, iliac, brachial). This is done to allow introduction of the large-diameter endovascular devices into the arterial system under direct vision. Catheterization services are separately reported with the appropriate catheterization code(s): 36200-36218, 36140.

Codes 33880 and 33881 are repectively cross-referenced to the radiological supervision and interpretation codes 75956 and 75957 to report all fluoroscopic guidance in the delivery of the endovascular components and intraprocedural arterial angiography (eg, position confirmation, endoleak detection, runoff, and angiography evaluation of the thoracic aorta and its branches for diagnostic imaging prior to deployment of the primary endovascular devices provided in conjunction with these endovascular repair services).

For the repair of the distal aorta, not involving coverage of the subclavian artery, 33881 is reported. This procedure includes placement of the initial device and all subsequent distally placed extension prostheses. Should proximal placement of an extension prosthesis be required, 33883 is reported for placement of the initial extension prosthesis placed in the proximal segment, in addition to 33881. If insertion and placement of further extension prosthesis in the proximal segments are required, add-on code 33884 is reported for the placement of each additional proximal segment after the initial proximal graft. However, an exclusionary note instructs that when extension prosthesis placement results in extending the prosthesis to include coverage of the left subclavian origin, these services are reported only with code 33880.

As all distal prosthesis extensions placed in conjunction with endovascular thoracic aorta repair are included in codes 33880 and 33881, separate reporting for placement of additional distal extensions is reportable only when performed at a separate session. This is occasionally necessary during postoperative follow-up care when the presence of an endoleak becomes evident, the endovascular components shift with the threat of an endoleak, or the aneurysm has extended distally. Under these circumstances, the placement of further distal prosthesis extensions to extend coverage of the original components is reported with 33886. An instructional cross-reference has been added to indicate that 33886 is reported one time, regardless of the number of required extensions placed for treatment. An exclusionary parenthetical further illustrates the secondary nature of this procedure providing clear instructions that this service cannot be reported in conjunction with initial thoracic aorta device placement.

Code 33889 is reported for subclavian artery ligation and anastomosis to the carotid artery. In these circumstances when it is anticipated that the endovascular repair will require coverage of the subclavian artery origin, it is necessary, for preservation of blood flow to the arm, that the subclavian artery be ligated and anastomosed to the carotid artery. An exclusionary parenthetical note instructs that arterial transposition code 36594 is not additionally reported.

Cross-neck carotid-carotid bypass using synthetic conduit is reported with code 33891 when the thoracic aorta aneurysm is proximal to the origin of the left common carotid artery. Coverage of the carotid origin with the endovascular graft is required. In order to retain vascular flow when the endoprosthesis requires deployment across (therefore occluding) the origin of this vessel, a cross-neck carotid-carotid bypass is performed using synthetic conduit to maintain blood flow to the brain. An exclusionary parenthetical note instructs that the bypass graft codes 35509 (vein) and 35601 (other than vein) are not additionally reported. As indicated in the guidelines, codes 33889 and 33891 are separately reported in addition to the endovascular graft placement codes.

Clinical Example (33880)

A 68-year-old male with hypertension, a 50-pack-per-year smoking habit, and previous myocardial infarction is found to have a 7.0-cm diameter descending thoracic aortic aneurysm that begins immediately beyond the origin of left subclavian artery. Risks and benefits of open surgical repair, endovascular repair, and watchful waiting have been discussed, and the patient has chosen endovascular repair. Perioperative risk evaluation, including cardiac workup, indicated suitability for the endovascular approach. Imaging studies (typically a combination of computed tomography scan, magnetic resonance imaging, and/or angiography) demonstrate that the aneurysm is within acceptable parameters for endovascular repair if the left subclavian artery origin is covered by the endoprosthesis. Endovascular repair of the descending thoracic aortic aneurysm is performed. The proximal extent of the endoprosthesis covers the left subclavian artery origin.

Note: The proposed new code includes all distal extensions required to complete the typical repair. Left subclavian to carotid transposition is separately reportable. This code follows endovascular repair guidelines such that open arterial exposure, arterial catheterization, and radiological supervision and interpretation are separately reported.

Description of Procedure (33880)

Reporting 33880 will follow the detailed coding guidelines in the CPT introductory notes for endovascular repairs. It is important to note that 33880 includes placement of as many distal extension components as required to complete the repair. The intraservice work begins after achieving arterial exposure and after initial catheter and guidewire placement has been completed. The intraservice work includes the following steps.

The surgeon performs a road-mapping arteriogram with specific attention to great vessel artery origins and the celiac origin. The aortic arch is imaged in multiple projections to determine the exact orthogonal coordinates to deploy the prosthesis. The surgeon waits for anesthesia to insert and adjust transesophageal echocardiogram, if employed. A final out-of-body examination of the endovascular components for correct models, diameters, lengths, etc, is completed. Soft J-wires are exchanged for superstiff wires. The initial component is unpackaged, inspected for damage, and prepared for insertion. The patient is anticoagulated with IV heparin. The initial component and carrier are loaded onto superstiff wire and advanced to the femoral artery. The tip of the carrier is introduced into the arteriotomy. The proximal vascular clamp is opened and the leading edge of the device is advanced into the artery. Rubber constrictor loops are used to limit blood loss. Under fluoroscopic guidance, the first component and carrier are directed through the external iliac. The first component and carrier are advanced into the common iliac, abdominal aorta, and thoracic aorta up to the arch. The surgeon advances with extreme care at the arch so that the nose cone lies in the ascending aorta and leading edge across the left subclavian origin. The arteriography is repeated as needed to absolutely confirm great vessel origins with the leading edge of the device. The surgeon asks the anesthesiologist to lower the patient's blood pressure and they wait for the desired effect. Deployment is begun. Contrast injections are performed in multiple planes to allow final exact positioning. The surgeon makes the final precise adjustments to align the leading edge of the component in the arch across the left subclavian origin. The initial component is deployed with constant attention to exact positioning. The carrier is advanced to recapture the nose cone. The carrier and nose cone are retracted with care not to disturb the first component. The carrier and nose cone are backed through the descending aorta and through the iliac arteries with care not to disrupt the iliacs. The first component carrier is removed from the femoral artery and the artery is reclamped. A compliant balloon is introduced under fluoro guidance, advanced through the iliac artery, abdominal aorta, and thoracic aorta to the arch. The surgeon warns the anesthesiologist that the aortic arch is about to be occluded. The compliant balloon is inflated under constant fluoroxopic observation to expand and seat the first component. The compliant balloon is deflated and backed carefully out of the first component. A multi-sidehole catheter is advanced into the aortic arch. Contrast is injected and the graft is imaged to confirm accurate placement. The surgeon prepares and loads the second component onto superstiff wire in groin. The second component is advanced into the femoral artery through the iliacs and the abdominal aorta into the thoracic aorta. The surgeon observes fluoroscopically while carefully invaginating the second component into the first. The overlap is adjusted.

The catheter is advanced and contrast is injected to ensure that the distal edge has not covered the celiac. Final leading and following edge adjustments are made with imaging. The second component is deployed. The carrier is retracted carefully without disrupting the deployed components or iliac artery. The carrier is removed from the groin and blood loss is minimized. The catheter is advanced and contrast is injected to assess the positioning of the second component, endoleak, etc. The surgeon determines the need for additional distal components. All of these steps are repeated in sequence with sufficient components to complete a hemostatic distal anastomosis above the celiac. A compliant balloon is introduced for final expansion and seating of all additional components. The final arteriogram determines the appropriate coverage, patency of major arteries, and absence of endoleaks. The introducers are removed, using fluoroscopic guidance to prevent the disruption of the graft position. The surgeon performs completion pressure measurements. Catheters, wires, and sheaths are removed using fluoroscopic guidance.

Clinical Example (33881)

A 68-year-old male with hypertension, a 50-pack-per-year smoking habit, and previous myocardial infarction is found to have a 7.0-cm diameter descending thoracic aortic aneurysm that begins several centimeters beyond the left subclavian artery origin. Risks and benefits of open surgical repair, endovascular repair, and watchful waiting have been discussed, and the patient opted for endovascular repair. Perioperative risk evaluation including cardiac workup indicated suitability for an endovascular approach. Imaging studies (typically a combination of computed tomography scan, magnetic resonance imaging, and/or angiography) demonstrate that the aneurysm is within acceptable parameters for endovascular repair. Endovascular repair of his descending thoracic aortic aneurysm is performed. The proximal portion of the endoprosthesis does not cover the left subclavian artery origin.

Note: The proposed new code includes all distal extensions required to complete the typical repair. This code follows endovascular repair guidelines such that open arterial exposure, arterial catheterization, and radiological supervision and interpretation are separately reported.

Description of Procedure (33881)

Reporting 33881 will follow the detailed coding guidelines in the CPT introductory notes for endovascular repairs. It is important to note that 33881 includes deployment of as many distal extension components as required to complete the repair. The intraservice work begins after achieving arterial exposure and after initial catheter and guidewire placement has been completed. The intraservice work includes the following steps.

The surgeon performs a road-mapping arteriogram with specific attention to great vessel artery origins and the celiac origin. The aortic arch and descending thoracic aorta are imaged in multiple projections to determine exact orthogonal coordinates. The surgeon waits for anesthesia to insert and adjust transesophageal echocardiogram, if employed. A final out-of-body examination of endovascular components for correct models, diameters, lengths, etc, is performed. Soft J-wires are exchanged for superstiff wires. The initial component is unpackaged, inspected for damage, and prepared for insertion. The patient is anticoagulated with IV heparin. The initial component and carrier are loaded onto superstiff wire and advance to the femoral artery. The tip of the carrier is introduced into the arteriotomy. The proximal vascular clamp is opened and the leading edge of the device is advanced into the artery. Rubber constrictor loops are used to limit blood loss. Under fluoroscopic guidance, the first component and carrier are directed through the external iliac. The first component and carrier are advanced into the common iliac, abdominal aorta, and thoracic aorta up to arch. The surgeon advanced with extreme care so the nose cone lies in the arch with the leading edge of the component just beyond the left subclavian origin. The arteriography is repeated as needed to absolutely confirm great vessel origins with the leading edge of the device. The surgeon asks the anesthesiologist to lower the patient's blood pressure and they wait for the desired effect. Deployment is begun. Contrast injections in multiple planes are made to allow final exact positioning. The surgeon makes the final precise adjustments to align the leading edge of the component just beyond left subclavian origin. The initial component is deployed with constant attention to exact positioning. The carrier is advanced to recapture the nose cone. The carrier and nose cone are retracted with care not to disturb the first component. The carrier and nose cone are backed through the descending aorta and through the iliac arteries with care not to disrupt the iliacs. The first component carrier is removed from the femoral artery and the artery is reclamped. A compliant balloon is introduced under fluoro guidance and advanced through the iliac artery, abdominal aorta, and thoracic aorta into the component. The surgeon warns the anesthesiologist that the aortic arch is about to be occluded. The compliant balloon is inflated under constant fluoroxopic observation to expand and seat the first component. The compliant balloon is deflated and backed carefully out of the first component. A multi-sidehole catheter is advanced into the aortic arch. Contrast is injected and the graft is imaged to confirm accurate placement. The surgeon prepares and loads the second component onto the superstiff wire in the groin. The second component is advanced into the femoral artery, through the iliacs and abdominal aorta into the thoracic aorta. The surgeon observes fluoroscopically while carefully invaginating the second component into the first. The overlap is adjusted. The multi-sidehole catheter is advanced and contrast is injected to ensure that the distal edge has not covered the celiac. Final leading and following edge adjustments are made with imaging. The second component is deployed. The carrier is retracted carefully without disrupting the deployed components or iliac artery. The carrier is removed from the groin and blood loss is minimized. The multi-sidehole catheter is advanced and contrast is injected to assess the positioning of the second component, endoleak, etc. The surgeon determines the need for additional distal components. All of these steps are repeated in sequence with sufficient components to complete a hemostatic distal anastomosis above the celiac. A compliant balloon is introduced for final expansion and seating of all additional components. The final arteriogram determines the appropriate coverage, patency of major arteries, and absence of endoleaks. The introducers are removed, using fluoroscopic guidance to prevent disruption of the graft position. The surgeon performs completion pressure measurements. Catheters, wires, and sheaths are removed using fluoroscopic guidance.

Clinical Example (33883)

A 68-year-old male with hypertension, a 50-pack-per-year smoking habit, and previous myocardial infarction underwent endovascular repair of the descending thoracic aortic aneurysm 1 year ago. On the follow-up computed tomography (CT) scan, he is found to have a proximal endoleak. Risks and benefits of endovascular endoleak repair have been discussed, and he opted to proceed. Perioperative risk evaluation, including cardiac workup, indicated suitability for endovascular repair. Imaging studies (typically a combination of CT scan, magnetic resonance imaging, and/or angiography) demonstrate that the endoleak is suitable for an endovascular approach. A proximal endovascular extension is deployed.

Description of Procedure (33883)

Reporting 33883 will follow the detailed coding guidelines in the CPT introductory notes for endovascular repairs. It is important to note that 33883 will most often be performed as a complex stand-alone procedure for endovascular repairs that develop late type I endoleaks. The intraservice work begins after achieving arterial exposure and initial catheter and guidewire placements. Intraservice work includes the following steps.

The surgeon performs a road-mapping arteriogram with specific attention to great vessel artery origins. The aortic arch is imaged in multiple projections to determine exact orthogonal coordinates to deploy the prosthesis. The surgeon waits for anesthesia to insert transesophageal echocardiogram (TEE), if employed. A final out-of-body examination of the endovascular components for correct models, diameters, lengths, etc, is completed. Soft J-wires are exchanged for superstiff wires. The component is unpackaged, inspected for damage, and prepared for insertion. The patient is anticoagulated with IV heparin. The proximal extension is loaded onto the superstiff wire and advanced to the femoral artery. The tip of the main device is introduced into the arteriotomy. The proximal vascular clamp is opened and the leading edge is advanced into the artery. Rubber constrictor loops are used to limit blood loss. Under fluoroscopic guidance, the proximal extension device is directed through the external iliac. The device is advanced into the common iliac and abdominal aorta to the descending thoracic aorta. The surgeon guides the device under fluoroscopy into and through the previously placed components. The nose cone of the carrier is directed carefully around the aortic arch so the tip lies in the ascending aorta. The arteriography is repeated in multiple projections to ensure the leading edge of the device is appropriate to the great vessel origins. The surgeon checks fluoroscopically in multiple projections to ensure that the trailing edge overlaps the previous component adequately. The surgeon asks the anesthesiologist to check the position with TEE, if used, and to lower the patient's blood pressure and wait for the desired effect.

Deployment is begun. Contrast is injected in multiple planes for final pre-deployment assessment. Final precise adjustments are made to align the leading edge of the component to the required position with the great vessel origins. Deployment is completed. The carrier is advanced to the nose cone, both are retracted over the wire while the surgeon avoids displacing new or old endovascular components. The carrier is retracted through the abdominal aorta and iliacs. The vascular clamp is opened and the carrier and nose cone are removed from the arterial system. A compliant balloon is backloaded and introduced. The surgeon guides the balloon under fluoroscopy through the pelvis, abdominal, and descending thoracic aorta. The balloon is guided into the newly deployed component with care not to disrupt it. The balloon position is checked in multiple fluoroscopic projections to avoid great vessel injury. The surgeon warns the anesthesiologist that the aorta will be occluded and recommends reduction of the blood pressure, as needed. The balloon is inflated and fully expanded, allowing the component to be seated. Contrast injections are performed in multiple planes to evaluate for position and possible leaks. The balloon steps and/or other maneuvers are repeated as required to treat the leaks. A final arteriogram determines the appropriate coverage, patency of major arteries, and absence of endoleaks. The introducers are removed using fluoroscopic guidance to prevent disruption of the graft position. **Note:** All of the balloon angioplasty steps are included in the work of this service.

Clinical Example (33884)

A 68-year-old male with hypertension, a 50-pack-per-year smoking habit, and previous myocardial infarction underwent endovascular repair of the descending thoracic aortic aneurysm 1 year ago. On the follow-up computed tomography (CT) scan, he is found to have a proximal endoleak. Placement of one proximal extension prosthesis has been performed, but the endoleak persists. An additional proximal extension is required.

Description of Procedure (33884)

The intraservice work of 33884 begins after the initial proximal extension (33883) has been deployed. Reporting 33884 also follows the detailed coding guidelines in the CPT introductory notes for endovascular repair. Arterial exposure and initial catheter and guidewire placement have already been performed. Intraservice work includes the following steps.

The surgeon performs a road-mapping arteriogram with specific attention to great vessel artery origins and prior components. The aortic arch is imaged in multiple projections to determine exact orthogonal coordinates to deploy additional prosthesis. The surgeon waits for anesthesia to insert transesophageal echocardiogram (TEE), if employed. A final examination of the endovascular components for correct model, size, etc, is completed. The physician ensures that the superstiff guidewire is in the appropriate position. The component is unpackaged, examined for defects, and prepared for insertion. The surgeon ensures that anticoagulation remains adequate. The proximal extension component is loaded onto the superstiff wire and advanced to the femoral artery. The tip of the device is introduced into the arteriotomy. A proximal vascular clamp is opened and the nose cone is advanced into the artery. The surgeon uses rubber constrictor loops to limit blood loss. Under fluoroscopic guidance, he or she directs the proximal component through the external iliac. The component is advanced into the common iliac, abdominal aorta, and descending thoracic aorta. The new component is guided under fluoroscopic guidance into and through the previously placed devices. The new component is directed carefully around the aortic arch so the tip and nose cone lie in the ascending aorta. The arteriography is repeated in multiple projections to ensure that the leading edge of the component is appropriate to great vessel origins. The surgeon checks fluoroscopically in multiple projections to ensure the trailing edge overlaps the previous component adequately. The surgeon asks the anesthesiologist to check the position with TEE (if used). The anesthesiologist is asked to lower the patient's blood pressure and they wait for the desired effect. Deployment is begun. Contrast is injected for a final pre-deployment assessment. Final precise adjustments are made to align the leading edge to the required position at the great vessel origins. Deployment is completed. The carrier is advanced to the nose cone and both are retracted over the wire while the surgeon avoids displacing the new or old endovascular components. The carrier is retracted through the abdominal aorta and iliacs. The vascular clamp is opened and the carrier and nose cone are removed from the arterial system. The surgeon backloads and introduces a compliant balloon. The balloon is guided under fluoroscopy through the pelvis, abdominal, and descending thoracic aorta. Next, the balloon is guided into the newly deployed component with care not to disrupt it. The surgeon checks the balloon position in multiple fluoroscopic projections to avoid great vessel injury. He or she also warns the anesthesiologist that the aorta will be occluded and that the patient's blood pressure should be reduced as needed. The balloon is inflated to fully expand and the component is seated. Contrast injections are performed in multiple planes to evaluate for position and possible leaks. The balloon steps and/or other maneuvers are repeated as required to treat leaks. A final arteriogram helps to determine appropriate coverage, patency of major arteries, and the absence of endoleaks. The surgeon removes introducers, using fluoroscopic guidance to prevent disruption of graft position. Note that all of these steps are included in the work of this service. No additional codes are reportable.

Clinical Example (33886)

A 68-year-old male with hypertension, a 50-pack-per-year smoking habit, and previous myocardial infarction underwent endovascular repair of a descending thoracic aortic aneurysm 1 year ago. On the follow-up computed tomography scan, he is found to have a distal endoleak. Placement of a distal extension is undertaken to seal the leak.

Note: This code cannot be reported during the primary thoracic aortic repair. Distal stents placed during thoracic aortic endovascular repair are included in the primary code. This code is only reportable if distal extensions are required at some date after the primary thoracic aortic repair has been completed. This differs from the abdominal aortic endovascular reporting conventions.

Description of Procedure (33886)

Reporting 33886 will follow detailed coding guidelines in the CPT introductory notes for endovascular repairs. Intraservice work begins after achieving arterial exposure and following initial catheter and guidewire placements. Intraservice work includes the following steps.

The surgeon performs a road-mapping arteriogram with specific attention given to device placement and the location of the distal endoleak. He or she images the descending thoracic aorta in multiple projections to determine the exact orthogonal coordinates to deploy the prosthesis. The anesthesiologist inserts transesophageal echocardiogram (TEE), if employed. A final out-of-body examination of the endovascular components is carried out to determine correct models, diameters, lengths, etc. Soft J-wires are exchanged for superstiff wires. The component is unpackaged, inspected for damage, and prepared for insertion. The patient is anticoagulated with IV heparin. The distal extension is loaded onto the superstiff wire and advanced to the femoral artery. The tip of the main device is introduced into the arteriotomy. A proximal vascular clamp is opened and the leading edge is advanced into the artery. The surgeon uses rubber constrictor loops to limit blood loss. Under fluoroscopic guidance, he or she directs the distal extension device through the external iliac. The nose cone of the device is advanced into the common iliac, abdominal aorta, and descending thoracic aorta. Under fluoroscopy, the device is guided into the previously placed components. Arteriography is repeated in multiple projections to ensure that the leading edge of the extension overlaps the existing device adequately. The surgeon checks fluoroscopically in multiple projections to ensure that the trailing edge of the new component does not cover the celiac origin. The anesthesiologist check the position with TEE, if used. The surgeon asks the anesthesiologist to lower the patient's blood pressure and they wait for the desired effect. Deployment is begun. Contrast is injected in multiple planes for final pre-deployment assessment. Final precise adjustments are made to align the leading and trailing edges of the component to the required position. Deployment is completed. The carrier is advanced to the nose cone and both are retracted over the wire while the surgeon avoids displacing the new or old endovascular components. The carrier is retracted through the abdominal aorta and iliacs. The vascular clamp is opened and the carrier and nose cone are removed from the arterial system. The surgeon backloads and introduces a compliant balloon. Under fluoroscopy, he or she guides the balloon through the pelvis, abdominal, and descending thoracic aorta. The balloon is guided into the newly deployed component with care not to disrupt it. The balloon's position is checked in multiple fluoroscopic projections to avoid injury to the patient. The surgeon warns the anesthesiologist that the aorta will be occluded and that blood pressure should be reduced as needed. The balloon is inflated to fully expand and seat the component. Contrast injections are performed in multiple planes to evaluate for position and possible leaks. The balloon steps and/or other maneuvers are repeated as required to treat the leaks.

All of these steps are repeated in sequence if more than one component is needed. A final arteriogram is conducted to determine the appropriate coverage, patency of major arteries, and absence of endoleaks. The introducers are removed using fluoroscopic guidance to prevent disruption of the graft position. **Note:** All of these balloon angioplasty steps are included in the work of this service.

Clinical Example (33889)

A 65-year-old female with hypertension, a 50-pack-per-year smoking habit, and previous myocardial infarction is found to have a 7-cm descending thoracic aortic aneurysm. The aneurysm originates immediately adjacent to her left subclavian artery origin, and in order to achieve a hemostatic proximal seal zone the endoprosthesis will need to be deployed across and, therefore, occlude the origin of this artery. To maintain blood flow to her left arm, a subclavian to carotid transposition is performed.

Description of Procedure (33889)

The intraservice work of 33889 begins with skin incision on the neck extending toward the left arm in the supraclavicular space. Access to the carotid and subclavian arteries is achieved by dissecting through soft tissue and mobilizing a plethora of nerves and veins, all very carefully. The common carotid artery is cleared for 5 to 6 cm, and the left subclavian is dissected under the clavicle as closely as possible to its origin on the aorta. Soft rubber loops are passed proximally and distally around both arteries. Once adequate exposure is achieved and intravenous heparin anticoagulation is administered, proximal and distal vascular clamps are applied to the subclavian near its origin. The artery is divided between clamps and the proximal stump is oversewn with fine polypropylene sutures. The proximal clamp is removed, and additional sutures are placed as required to achieve hemostasis.

Vascular clamps are applied to the common carotid artery. The left subclavian, now free from its original origin, is mobilized and extended to meet the side of the common carotid. An arteriotomy is fashioned at an appropriate site on the carotid, and the end of subclavian artery is anastomosed to the side of the carotid using fine polypropylene sutures. All vascular clamps are removed, and additional sutures are placed as needed to achieve hemostasis. All pulses are checked and confirmed with Doppler. The wound is irrigated copiously and closed in layers.

Clinical Example (33891)

A 65-year-old female with hypertension, a 50-pack-per-year smoking habit, and previous myocardial infarction is found to have a 7-cm descending thoracic aortic aneurysm. The aneurysm originates immediately beyond her left common carotid artery origin. In order to achieve a hemostatic proximal seal zone, the endoprosthesis will need to be deployed across and, therefore, occlude the origin of this vessel. To maintain blood flow to her brain, a cross-neck carotid-carotid bypass is performed using synthetic conduit.

Description of Procedure (33891)

The intraservice work of 33891 begins with bilateral neck skin incisions. Access to the common carotid arteries is achieved by dissecting through soft tissue and mobilizing a plethora of nerves and veins, all very carefully. Each common carotid artery is cleared for 5 to 6 cm. Soft rubber loops are passed proximally and distally around both arteries. Very careful dissection is performed to create a soft tissue tunnel from one side of the neck to the other behind the pharynx. An appropriately sized synthetic conduit is passed through the tunnel. Once adequate exposure is achieved and intravenous heparin anticoagulation is administered, proximal and distal vascular clamps are applied to the right common carotid artery. The artery is opened longitudinally and the proximal anastomosis of the bypass is sewn with fine polypropylene sutures. The anastomosis is flushed to remove debris prior to completion of the suture line. Extreme care is taken to avoid air or other embolus from traveling up the carotid artery. A vascular clamp is applied to the graft, and clamps are then removed from the carotid. Anastomotic leaks are sealed with additional sutures. The left common carotid artery is clamped. An arteriotomy is created, and the distal anastomosis is sewn with the end of the bypass conduit applied to the side of the carotid artery. The anastomosis is flushed to remove debris and the suture line completed. Extreme care is taken to prevent emboli from traveling up the carotid artery into the brain. Clamps are removed and leaks are sealed with additional sutures. All pulses are checked and flow is confirmed with a Doppler. The left common carotid artery just proximal to the anastomosis may be suture ligated at this point to help maintain patency of the carotid-carotid bypass graft. The wounds are irrigated copiously and closed in layers.

PULMONARY ARTERY

33917 Repair of pulmonary artery stenosis by reconstruction with patch or graft

▶(33918, 33919 have been deleted. To report, see 33925, 33926)◀

33920 Repair of pulmonary atresia with ventricular septal defect, by construction or replacement of conduit from right or left ventricle to pulmonary artery

33922 Transection of pulmonary artery with cardiopulmonary bypass

+33924 Ligation and takedown of a systemic-to-pulmonary artery shunt, performed in conjunction with a congenital heart procedure (List separately in addition to code for primary procedure)

(Use 33924 in conjunction with 33470-33475, 33600-33619, 33684-33688, 33692-33697, 33735-33767, 33770-33781, 33786, ▶33920◀-33922)

●33925 Repair of pulmonary artery arborization anomalies by unifocalization; without cardiopulmonary bypass

●33926 with cardiopulmonary bypass

▶(Do not report 33925, 33926 in conjunction with 33697)◀

Rationale

Codes 33918 and 33919 have been deleted and two codes, 33925 and 33926, have been established to more accurately describe the repair of pulmonary artery arborization anomalies by unifocalization with cardiopulmonary bypass and without cardiopulmonary bypass.

Deleted codes 33918 and 33919 included reference to ventricular septal defect. With the inclusion of this verbiage, the descriptor did not accurately reflect the procedure that is typically performed in repair of pulmonary artery arborization defects. In most cases, treatment of children with arborization abnormalities of the branch pulmonary arteries requires that the arteries be brought to a more central confluence (unifocalization) prior to complete repair of the heart defects. This unifocalization is most typically performed as a staged procedure (first one side, then the other, if necessary) through a thoracotomy incision without the use of cardiopulmonary bypass. A systemic-to-pulmonary artery shunt may be constructed at the same time. It is uncommon for the cardiac part of the defect (pulmonary atresia with ventricular septal defect) to be dealt with at this operation.

For pulmonary arborization defect repairs performed on neonates and infants up to a present body weight of 4 kg, it would be appropriate to append modifier 63 to the procedure to capture the significantly increased complexity and physician work commonly associated with these patients.

Clinical Example (33925)

A 3-month-old child presents with cyanosis and is found to have a tetralogy of Fallot with pulmonary atresia, diminutive central pulmonary arteries, and several large aorto-pulmonary collaterals that supply more than 50% of the lung mass.

Description of Procedure (33925)

This operation is typically done through thoracotomy or sternotomy, and colateral vessels (MAPCAs) are dissected out and mobilized at their origin from the descending aorta. The intraparenchymal or hiler pulmonary artery segment, which is most appropriate for MAPCA implantation, is mobilized and branch vessels are controlled. The MAPCA or MAPCAs are divided off the aorta and the aortic end is oversewn. The distal end of the MAPCA(s) is sewn to the appropirate segment(s) of the true pulmonary artery. Clamps on the pulmonary artery branches and the MAPCA are released and hemostasis is obtained. Chest tubes are placed and the incision is closed. Careful monitoring of the oxygen saturation is maintained throughout the procedure.

Clinical Example (33926)

A 6-month-old child is referred with cyanosis and echocardiogram, and catheterization shows a tetralogy of Fallot with pulmonary atresia. The central pulmonary arteries are discontinuous, and the blood supply to the left lung comes from a ductus-like collateral vessel. The right lung is supplied by three large collateral vessels arising from the descending aorta.

Description of Procedure (33926)

This operation is typically done through mediansternotomy, and colateral vessels (MAPCAs) are dissected out and mobilized at their origin from the descending aorta or brachiocephalic vessels. The patient is placed on cardiopulmonary bypass with aortic and venous cannulation. The intraparenchymal or hiler pulmonary artery segment, which is most appropriate for MAPCA implantation, is mobilized and branch vessels are controlled. The MAPCA or MAPCAs are divided off the aorta and the aortic end is oversewn. The distal end of the MAPCA(s) is sewn to the appropriate segment(s) of the true pulmonary artery. Clamps on the pulmonary artery branches and the MAPCA are released and hemostasis is obtained. The patient is weaned from cardiopulmonary bypass and after removal of the venous cannulas protamine is given. After hemostasis is achieved, the arterial cannula is removed and the cannulation site is repaired. Chest tubes are placed and the incision is closed. Careful monitoring of oxygen saturation is maintained throughout the postbypass period.

Arteries and Veins

ENDOVASCULAR REPAIR OF ABDOMINAL AORTIC ANEURYSM

▲34833 Open iliac artery exposure with creation of conduit for delivery of aortic or iliac endovascular prosthesis, by abdominal or retroperitoneal incision, unilateral

(For bilateral procedure, use modifier 50)

(Do not report 34833 in addition to 34820)

▲34834 Open brachial artery exposure to assist in the deployment of aortic or iliac endovascular prosthesis by arm incision, unilateral

(For bilateral procedure, use modifier 50)

Rationale

Consistent with the conversion of the endovascular repair of the descending thoracic aortic aneurysm Category III codes to Category I codes, 34833-34834 have been editorially revised to broaden the description of these codes to allow use of these open exposure codes with codes 33880-33891 for endovascular repair of the thoracic aorta.

Clinical Example (34833)

A 65-year-old female smoker with hypertension, chronic obstructive pulmonary disease (COPD), and previous myocardial infarction (MI) has a 7-cm infrarenal aortic aneurysm. Her iliac arteries are very small in caliber and heavily calcified. Placement of an iliac conduit will be required to enable endovascular aortic aneurysm repair.

Description of Procedure (34833)

Every patient requires individualized assessment and surgical approach, and every surgeon has his or her own "best" method to accomplish an operation. Realizing that, a typical case may include the following steps.

A skin incision is made. Access to the iliac artery is achieved via a transabdominal or retroperitoneal approach. All soft tissue, bowels, ureters, and veins are carefully mobilized as the iliac artery is approached. The artery is cleared for 5 to 6 cm, and vessel loops are passed around the vessel proximally and distally. Once adequate exposure is achieved and intravenous heparin anticoagulation is administered, proximal and distal vascular clamps are applied. A longitudinal arteriotomy is made. The conduit (a large-diameter tubular segment of synthetic bypass graft) is brought onto the field, tailored to the appropriate size, and an anastomosis of conduit to the iliac artery is sutured with fine polypropylene. The conduit is clamped and vascular clamps are removed from the iliac artery. The suture line is checked for hemostasis and additional sutures are applied as required.

Endovascular repair (separately reportable) is undertaken with the prostheses introduced through the newly formed conduit.

Once endovascular repair is complete, closure of the conduit is achieved in one of two ways. The unattached distal end of the conduit may be sewn to the more distal external iliac artery, thereby leaving the conduit in place as a common channel to external iliac bypass graft. Alternatively, the conduit can be transected close to the iliac artery and oversewn with a polypropylene suture. Hemostasis is achieved. The wound is irrigated and closed in layers.

Clinical Example (34834)

A 65-year-old female smoker with hypertension, COPD, and previous MI has a 7-cm infrarenal aortic aneurysm. Her iliac arteries are tortuous. Exposure of the brachial artery is performed to insert a guide to enable endovascular aortic aneurysm repair.

Description of Procedure (34834)

Every patient requires individualized assessment and surgical approach, and every surgeon has his or her own "best" method to accomplish an operation. Realizing that, a typical case may include the following steps.

A skin incision is made. Access to the brachial artery is achieved via an upper arm incision. All soft tissue, nerves, and veins are carefully mobilized as the brachial artery is approached. The artery is cleared for 5 to 6 cm, and soft vessel loops are passed around the artery proximally and distally. Once adequate exposure is achieved and intravenous heparin anticoagulation administered, proximal and distal vascular clamps are applied and removed as required for subsequent introduction of wires, sheaths, and catheters.

The endovascular procedure is performed (and separately reported).

Upon completion of the endovascular procedure, vascular clamps are reapplied. The large hole in the brachial artery is irrigated, the edges are trimmed as needed, and it is closed with fine polypropylene sutures. The suture line is checked for hemostasis and additional sutures are applied as required. The wound is irrigated and closed in layers.

DIRECT REPAIR OF ANEURYSM OR EXCISION (PARTIAL OR TOTAL) AND GRAFT INSERTION FOR ANEURYSM, PSEUDOANEURYSM, RUPTURED ANEURYSM, AND ASSOCIATED OCCLUSIVE DISEASE

Procedures 35001-35152 include preparation of artery . . .

(For direct repairs associated with occlusive disease only, see 35201-35286)

(For intracranial aneurysm, see 61700 et seq)

(For endovascular repair of abdominal aortic aneurysm, see 34800-34826)

(For endovascular repair of iliac artery aneurysm, see 34900)

(For thoracic aortic aneurysm, see 33860-33875)

▶(For endovascular repair of descending thoracic aorta, involving coverage of left subclavian artery origin, use 33880)◀

✍ Rationale

Consistent with the conversion of the endovascular repair of the descending thoracic aortic aneurysm Category III codes to Category I codes, the cross-reference following the guidelines for direct repair of an aneurysm has been revised to reflect the renumbering of these codes.

BYPASS GRAFT

Other Than Vein

35601 Bypass graft, with other than vein; carotid

35606 carotid-subclavian

▶(For open transcervical common carotid-common carotid bypass performed in conjunction with endovascular repair of descending thoracic aorta, use 33891)◀

(For open subclavian to carotid artery transposition performed in conjunction with endovascular thoracic aneurysm repair ▶by neck incision, use 33889◀)

✍ Rationale

Consistent with the conversion of the endovascular repair of the descending thoracic aortic aneurysm Category III codes to Category I codes, the cross-reference following code 35606 has been revised to include a reference to 33889 for bypass graft procedures performed in conjunction with endovascular descending thoracic aortic aneurysm repairs. A second cross-reference has been added to direct the user to 33891 for performance of transcervical common carotid bypass performed with endovascular repair of the descending thoracic aorta.

ARTERIAL TRANSPOSITION

35691 Transposition and/or reimplantation; vertebral to carotid artery

35694 subclavian to carotid artery

(For open subclavian to carotid artery transposition performed in conjunction with endovascular ►repair of descending thoracic aorta, use 33889◄)

Rationale

Consistent with the conversion of the endovascular repair of the descending thoracic aortic aneurysm Category III codes to Category I codes, the cross-reference following code 35694 has been revised to include a reference to 33889 for carotid artery transposition procedures performed in conjunction with endovascular descending thoracic aortic aneurysm repairs.

VENOUS

Central Venous Access Procedures

Other Central Venous Access Procedures

36597 Repositioning of previously placed central venous catheter under fluoroscopic guidance

(For fluoroscopic guidance, use 76000)

●**36598** Contrast injection(s) for radiologic evaluation of existing central venous access device, including fluoroscopy, image documentation and report

►(Do not report 36598 in conjunction with 76000)◄

►(Do not report 36598 in conjunction with 36595, 36596)◄

►(For complete diagnostic studies, see 75820, 75825, 75827)◄

Rationale

Code 36598 was established to report performance of a contrast injection for radiological evaluation of an existing venous access device provided in the evaluation of malfunctioning central venous access devices, commonly provided in the maintenance of central venous access for patients. The injection, fluoroscopy, image documentation, and report are included in this code, and not separately reported.

Code 36598 is intended to report the evaluation of the position and function of an existing central venous access device. For this procedure, it is typically only necessary to inject a small amount of contrast. The associated imaging is limited in this procedure to the catheter and those structures immediately beyond (ie, vena cava, extremity vein).

Cross-references to imaging code 76000 and the diagnostic study codes 75820, 75825, and 75827 indicate that these codes are not reported for the imaging. The exclusionary parenthetical that refers to 76000 supports the inclusion of "fluoroscopy" in the descriptor, which would therefore not be separately reported. The cross-reference for diagnostic study codes 75820, 75825, and 75827 directs reporting these codes only for complete diagnostic studies of the vena cava and extremity veins, and would be reported only for those circumstances where these structures required a more extensive study. The exclusionary parenthetical to 36595 and 36596 indicates that 36598 would not be separately reported in addition to these codes used to report removal of intracatheter and pericatheter obstructive material from the central venous device.

Clinical Example (36598)

A 45-year-old patient with Hodgkin's lymphoma is undergoing several weeks of chemotherapy, and a Hickman catheter was previously placed to allow for ongoing intravenous chemotherapy and frequent blood draws. After 2 months, however, the oncology staff is no longer able to draw blood from the catheter. It is not clear whether the catheter tip remains in the vein, and the oncology staff is unable to administer the chemotherapy without knowing the location of the catheter tip. The patient is referred for imaging of the catheter to determine its position, patency, and if anything can be done to restore the ability to draw blood from the catheter.

Description of Procedure (36598)

The physician performs a quick physical inspection of the catheter site. If the catheter is not dislodged or kinked, the physician exposes and preps the external port of the catheter in sterile fashion. Fluoroscopic evaluation of the catheter is performed by the physician, confirming that the tip of the catheter lies in the central vein as intended and has not migrated into the heart or been pulled back into a peripheral vein or out of the vein. Fluoroscopy also determines if the catheter has been fractured or kinked. The physician aspirates the catheter and indwelling anticoagulant is discarded if possible. Contrast is injected by the physician with imaging of the catheter tip and the vein where the catheter tip is positioned. If necessary, imaging is performed along the course of the catheter to determine if there is a leak in the catheter. (Once imaging is completed, any procedures that are done to try to restore function of the catheter, if necessary, are coded separately.) The catheter is flushed with saline and may be locked with anticoagulant solution.

TRANSCATHETER PROCEDURES

Codes for catheter placement and the radiologic supervision and interpretation should also be reported, in addition to the code(s) for the therapeutic aspect of the procedure.

▶*Mechanical Thrombectomy*◀

▶Code(s) for catheter placement(s), diagnostic studies, and other percutaneous interventions (eg, transluminal balloon angioplasty, stent placement) provided are separately reportable.◀

▶Codes 37184-37188 specifically include intraprocedural fluoroscopic radiological supervision and interpretation services for guidance of the procedure.◀

▶Intraprocedural injection(s) of a thrombolytic agent is an included service and not separately reportable in conjunction with mechanical thrombectomy. However, subsequent or prior continuous infusion of a thrombolytic is not an included service and is separately reportable (see 37201, 75896, 75898).◀

►For coronary mechanical thrombectomy, use 92973.◄

►For mechanical thrombectomy for dialysis fistula, use 36870.◄

►*Arterial Mechanical Thrombectomy*◄

►Arterial mechanical thrombectomy may be performed as a "primary" transcatheter procedure with pretreatment planning, performance of the procedure, and postprocedure evaluation focused on providing this service. Primary mechanical thrombectomy is reported per vascular family using 37184 for the initial vessel treated and 37185 for second or all subsequent vessel(s) within the same vascular family. To report mechanical thrombectomy of an additional vascular family treated through a separate access site, use modifier 51 in conjunction with 37184-37185.◄

►Do NOT report 37184-37185 for mechanical thrombectomy performed for treatment of thrombus or embolus complicating other percutaneous interventional procedures. See 37186 for these procedures.◄

►Arterial mechanical thrombectomy is considered a "secondary" transcatheter procedure for removal or retrieval of short segments of thrombus or embolus when performed either before or after another percutaneous intervention (eg, percutaneous transluminal balloon angioplasty, stent placement). Secondary mechanical thrombectomy is reported using 37186. Do NOT report 37186 in conjunction with 37184-37185.◄

►*Venous Mechanical Thrombectomy*◄

►Use code 37188 to report the initial application of venous mechanical thrombectomy. To report bilateral venous mechanical thrombectomy performed through a separate access site(s), use modifier 50 in conjunction with 37188. For repeat treatment on a subsequent day during a course of thrombolytic therapy, use 37188.◄

►*Arterial Mechanical Thrombectomy*◄

⊙●**37184** Primary percutaneous transluminal mechanical thrombectomy, noncoronary, arterial or arterial bypass graft, including fluoroscopic guidance and intraprocedural pharmacological thrombolytic injection(s); initial vessel

►(Do not report 37184 in conjunction with 76000, 76001, 90774, 99143-99150)◄

✚⊙●**37185** second and all subsequent vessel(s) within the same vascular family (List separately in addition to code for primary mechanical thrombectomy procedure)

►(Do not report 37185 in conjunction with 76000, 76001, 90775)◄

✚⊙●**37186** Secondary percutaneous transluminal thrombectomy (eg, nonprimary mechanical, snare basket, suction technique), noncoronary, arterial or arterial bypass graft, including fluoroscopic guidance and intraprocedural pharmacological thrombolytic injections, provided in conjunction with another percutaneous intervention other than primary mechanical thrombectomy (List separately in addition to code for primary procedure)

►(Do not report 37186 in conjunction with 76000, 76001, 90775)◄

▶*Venous Mechanical Thrombectomy*◀

⊙●**37187** Percutaneous transluminal mechanical thrombectomy, vein(s), including intraprocedural pharmacological thrombolytic injections and fluoroscopic guidance

▶(Do not report 37187 in conjunction with 76000, 76001, 90775)◀

⊙●**37188** Percutaneous transluminal mechanical thrombectomy, vein(s), including intraprocedural pharmacological thrombolytic injections and fluoroscopic guidance, repeat treatment on subsequent day during course of thrombolytic therapy

▶(Do not report 37188 in conjunction with 76000, 76001, 90775)◀

Rationale

Code 37209 has been revised, and five codes, guidelines, and cross-references have been established to report percutaneous thrombus (blood clot) removal in peripheral vessels. Thrombus removal is performed for patients with acute limb ischemia, pulmonary embolus, or venous occlusion due to thrombus or embolus. These codes and guidelines are distinguished by provision of arterial or venous therapy.

Mechanical thrombectomy is the removal of thrombus from a vessel for restoration of circulation. In contrast, percutaneous transluminal angioplasty (PTA) (35470) is the process of opening a narrowed or occluded segment of vessel. The narrowing or occulsion typically is due to plaque or intimal hyperplasia. PTA treats the diseased vessel wall, but does not remove the thrombus from a vessel. Therefore, PTA and mechanical thrombectomy are procedures that are distinct from one another.

The previously existing codes within the CPT codebook described procedures that alter the anatomy of the peripheral vessel by modification of the arterial wall or removal of a portion of the plaque. These codes did not describe the removal of a thrombus within the lumen of the vessel. The new mechanical thrombectomy codes describe a procedure using a unique method of fragmenting and/or removing clots from the peripheral vessel. Since there are a significant number of cases of embolization or thrombosis where only mechanical thrombectomy is required with no underlying lesions requiring angioplasty, separate codes have been added to report these procedures. There are instances where other therapeutic procedures are provided in conjunctiom with mechanical thrombectomy. For example, after removal of a thrombus from a vessel with mechanical thrombectomy, an underlying atherosclerotic stenosis is revealed. In such a case, PTA would be performed and reported as a separate component of work because it is a different procedure for treatment of a different pathology.

Mechanical thrombectomy is performed using devices specific for mechanically breaking up, macerating, and/or removing thrombus from a vessel. Mechanical thrombectomy may also partially break up (debulk) a clot prior to thrombolytic infusion therapy, increasing the surface area upon which a lytic drug may directly act, thereby reducing the time of treatment and the overall dose of drug required to break up the thrombus. Therefore, mechanical thrombectomy is occasionally performed in addition to pharmacological thrombolysis for restoration of flow to the vessel occluded or compromised by thrombus in certain clinical circumstances (eg, extensive residual thrombus over a significant vessel length) and is frequently used as a "debulking" procedure, particularly in veins. If mechanical thrombectomy is done in conjunction with pharmacological thrombolysis, the catheters used for lysis are generally positioned through percutaneous vessel access(s) previously established for mechanical thrombectomy directly into the thrombus for institution of pharmacologic thrombolytic therapy. Pharmacological thrombolysis may be more rapidly and extensively effective if a large portion of the thrombus has been mechanically removed prior to the institution of thrombolysis. Pharmacologic thrombolysis, reported with code 37201, is performed by direct delivery of a thrombolytic drug into the thrombus.

When performed in conjunction with pharmacologic thrombolysis, the necessary catheter exchange during thrombolytic therapy, which may last for several hours or days, is separately reportable. Catheter exchanges are done during thrombolysis to "chase" the thrombus (ie, to position the catheter so that the lytic dose is directed precisely into the thrombus, and this target may change as the thrombus lyses) or, if the indwelling infusion catheter is dislodged during the therapy, prevent delivery of the drug directly to the thrombus. Catheter exchanges are variably necessary for these procedures and require additional trips to the interventional suite, often on different days. Therefore, this service is separately reportable. In tandem with the addition of the Mechanical Thrombectomy codes, code 37209, which previously specified "arterial" catheter exchange during thrombolysis, has been editorially revised to expand the use of the code for arterial and venous catheter exchange with the addition of "intravascular" because catheter exchange during venous thrombolytic therapy requires the same effort as arterial therapy. These codes are further identified with the moderate sedation bull's-eye symbol to indicate that conscious sedation is included in these codes and, therefore, not separately reported.

The guidelines for mechanical thrombectomy are organized within a main section that defines the services included in mechanical thrombectomy (intraprocedural fluoroscopic supervision and interpretation for guidance of the procedure, thrombolytic agent injection). Also indicated are the diagnostic studies and other interventions that are separately reported (ie, percutaneous transluminal balloon angioplasty, stent placement, subsequent or prior continuous infusions of thrombolytic agents). Separate guideline sections for arterial and venous therapy have also been added to provide instructions specific to these routes of access. Cross-references following the mechanical thrombectomy guidelines direct the user to other mechanical thrombectomy codes (92973 for coronary and 36870 for dialysis fistula).

The arterial mechanical thrombectomy codes differentiate between "primary" and "secondary" mechanical thrombectomy. The arterial mechanical thrombectomy guidelines define what is meant by primary and secondary mechanical thrombectomy. The differentiation between primary and secondary mechanical thrombectomy is **not** dependent upon whether mechanical thrombectomy is the only percutaneous procedure provided. Both primary and secondary mechanical thrombectomy can be provided in conjunction with other percutaneous interventions. Primary arterial mechanical thrombectomy indicates that pre-treatment planning, performance of the procedure, and post-procedure evaluation focused on providing this service. Primary mechanical thrombectomy may precede another percutaneous intervention, with the decision regarding the need for other services not made until after mechanical thrombectomy has been performed. Once the thrombus has been removed, an underlying lesion responsible for the thrombosis may be identified. PTA and/or stenting or thrombolytic infusion services to treat the underlying lesion may follow the performance of primary mechanical thrombectomy. Mechanical thrombectomy is considered primary, as the need for these other services was not known prior to mechanical thrombectomy. Occasionally, the performance of primary mechanical thrombectomy may follow another percutaneous intervention. Performance of mechanical thrombectomy after a course of thrombolytic infusion therapy would be the most common example of primary mechanical thrombectomy following another percutaneous intervention.

Secondary arterial mechanical thrombectomy, also commonly referred to as "rescue" mechanical thrombectomy, is always performed in conjunction with another percutaneous intervention (eg, percutaneous transluminal balloon angioplasty, stent placement). These circumstances include those in which a small amount of clot is present in the lesion and needs to be removed prior to PTA/stent or the thrombus/embolus has complicated a PTA/stent procedure, requiring removal of the thrombus/embolus to complete the procedure.

For secondary mechanical thrombectomy, pre-treatment planning, performance of the procedure, and postprocedure evaluation are not focused on providing this service. Secondary arterial mechanical thrombectomy is reported using add-on code 37186 and is not reportable at the same session as 37184 or 37185.

In summary, three new codes have been established to report arterial mechanical thrombectomy: primary thrombectomy in the initial vessel of an arterial family (37184); primary thrombectomy in a second vessel of the same vascular family (37185); and secondary thrombectomy (37186).

The use of venous mechanical thrombectomy is not quite as variable as that of arterial mechanical thrombectomy and two codes are believed to effectively capture these services. Venous mechanical thrombectomy may be the only intervention in the treatment of venous thrombus or it may be provided in conjunction with thrombolytic infusion therapy. Code 37187 is used to report venous mechanical thrombectomy either by itself or in conjunction with other percutaneous interventions.

Occasionally, it is necessary to repeat venous mechanical thrombectomy during a course of thrombolytic therapy. For example, mechanical thrombectomy may initially be used to "debulk" venous thrombus (37187), followed by pharmacological thrombolysis (separately reportable using code procedural 37201) and, if the thrombus is particularly resistant, it may be necessary to repeat venous mechanical thrombectomy after pharmacologic thrombolytic infusion. Code 37188 is used to report "repeat" venous mechanical thrombectomy during a course of pharmacological thrombolysis.

As with arterial mechanical thrombectomy coding, any additional percutaneous interventions provided to treat underlying and/or distinct pathology(ies) is/are separately reportable. Diagnostic and catheterization services are also separately reportable. Existing coding conventions are followed when multiple services are provided through the same catheter (please see the introductory text for the Vascular Injection Procedure section of the CPT codebook for more information).

Unlike most transcatheter procedures, there are not separate radiological supervision and interpretation codes to report imaging services provided in conjunction with mechanical thrombectomy. Arteriography and/or venography related to guidance and monitoring of the mechanical thrombectomy and completion study(s) for this service performed on the same day are included in codes 37184-37188. However, diagnostic arteriography or venography done to diagnose the problem before therapy is begun is separately reportable and completion angiography (75898) provided to conclude infusion therapy that may be provided in conjunction with mechanical thrombectomy is separately reportable if provided at a distinct and separate session and/or on a subsequent date of service. Exclusionary cross-references in Arterial and Venous Mechanical Thrombectomy guidelines sections have been included to indicate that fluoroscopy is considered an inclusive service and codes 76000, 76001 are not separately reportable. Additionally, intra-procedural injection(s) of lytic is/are included, and not separately reported.

Clinical Example (37184)

The patient is a 75-year-old female with a history of recent stroke who presents with acute onset of lower limb ischemia, beginning earlier the same day. At presentation to the emergency department, the foot is cool and pale. There is no rest pain, but a light hypesthesia of the forefoot is noted. The patient has a history of previous synthetic femoral-popliteal bypass graft in the left leg. Physical exam reveals a normal left femoral pulse, but no pulse is palpable in the bypass graft, the popliteal artery, or pedal or tibial arteries. The emergency department physician refers the patient to the vascular specialist on-call, who orders an emergent diagnostic angiogram (reported separately), which demonstrates a patent common femoral artery and profunda femoral artery, but total occlusion of the femoral popliteal bypass graft is confirmed. There is reconstitution of the popliteal artery below the level of the distal anastomosis, and delayed run-off is identified in the personal and posterior tibial arteries. After considering all treatment options, the physician decides to use an endovascular approach for treatment. Because of the history of recent stroke, the patient is felt to be a poor surgical candidate and is not a candidate for pharmacologic thrombolysis. Mechanical thrombectomy is offered to try to re-establish flow to the foot.

Description of Procedure (37184)

The physician orders the medications for conscious sedation. He or she punctures the common femoral artery in an antegrade fashion, and a wire is used to select the occluded bypass graft (separately reported). Under fluoroscopy, the guidewire is positioned across the occlusion and an appropriate-sized sheath is placed at the groin. Heparin is administered. The mechanical thrombolysis device is advanced over the wire into the thrombus and into the lower limit of the occlusion. The physician positions the device optimally under fluoroscopy. The device is activated and passed across the site (often several times), macerating the thrombus. All fluoroscopy and angiograms performed to guide the therapy and monitor the progress of the therapy are included. If residual thrombus is documented, the mechanical thrombolytic device is again activated for further thrombus removal. A lytic agent may be administered as necessary. Fluoroscopy is again used to direct the device. If a small fragment of thrombus is not removed by the thrombectomy device, it may be removed with aspiration through the sheath or through a large bore catheter placed to the remaining thrombus.

The physician performs a final completion angiogram to confirm that the entire volume of occlusive material has been removed and that flow has been restored. The mechanical thrombectomy device, catheters, and guidewires are removed. Compression is applied to achieve hemostasis.

Clinical Example (37185)

The patient is a 75-year-old female with a history of recent stroke who presents with acute onset of lower limb ischemia, beginning earlier the same day. At presentation to the emergency department, the foot is cool and pale. There is no rest pain, but a light hypesthesia of the forefoot is noted. The patient has a history of previous synthetic femoral-popliteal bypass graft in the left leg. Physical exam reveals a normal left femoral pulse, but no pulse is palpable in the bypass graft, the popliteal artery, or pedal or tibial arteries. The emergency department physician refers the patient to the vascular specialist on-call, who orders an emergent diagnostic angiogram (reported separately), which demonstrates a patent common femoral artery and profunda femoral artery, but total occlusion of the femoral popliteal bypass graft is confirmed. There is reconstitution of the popliteal artery several centimeters below the level of the distal anastomosis with thrombus extending below the graft into the native popliteal artery. After thrombectomy of the bypass graft (coded separately) a distal embolus occluding the common peroneal trunk is noted requiring additional mechanical thrombectomy.

Description of Procedure (37185)

Once the femoral popliteal graft has been cleared of the thrombus using mechanical thrombectomy as described in the clinical example for code 37184, a wire is used by the physician to cross the thrombus extending into the native popliteal artery and through the embolus in the common peroneal artery. The mechanical thrombectomy device is advanced by the physician into the common peroneal trunk, activated, and pulled back through the thrombus in the common peroneal trunk and in the popliteal artery. Fluoroscopy is used to position the device optimally. All fluoroscopy and angiograms performed to guide the therapy and monitor the progress of the therapy are included. If residual thrombus is documented, the mechanical thrombolytic device is again activated for further thrombus removal. Fluoroscopy is again used to direct the device. A bolus of 1 mg tissue plasminogen activator (t-PA) is also given by the physician to help clear any small fragments, which could have embolized more distally. If a small fragment of thrombus is not removed by the thrombectomy device, it may be removed by the physician with aspiration through the sheath or through a large-bore catheter placed to the remaining thrombus. A final completion angiogram is performed to confirm that the entire occlusive material has been removed and that flow has been restored.

Clinical Example (37186)

The patient is a 75-year-old female who presents with rest pain of the left lower extremity. Work-up documents decreased perfusion to the limb, and non-invasive studies suggest superficial femoral arterial stenosis or occlusion. A diagnostic angiogram (reported separately) shows a focal high-grade stenosis of the distal superficial femoral artery (SFA). All potential therapies are considered, and the patient is referred for SFA, percutaneous transluminal angioplasty (PTA), and/or stent. The procedure is performed percutaneously with balloon angioplasty of the lesion done (reported separately). Follow-up angiography shows patency of the PTA site but stagnant column of contrast with no run-off, and distal imaging shows a filling defect at the popliteal artery bifurcation. The foot is cool and pale with no palpable pulse. Reconstitution of the trifurcations vessels is documented, with only the short focal occlusion representing the distal embolus found. Mechanical thrombectomy of the popliteal is employed.

Note: Code 37186 is intended for removal or retrieval of short segments of a thrombus or embolus treated either before or after (but during the same operative session) another percutaneous intervention such as PTA or stent placement, where a small amount of clot is present in the lesion and needs to be removed prior to PTA or stent placement or where the thrombus or embolus has complicated a PTA or stent procedure, requiring removal of the thrombus or embolus to complete the procedure. The primary intervention(s) is reported separately.

Description of Procedure (37186)

Wire access is maintained across the PTA site to ensure that further catheters are not passed subintimally. The existing sheath is upsized to allow placement of a larger-bore catheter. A bolus of tPA is given into the distal popliteal artery, and additional heparin is given intravenously. Over a wire, a guiding catheter is advanced into the popliteal artery distally, taking care not to dislodge the distal embolus. The tip of the guiding catheter is carefully placed at the level of the embolus, and a 30 cc syringe is attached to the catheter, placing suction to the embolus. The embolus is engaged within the tip of the guiding catheter and, with continued suction continuously applied, the guiding catheter is removed through the sheath at the vessel access, pulling the embolus from the vessel. Follow-up angiography is done. If the embolus was completely removed, final angiography and physical exam are done prior to removal of the sheath. If there is persistent embolus, further passes with the same guiding catheter or with another catheter or device are done to allow complete removal of the embolus before the sheaths are removed and hemostasis is obtained.

Clinical Example (37187)

A 42-year-old woman with no significant past medical history presents to the emergency department with a 2-day history of left lower extremity pain and swelling. She has no history of injury to the leg, does not smoke, and exercises regularly. She is on no medications. Physical examination reveals severe swelling of the entire left lower extremity. The right lower extremity exam is normal. The pulses in both extremities are palpable throughout. The remainder of the physical exam is unremarkable. The emergency department physician refers the patient to the vascular specialist on call, who orders a Doppler ultrasound examination that reveals acute occlusive thrombus in the left deep venous system beginning at the level of the popliteal vein and extending to the visualized portion of the left external iliac vein. The patient is admitted to the hospital. Initial treatment consists of intravenous heparin for anticoagulation, and a workup for hypercoagulability ensues. Over the course of the next 24 hours, the patient experiences minimal symptomatic improvement. After considering all treatment options, the physician discusses treatment options with the patient, family, and referring physician and chooses an endovascular approach. Because there has been little improvement with systemic anticoagulation and to try to decrease the incidence of post-thrombotic chronic venous disease, mechanical thrombectomy of the large iliofemoral deep vein thrombosis possibly followed by pharmacologic thrombolysis (separately reportable if provided) is offered.

Description of Procedure (37187)

The physician orders the medications for conscious sedation. The popliteal vein is assessed with ultrasound imaging and punctured in a retrograde fashion with direct ultrasound visualization (separately coded using appropriate catheterization code). The physician advances a guidewire, under fluoroscopic guidance, and a sheath is placed into the popliteal vein. Separately reportable diagnostic venography is performed with attention to the profunda and saphenous system. The physician activates and advances the mechanical thrombolysis device over the wire to macerate the thrombus. (This is often performed numerous times.) All fluoroscopy and venograms performed to guide the therapy and monitor the progress of the therapy are included. Venography is performed demonstrating residual thrombus. This scenario is repeated with multiple passes of the device being performed with the device activated with each pass, and repeat venography is performed intermittently to determine the progress of thrombus removal. Venography demonstrates residual thrombus and occlusion at the level of the left common iliac vein origin. Attempts to advance a wire across the occlusion are not successful. In order to treat the residual thrombus and to facilitate treatment of the occlusion (separately reportable), pharmacologic thrombolysis is begun with the diagnostic catheter exchanged for a multi-sided hole infusion catheter that is positioned under fluoroscopic guidance along the length of the residual thrombus to the level of the occlusion. The catheter and sheath are secured in position.

Clinical Example (37188)

Venography reveals persistent residual thrombus of the left external iliac vein in a 42-year-old woman who presented 3 days ago with acute occlusive thrombus in the left deep venous system, beginning at the level of the popliteal vein and extending to the visualized portion of the left external iliac vein. Mechanical thrombectomy was performed 2 days ago, macerating a significant portion of the thrombus (reported separately), which was followed by pharmacologic thrombolysis therapy (reported separately). Treatment options including the benefits and potential complications of repeat mechanical thrombectomy are discussed with the patient, family, and referring physician. In an effort to reduce the patients exposure to and overall dose of thrombolytic agent required to completely resolve the thrombus, the physician elects to repeat mechanical thrombectomy.

Description of Procedure (37188)

The physician orders medications for conscious sedation. The popliteal vein is accessed through the existing catheter that was placed for pharmacologic thrombolysis therapy. Under fluoroscopic guidance, a guidewire is advanced and a sheath is placed into the distal external iliac vein. The mechanical thrombolysis device is advanced over the wire and activated to macerate the residual thrombus, often several times. All fluoroscopy and venograms performed to guide the therapy and monitor the progress of the therapy are included. Venography is performed, demonstrating persistent residual thrombus. This scenario is repeated with multiple passes of the device being performed with the device activated with each pass and repeat venography performed intermittently to determine the progress of thrombus removal. A final completion venogram is performed to confirm that all occlusive material has been removed and that flow has been restored. The mechanical thrombectomy device, catheters, and guidewires are removed and compression is applied for hemostasis.

▶*Other Procedures*◀

37195 Thrombolysis, cerebral, by intravenous infusion

37205 Transcatheter placement of an intravascular stent(s), (except coronary, carotid, and vertebral vessel), percutaneous; initial vessel

(For radiological supervision and interpretation, use 75960)

(For coronary stent placement, see 92980, 92981▶; intracranial, use 61635◀)

Rationale

In tandem with the establishment of code 61635 to report transcatheter intracranial stent placement, the cross-reference following 37205 has been revised to refer to the new intracranial code.

▲37209 Exchange of a previously placed intravascular catheter during thrombolytic therapy

(For radiological supervision and interpretation, use 75900)

Rationale

In tandem with the addition of the Mechanical Thrombectomy codes, code 37209, which previously specified "arterial" catheter exchange during thrombolysis, has been editorially revised to expand the use of the code for arterial and venous catheter exchange with the addition of "intravascular," as catheter exchange during venous thrombolytic therapy requires the same effort as arterial therapy. These codes are further identified with the moderate sedation bull's-eye symbol to indicate that conscious sedation is included in these codes and are not separately reported.

Clinical Example (37209)

A 58-year-old man is undergoing thrombolytic therapy for a thrombosed left femoral-popliteal graft. Urokinase has been infusing into the proximal portion of the graft for 14 hours via a catheter placed from the right groin. There has been some clinical improvement. A routine follow-up angiogram has shown clearing of the clot in the graft but there has been embolization of the thrombus to the tibial trifurcation. In order to treat the distal occlusion, a guide wire is manipulated into the distal popliteal artery and the infusion catheter is exchanged for a new catheter, which has its tip positioned within the distal thrombus. The catheter is secured in the right groin, covered with a sterile dressing, and the infusion is continued.

Description of Procedure (37209)

The patient is positioned on the table; the groin is prepped; all dressings are removed; and Providone-Iodine solution is applied. The guidewire is inserted through the catheter, and manipulated into a distal position. The existing catheter is pulled over the guidewire and a new catheter is placed over the guidewire to a new distal position. The catheter and guidewire are manipulated into a final selective position. With confirmation of the catheter location by injection of contrast material, the new catheter is secured in place in the groin with the application of sterile dressing and re-initiation of infusion.

LIGATION

37700 Ligation and division of long saphenous vein at saphenofemoral junction, or distal interruptions

▶(Do not report 37700 in conjunction with 37718, 37722)◀

(For bilateral procedure, report 37700 with modifier 50)

●37718 Ligation, division, and stripping, short saphenous vein

▶(For bilateral procedure, use modifier 50)◀

▶(Do not report 37718 in conjunction with 37735, 37780)◀

▶(37720 has been deleted)◀

●37722 Ligation, division, and stripping, long (greater) saphenous veins from saphenofemoral junction to knee or below

▶(For ligation and stripping of the short saphenous vein, use 37718)◀

▶(For bilateral procedure, report 37722 with modifier 50)◀

▶(Do not report 37722 in conjunction with 37700, 37735)◀

►(37730 has been deleted. For ligation, division, and stripping of the greater saphenous vein, use 37722. For ligation, division, and stripping of the short saphenous vein, use 37718)◄

37735 Ligation and division and complete stripping of long or short saphenous veins with radical excision of ulcer and skin graft and/or interruption of communicating veins of lower leg, with excision of deep fascia

►(Do not report 37735 in conjunction with 37700, 37718, 37722, 37780)◄

(For bilateral procedure, report 37735 with modifier 50)

Rationale

Codes 37720 and 37730 have been deleted; two codes 37718 and 37722 and instructional or exclusionary cross-references have been established to appropriately describe open surgical ablation procedures of the saphenous vein.

Codes 37718 and 37722 have been added to describe the excision of long (37722) and short (37718) saphenous veins. The indications for ligation, division, and stripping of the long (greater) or short saphenous veins include symptoms such as swelling, pain, lipodermatosclerotic venous skin changes, and/or venous ulcer formation. These are typically coupled with identification of superficial venous valvular incompetence.

The inclusion in the code descriptors of 37720 and 37730 of the phrase "complete stripping" was found to be problematic. When originally included within the CPT codebook, code 37720 described the practice in which physicians, who performed greater saphenous vein stripping, typically removed the vein from the saphenofemoral venous confluence in the groin to the level of the ankle. Clinical outcomes research subsequently identified a high incidence of saphenous nerve injury when the greater saphenous vein is stripped out of the calf. Also, when venous insufficiency symptoms such as swelling, pain, lipodermatosclerosis, and venous ulceration are due to malfunction of the superficial system, pathophysiologic studies identified incompetence of the thigh portion of the greater saphenous as the main contributor. The deletion of code 37730 within the CPT codebook was necessary to eliminate the possibility of multiple coding that could occur with the addition of the two new codes to report long and short saphenous vein removal.

Current practice finds that the procedure that has become standard is that for which the greater saphenous is stripped from the saphenofemoral junction only to the knee; the procedure has excellent clinical efficacy with a minimized risk of saphenous nerve injury. Due to clinical practice preference for this reduced procedure and the inclusion of "complete" in the descriptor, it was necessary to delete 37720.

Since codes 37718 and 37722 are unilateral procedures, instructional cross-references have been added to instruct the use of modifier 50 for bilateral procedures. In the unusual situation where both the greater saphenous and the short saphenous veins are excised, code 37718 plus 37722 with modifier 51 appended would be reported. Cluster excision (37785) is co-reportable with stripping of the greater or short saphenous veins (37722, 37718) when both procedures are performed during the same operation. Exclusionary cross-references instruct that 37700 (ligation and division of long saphenous vein), a component procedure of the new codes, is not appropriately reported in addition to 37718 and 37722 because the new codes include vein removal in addition to ligation and division. Exclusionary cross-references also preclude reporting 37735 (ligation, division, or complete stripping or radical excision of ulcer and skin graft or interruption of communicating veins of the lower leg or excision of deep fascia), a component procedure of the new codes, in addition to 37718 and 37722 because ligation and stripping of long or short saphenous vein are also procedures within the 37735 bundle. Code 37780 (ligation or division of the short saphenous vein) has also been added to the exclusionary parenthetical following codes 37718 and 37735 as a component of these procedures.

Clinical Example (37718)

A 66-year-old man suffered spontaneous development of a large skin ulcer on the posterior aspect of his calf, just above the ankle. He has normal arterial pulses. A venous duplex exam revealed incompetence of his short saphenous vein with extensive reflux. Valve function in his deep veins and the greater saphenous vein was normal. The patient's ulcer healed after 6 weeks of therapy, including medicated compression dressings and leg elevation. An open surgical procedure, ligation, division, and stripping of the short saphenous vein is performed to prevent recurrence.

Description of Procedure (37718)

A skin incision adjacent to popliteal skin crease is made over the saphenopopliteal junction. The physician dissects through the soft tissue to find the short saphenous vein. A positive identification of saphenopopliteal junction is made to ensure that the correct vein has been reached. The physician identifies, dissects, and divides the venous branches in the region between the silk sutures. Several centimeters of the short saphenous are cleared, and the branches are found and ligated. A skin incision is made over the short saphenous vein on posterior aspect of the calf, near the ankle. The physician dissects through the soft tissue to find the short saphenous vein. Several centimeters of the short saphenous are cleared and the branches ligated. The physician divides the saphenous between the clamps and ties the lower end. He or she opens the clamp on the transected saphenous and inserts a stripper. The stripper is carefully manipulate upwards within the vein to the popliteal region. The physician identifies the end of the stripper in the saphenous at the saphenopopliteal junction. The short saphenous is divided between the clamps adjacent to the saphenopopliteal junction. The upper end of the saphenous vein is sutured and the physician tests for hemostasis. The stripper is passed out through the transected end of the short saphenous. The physician attaches the stripper head and ties the end of the vein to the stripper. With extreme care, the stripper is pulled downwards through the calf and strips the vein. Pressure is held on the calf to control bleeding. When the bleeding stops, all wounds are irrigated with saline. The physician checks again for hemostasis. Both wounds are closed in multiple layers.

Clinical Example (37722)

A 66-year-old man suffered spontaneous development of a large skin ulcer on the medial aspect of his calf, just above the ankle. He has normal arterial pulses. A venous duplex exam revealed incompetence of his greater saphenous vein with extensive reflux. Valve function in his deep veins was normal. The patient's ulcer healed after 6 weeks of therapy, including medicated compression dressings and leg elevation. Ligation, division, and stripping of his greater saphenous vein is performed to prevent recurrence.

Description of Procedure (37722)

A skin incision is made adjacent to the groin crease, over the saphenofemoral junction. The physician dissects through the soft tissue to find the greater saphenous vein. He or she makes a positive identification of the saphenofemoral junction to ensure that the correct vein has been accessed. The physician identifies, dissects, and divides the venous branches between silk sutures. Several centimeters of the greater saphenous are cleared and the branches are found and ligated. A second skin incision is made over the saphenous vein at or just below the knee. The physician dissects through the soft tissue to find the greater saphenous vein. Several centimeters of greater saphenous are cleared and the branches are ligated. The physician divides the saphenous between the clamps and ties the lower end. The clamp on the transected saphenous is opened and the stripper is inserted. The stripper is manipulated carefully upwards within the saphenous vein through the thigh. The physician identifies the end of the stripper within the saphenous vein at the saphenofemoral junction. He or she divides the greater saphenous between the clamps adjacent to the saphenofemoral junction. The upper end of the transected saphenous vein is sutured at the saphenofemoral junction. The physician tests for hemostasis and adds more sutures as needed. Through the open end of the saphenous vein, the stripper is passed. The stripper head is attached and the end of the vein is tied to the stripper. With extreme care, the physician pulls the stripper downwards through the thigh and strips the vein. Pressure is held on the thigh to control bleeding. When the bleeding stops, all wounds are irrigated with saline. Again, the physician checks for hemostasis. Both wounds are closed in multiple layers.

Digestive System

Salivary Gland and Ducts

INCISION

►(For drainage of abscess, see 42310, 42320)◄

►(42325, 42326 have been deleted)◄

►(For sialolithotomy, see 42330)◄

✍ Rationale

Codes 42325 and 42326 have been deleted because these codes were found to be used infrequently in reporting data.

EXCISION

42409 Marsupialization of sublingual salivary cyst (ranula)

Esophagus

ENDOSCOPY

For endoscopic procedures, code appropriate endoscopy of each anatomic site examined.

Surgical endoscopy always includes diagnostic endoscopy.

⊙43200 Esophagoscopy, rigid or flexible; diagnostic, with or without collection of specimen(s) by brushing or washing (separate procedure)

⊙43235 Upper gastrointestinal endoscopy including esophagus, stomach, and either the duodenum and/or jejunum as appropriate; diagnostic, with or without collection of specimen(s) by brushing or washing (separate procedure)

⊙43239 with biopsy, single or multiple

(For upper gastrointestinal endoscopy with suturing of the esophagogastric junction, use Category III code 0008T)

►(For upper gastrointestinal endoscopy with injection of implant material into and along the muscle of the lower esophageal sphincter, use Category III code 0133T)◄

✍ Rationale

In tandem with the establisment of Category III code 0133T, a cross-reference has been added to the upper gastrointestinal endoscopy section to refer the user to the new code for reporting implant material injection to the esophageal sphincter.

Stomach

EXCISION

►(43638, 43639 have been deleted)◄

►(For vagotomy with partial gastrectomy, see 43635)◄

►(For vagotomy with or without gastrostomy, see 43640)◄

✍ Rationale

Codes 43638 and 43639 were deleted because these procedures are considered to be obsolete when performed as described and inclusive when performed as the larger procedures of partial esophogectomy codes 43122 and 43123.

▶BARIATRIC SURGERY◀

▶Bariatric surgical procedures may involve the stomach, duodenum, jejunum, and/or the ileum.◀

▶*Laparoscopy*◀

▶Surgical laparoscopy always includes diagnostic laparoscopy. To report a diagnostic laparoscopy (separate procedure), use 49320.◀

▶Typical postoperative follow-up care (see Surgery Guidelines, CPT Surgical Package Definition) after gastric restriction using the adjustable gastric band technique includes subsequent band adjustment(s) through the postoperative period for the typical patient. Band adjustment refers to changing the gastric band component diameter by injection or aspiration of fluid through the subcutaneous port component.◀

●**43770** Laparoscopy, surgical, gastric restrictive procedure; placement of adjustable gastric band (gastric band and subcutaneous port components)

▶(For individual component placement, report 43770 with modifier 52)◀

●**43771** revision of adjustable gastric band component only

●**43772** removal of adjustable gastric band component only

●**43773** removal and replacement of adjustable gastric band component only

▶(Do not report 43773 in conjunction with 43772)◀

●**43774** removal of adjustable gastric band and subcutaneous port components

▶(For removal and replacement of both gastric band and subcutaneous port components, use 43659)◀

OTHER PROCEDURES

▲**43848** Revision, open, of gastric restrictive procedure for morbid obesity, other than adjustable gastric band (separate procedure)

▶(For adjustable gastric band procedures, see 43770-43774, 43886-43888)◀

43880 Closure of gastrocolic fistula

●**43886** Gastric restrictive procedure, open; revision of subcutaneous port component only

●**43887** removal of subcutaneous port component only

●**43888** removal and replacement of subcutaneous port component only

▶(Do not report 43888 in conjunction with 43774, 43887)◀

▶(For laparoscopic removal of both gastric band and subcutaneous port components, use 43774)◀

▶(For removal and replacement of both gastric band and subcutaneous port components, use 43659)◀

Rationale

A new section has been added to the CPT codebook to identify bariatric surgical procedures and the laparoscopic techniques that currently are used to treat obesity, which includes the application of a gastric restrictive band. The new section is complete with a new heading (Bariatric Surgery), subheading (Laparoscopy), guidelines, parenthetical notes, and codes. The guidelines provide instruction regarding the specific anatomic areas that may be involved and services that would ordinarily be included as part of the procedure(s) including diagnostic laparoscopy and typical postoperative follow-up care that includes band adjustments. These guidelines also define band adjustment (ie, changing the gastric band component diameter by injection or aspiration of fluid through the subcutaneous port component).

The codes included for these procedures comprise language that identifies different elements involved in providing this type of care, including laparoscopic placement of the adjustable band (43770), laparoscopic revision of the band (43771), laparoscopic removal of the band (43772), laparoscopic removal and replacement of the band component (43773), and laparoscopic removal of the band and subcutaneous port components (43774). In some cases, existing codes have been revised to reflect the changes (eg, 43848), identifying open procedures of a related nature. Parenthetic notes included in this section alert users to special circumstances and coding that may be necessary (eg, use of the modifier 52 with code 43770 for placement of individual component) as well as appropriate coding for replacement of the band and subcutaneous port.

Other codes have also been added for open procedures that involve gastric banding. These codes include the addition of an open surgical code for revision of the subcutaneous port component (43886), open removal of the subcutaneous port component (43887), and open removal and replacement of the subcutaneous port (43888). Parenthetical notes have been included to inform the user of restrictions regarding use and to direct the user to laparoscopic and other coding for these (and related) procedures.

Laparoscopic adjustable gastric banding is a widely performed operation for morbid obesity that entails placement of a silicone band using laparoscopic techniques around the upper stomach just below the gastroesophageal junction. The band is connected by way of hollow silicon tubing to an access port that is secured to the abdominal wall fascia. The access port allows the clinician to inject saline into the band. This expands the inner balloon of the band, causing external compression of the stomach resulting in increased appetite suppression, early satiety, and weight loss.

The need for a band adjustment is determined individually, based on the patient's weight loss, and feelings of satiety and hunger. Band patients are seen frequently in follow-up, so that serial adjustments can be performed to gradually and incrementally tighten the band until it is functioning optimally. If a patient is losing weight, food intake has been successfully restricted, and the patient is not hungry, then the band is not adjusted. If the patient is not losing weight, is hungry, and food intake is not restricted, then fluid is added to the band during an adjustment, to narrow the stoma. Adjustments to remove fluid volume may be necessary if the stoma is too narrow and the patient is having symptoms of obstruction (ie, vomiting, heartburn, or dysphagia).

As indicated in the guidelines, subsequent band adjustments are included as part of the postoperative period for this procedure and are not separately reportable.

Clinical Example (43770)

A 44-year-old woman presents with a body mass index of 48, hypertension, and poorly controlled diabetes. She has failed nonoperative obesity interventions and has elected gastric banding instead of gastric bypass surgery. She undergoes laparoscopic placement of an adjustable gastric band and subcutaneous port.

Description of Procedure (43770)

Under general anesthesia, surgical laparoscopy is performed. Pneumoperitoneum is established to distend the abdomen, and the laparoscope is introduced. Gas flow and intra-abdominal pressure are carefully monitored so as not to impair ventilation or venous return. Four to six trocar ports are sited through the anterior abdominal wall above the umbilicus. The viscera are inspected. An orogastric tube may be placed to decompress the stomach. The liver is retracted to expose the gastroesophageal junction. A path is made behind the upper stomach 2 cm below the gastroesophageal junction. The dissection plane may be guided by use of a per-oral gastric balloon catheter, which defines the location of the gastroesophageal junction, or by anatomical landmarks from the right crus of the diaphragm to the Angle of His. Excess visceral fat covering the upper stomach may need to be excised to prevent incorporation within the band, which would cause external compression and subsequent obstruction. The adjustable gastric band is introduced into the abdomen and pulled through the prepared retro-gastric path and around the upper stomach, just below the gastroesophageal junction. The band is locked. The band position is secured with strategically placed gastro-gastric sutures to prevent band slippage or gastric prolapse. The tubing attached to the band is tunneled through the abdominal wall. It is connected to an access port that is secured in or on the abdominal rectus muscle or other secure subcutaneous location. Hemostasis is obtained. The trocars are removed and all fascial and skin openings are closed as appropriate.

Clinical Example (43771)

A 45-year-old woman presents 15 months after surgical placement of adjustable gastric banding for a body mass index of 45. She has lost 85 lbs since surgery but has developed recent new onset symptoms of night-time gastroesophageal reflux that wake her from sleep. She also complains of decreased restriction and a capacity to eat more food. A contrast esophagram has confirmed band slippage or gastric prolapse. She undergoes laparoscopic revision of the adjustable gastric band.

Description of Procedure (43771)

Under general anesthesia, surgical laparoscopy is performed. A supraumbilical incision is made, and the peritoneum is grasped with sutures on the fascia. Insertion of the first trocar is handled cautiously in view of the prior surgery. Gas flow is initiated to distend the abdomen, and the laparoscope is introduced. Gas flow and intra-abdominal pressure are carefully monitored so as not to impair ventilation or venous return. Four to six trocar ports are sited through the anterior abdominal wall above the umbilicus. The viscera are inspected.

Pneumoperitoneum is maintained at 15 mm Hg throughout the procedure. An orogastric tube may be placed to decompress the stomach. The liver is retracted anteriorly to expose the upper stomach. Adhesions (which can be extensive) of the stomach to the undersurface of the liver are lysed with an ultrasonic scalpel. The band and its tubing are identified. The band is freed from the fibrin seal created by adhesions. The gastro-gastric sutures are cut and the securing gastric plication is released. The enlarged pouch is reduced by gentle retraction of the stomach tissue below the band in a caudad direction. This slides the stomach that has prolapsed upwards through the band back down through the band to its appropriate original position below. The band is re-positioned 1 to 2 cm below the gastroesophageal junction to create an appropriately small pouch. The gastric wall integrity is inspected. A leak test using methylene blue or air is performed to test for inadvertent gastrotomy. Any gastric wall injury is repaired with intra-corporeal sutures. A new gastro-gastric imbrication of the band is completed. Additional posterior-lateral sutures are added as necessary to secure the stomach-band position. Hemostasis is obtained. The trocars are removed, and all fascial and skin openings are closed as appropriate.

Clinical Example (43772)

A 45-year-old woman presents 15 months after surgical placement of adjustable gastric banding for a body mass index of 45. She has lost 85 lbs since surgery but has developed recent new onset symptoms of severe abdominal (epigastric) pain with dysphagia and vomiting. A contrast esophagram has confirmed a large band slippage or gastric prolapse. She undergoes laparoscopic removal of the adjustable gastric band.

Description of Procedure (43772)

Under general anesthesia, surgical laparoscopy is performed. Insertion of the first trocar is handled cautiously in view of prior surgery. Gas flow is initiated to distend the abdomen, and the laparoscope is introduced. Gas flow and intra-abdominal pressure are carefully monitored so as not to impair ventilation or venous return. Four to six trocar ports are placed in the anterior abdominal wall above the umbilicus. The viscera are inspected. Pneumoperitoneum is maintained at 15 mm Hg throughout the procedure. An orogastric tube may be placed to decompress the stomach. The liver is retracted anteriorly to expose the upper stomach. Adhesions (which can be extensive) of the stomach to the undersurface of the liver are lysed with an ultrasonic scalpel. The band and its tubing are identified. The band is freed from the fibrin seal created by adhesions. Some of the gastro-gastric suturing may be divided, taking care not to create a gastrotomy. The band is removed by cutting the buckle or the band next to the buckle. Gastric wall defects are identified and repaired in layers with sutures. Testing for leaks is performed with methylene blue, air insufflated though a nasogastric tube, or by intraoperative endoscopy. The tube connecting the band to the port is cut and the band with part of the tubing is removed from the abdomen. Hemostasis is obtained. The trocars are removed, and all fascial and skin openings closed as appropriate.

Clinical Example (43773)

A 45-year-old woman presents 15 months after surgical placement of adjustable gastric banding for a body mass index of 45. She has lost 85 lbs since surgery. She has had a known chronic slippage diagnosed by contrast esophagram and has now developed worsening symptoms of dysphagia and/or vomiting. She undergoes laparoscopic removal of the old adjustable gastric band and placement of a new adjustable gastric band.

Description of Procedure (43773)

Under general anesthesia, surgical laparoscopy is performed. Initial trocar insertion is handled in a cautious manner in view of prior surgery. Gas flow is initiated to distend the abdomen, and the laparoscope is introduced. Gas flow and intra-abdominal pressure are carefully monitored so as not to impair ventilation or venous return. Four to six trocar ports are placed in the anterior abdominal wall above the umbilicus. The viscera are inspected. Pneumoperitoneum is maintained at 15 mm Hg throughout the procedure. An orogastric tube may be placed to decompress the stomach. The liver is retracted anteriorly to expose the upper stomach. Adhesions (which can be extensive) of the stomach to the undersurface of the liver are lysed with an ultrasonic scalpel. The band and its tubing are identified. The band is freed from the fibrin seal created by adhesions.

The gastro-gastric sutures are cut and the securing gastric plication is released. The enlarged pouch is identified and attempts are made to reduce it by gentle retraction of the stomach tissue below the band in a caudad direction. The adhesions of the prolapsed stomach prevent adequate reduction of stomach into the correct position. Removal of the band to release the gastric prolapse is necessary. The band is cut along the side of the buckle to release the locking mechanism, or the band may be cut through the ring or shell section next to the buckle. The band portion is completely removed and a new band is placed in the correct position. This requires a new retrogastric dissection typically in a location above the original band placement and is time consuming due to scarring from the previous band. The gastric wall integrity is inspected. A leak test using methylene blue or air may be performed to test for inadvertent gastrotomy. Any gastric wall injury is repaired with intra-corporeal sutures. A new gastro-gastric imbrication of the band is completed. Additional posterior-lateral sutures may be added as necessary to secure the stomach-band position. The old band is removed from the abdomen; the tubing leading to the access port is cut and reconnected to the tubing of the newly placed band. Hemostasis is obtained. The trocars are removed, and all fascial and skin openings are closed as appropriate.

Clinical Example (43774)

A 40-year-old woman presents 18 months after surgical placement of adjustable gastric banding for a body mass index of 45. She has had inadequate weight loss. The band system is determined to be functioning appropriately. She undergoes laparoscopic removal of the adjustable gastric band and the subcutaneous port.

Description of Procedure (43774)

Under general anesthesia, surgical laparoscopy is performed. Insertion of the first trocar in handled in a cautious manner in view of prior surgery. Gas flow is initiated to distend the abdomen, and the laparoscope is introduced. Gas flow and intra-abdominal pressure are carefully monitored so as not to impair ventilation or venous return. Four to six trocar ports are sited through the anterior abdominal wall above the umbilicus. The viscera are inspected. Pneumoperitoneum is maintained at 15 mm Hg throughout the procedure. An orogastric tube may be placed to decompress the stomach. The liver is retracted anteriorly to expose the upper stomach. Adhesions (which can be extensive) of the stomach to the undersurface of the liver are lysed. The band and its tubing are identified. The band is freed from the fibrin seal created by adhesions. Some of the gastro-gastric suturing may be divided, taking care not to open into the stomach lumen. The band is removed by cutting the buckle or the band next to it. Gastric wall defects are identified and repaired. A methylene blue test or air leak test through a nasogastric tube or intraoperative endoscopy is performed. The tube connecting the band to the port is cut and the band is removed from the abdomen. An incision is made over the access port. The port sutures are released and the access port is removed. Hemostasis is obtained. The trocars are removed, and all fascial and skin openings are closed as appropriate.

Clinical Example (43848)

Four years ago, a 65-year-old female underwent vertical banded gastroplasty for morbid obesity. She was very compliant, and her weight decreased from 385 to 205 lbs. Within the last 3 months, she has suddenly gained 35 lbs and has developed severe gastroesophageal reflux symptoms. Barium swallow and upper GI endoscopy confirm break down of the staple line with restoration of gastric continuity. At re-operation, after difficult and extensive lysis of adhesions in the left upper quadrant, a 30-ml gastric pouch with a Roux-en-Y gastrojejunostomy is fashioned. The pouch is completely divided from the remainder of the stomach. She develops a wound hematoma, which becomes infected and requires bedside incision and drainage. The patient is discharged on the 14th postoperative day.

Description of Procedure (43848)

The patient is specially positioned with a footboard and taping of the ankles; strapping of the knees; preparing for a 50° tilt of the operating table; prepping and draping of the patient; and setting up the mechanical, table-mounted retractors. Lysis of adhesions is accomplished in the mid-abdomen and a 45-cm Roux limb is created. The severe adhesions between the left lobe of the liver and stomach and the distal esophagus, colon, and spleen are painstakingly taken down in a time-consuming manner. A pressure or volume-measured 30-ml pouch is created and divided from the remainder of the stomach. A 10-mm gastroenterostomy is created and a gastrostomy placed in the distal stomach. The wound is drained and closed in layers, and an intercostal block is placed to aid postoperative pulmonary mechanics. The wound and tubes are dressed.

Clinical Example (43886)

A 45-year-old woman presents 3.5 months after surgical placement of adjustable gastric banding for a body mass index of 45. Attempts to access the subcutaneous port component are unsuccessful. An abdominal radiograph reveals that the subcutaneous port component has flipped. She undergoes revision of the subcutaneous port.

Description of Procedure (43886)

Under general anesthesia, an incision is made over the access port. The subcutaneous fat and capsule around the port are divided. The port is found to be flipped over with the access portion facing the fascia. The securing suture is found to have been disrupted. The port is replaced into its original position with the silicone access portion facing up. The access port is secured to the anterior abdominal wall fascia with nonabsorbable sutures. Saline may be injected into the band for tightening via the access port during surgery. Hemostasis is obtained and the wound is closed.

Clinical Example (43887)

A 45-year-old woman presents 3 weeks after surgical placement of an adjustable gastric banding for a body mass index of 45. She has developed a wound infection at the subcutaneous port component site, which has failed to respond to antibiotic treatment. She undergoes removal of the subcutaneous port.

Description of Procedure (43887)

Under general anesthesia, an incision is made over the access port. The subcutaneous fat and capsule around the port are divided. The port sutures are released, the tubing connecting the access port to the band is divided, and the port is removed. The band is left intact, with the remaining tubing tied off and placed inside the peritoneal cavity. The wound is irrigated copiously and packed with gauze dressings. The dressings will need to be changed daily until the infection has cleared and the wound can be closed secondarily or heal by secondary intention.

Clinical Example (43888)

A 45-year-old woman presents 9 months after surgical placement of an adjustable gastric banding for a body mass index of 45. Band adjustments are ineffective at maintaining band diameter. A determination is made that there is a leak from the subcutaneous port component or tubing. She undergoes removal of the old subcutaneous port and placement of a new subcutaneous port.

Description of Procedure (43888)

Under general anesthesia, an incision is made over the access port. The subcutaneous fat and capsule around the port are divided. The port sutures are released, the tubing connecting the access port to the band is divided, and the port is removed. The band is left intact with the remaining tubing. A new access port is connected to the existing tubing, leading to the gastric band, using a tubing connector. The tubing is replaced into the peritoneal cavity. The access port is secured to the anterior abdominal wall fascia with nonabsorbable sutures. Saline may be injected into the band for tightening via the access port during the time of surgery. Hemostasis is obtained and the wound is closed.

Intestines (Except Rectum)

INCISION

44005 Enterolysis (freeing of intestinal adhesion) (separate procedure)

(Do not report 44005 in addition to 45136)

(For laparoscopic approach, use ►44180◄)

LAPAROSCOPY

Surgical laparoscopy always includes diagnostic laparoscopy. To report a diagnostic laparoscopy (peritoneoscopy) (separate procedure), use 49320.

►*Incision*◄

●44180 Laparoscopy, surgical, enterolysis (freeing of intestinal adhesion) (separate procedure)

►*Enterostomy—External Fistulization of Intestines*◄

●44186 Laparoscopy, surgical; jejunostomy (eg, for decompression or feeding)

●44187 ileostomy or jejunostomy, non-tube

►(For open procedure, use 44310)◄

●44188 Laparoscopy, surgical, colostomy or skin level cecostomy

►(For open procedure, use 44320)◄

►(Do not report 44188 in conjunction with 44970)◄

►(44200 has been deleted. To report, use 44180)◄

►(44201 has been deleted. To report, use 44186)◄

Rationale

New codes have been added to the Intestines (Except Rectum) and Rectum subsections of the Digestive System to identify laparoscopic performance of various services. These laparoscopic subsections are further sub-divided into areas of (1) Excision, (2) Repair, and (3) Enterostomy-External Fistulization of Intestines. Addition of these new sections follows the pattern used throughout the Digestive System section. To accommodate these changes, the descriptors of some of the existing codes have been revised to denote the specific procedures for which they are intended to be used (ie, the additions improve granularity of each of the codes for more specifc usage).

Clinical Example (44187)

A 58-year-old man, who recently underwent a supra-pubic prostatectomy, presents with rectal discharge of urine. His urinalysis is positive for fecal flora and sediment. He has a computed tomography-confirmed abscess in the prostate bed and communication between the rectum and the neck of the bladder at the urethral anastomosis and a contrast-confirmed recto-urethral fistula. At laparoscopy, to achieve fecal diversion, the terminal ileum is identified and brought out as an ileostomy through the skin in a preoperatively selected site.

Description of Procedure (44187)

Under general anesthesia, surgical laparoscopy is performed. A supraumbilical incision is made and a 12-mm port is placed. Gas flow is initiated to distend the abdomen, and the laparoscope is introduced. Gas flow and intra-abdominal pressure are carefully monitored so as not to impair ventilation or venous return. Two additional 5-mm ports are placed: one in the right paraumbilical region in the preoperative marked stoma site and one in the left iliac fossa, lateral to the rectus muscle. The abdomen is explored with the patient in steep Trendelenburg and left-side-down position. Through the right-sided port site, the bowel at the terminal ileum is gently grasped to ensure adequate mobilization of the terminal ileum to reach the anterior abdominal wall. The proximal and distal end is marked with one and two clips, respectively. The stoma site is created with the use of the Bovie and splitting the rectus muscle, working around the trocar in the stoma site. The bowel is delivered through the abdominal wall after releasing the pneumoperitoneum, which is then reestablished to inspect the abdomen to ensure hemostasis, bowel viability, and a tension-free ileostomy without unwanted twists. The trocars are removed, the fascial openings are closed as appropriate, and the individual wounds of the port sites are closed.

Clinical Example (44188)

A gravida 4 para 4 (G4P4) 78-year-old woman, who is undergoing preoperative chemotherapy and radiation therapy for a distal stage 3 rectal cancer located at 2 cm from the dentate line, presents with complaints of severe tenesmus, fecal incontinence, worsened by the diarrhea associated with the chemotherapy. Her perineum is severely excoriated and associated with severe ulcerative dermatitis. At laparoscopy, the left colon is mobilized and brought out as a colostomy through the skin in a preoperatively selected site to allow for relief from fecal incontinence and perineal irritation and completion of the neo-adjuvant treatment, prior to definitive resection.

Description of Procedure (44188)

Under general anesthesia, surgical laparoscopy is performed. A supraumbilical incision is made and carried down to the linea alba, which is grasped with clamps. Divided sutures are placed in the linea alba. The peritoneum is identified and divided. The port is placed. Gas flow is initiated to distend the abdomen, and the laparoscope is introduced. Gas flow and intra-abdominal pressure are carefully monitored so as not to impair ventilation or venous return. Three additional ports are placed, one in the left paraumbilical region, one in the right paraumbilical region, and one in the right iliac fossa, each lateral to the rectus muscle, each placed under direct vision. The abdomen is explored with the patient in steep Trendelenburg and right-side-down position. Adhesions of the sigmoid to the anterior abdominal wall are divided. The line of Toldt is divided to achieve mobilization and the left ureter is identified and reflected posteriorly out of harm's way. A trocar is placed in the previously marked stoma site. The proximal and distal ends of the loop are marked with one and two clips, respectively, and grasped. The stoma site is created around the trocar and enlarged to accept two fingers. After decompressing the pneumoperitoneum, the bowel is exteriorized and divided with a linear stapler cutter. The distal end is returned in the abdomen and the proximal end secured to the skin. The pneumoperitoneum is then reestablished to inspect the abdomen to ensure hemostasis, bowel viability, and a tension-free colostomy, without unwanted twists. The trocars are removed and the fascial openings are closed as appropriate, and the individual wounds of the port sites are closed.

▶*Excision*◀

▲44202 Laparoscopy, surgical; enterectomy, resection of small intestine, single resection and anastomosis

44212 colectomy, total, abdominal, with proctectomy, with ileostomy

(For open procedure, use 44155)

+●44213 Laparoscopy, surgical, mobilization (take-down) of splenic flexure performed in conjunction with partial colectomy (List separately in addition to primary procedure)

▶(Use 44213 in conjunction with 44204-44208)◀

▶(For open procedure, use 44139)◀

▶*Repair*◀

●44227 Laparoscopy, surgical, closure of enterostomy, large or small intestine, with resection and anastomosis

▶(For open procedure, see 44625, 44626)◀

▶*Other Procedures*◀

44238 Unlisted laparoscopy procedure, intestine (except rectum)

▶(44239 has been deleted. To report, use 45499)◀

Rationale

A new section has been created, new parenthetical notes added, and six new codes established to identify laparoscopic procedures for the large and small intestine. The new section includes procedures that identify jejunostomy (44186), non-tube ileostomy or jejunostomy (44187), colostomy or skin level cecostomy (44188), enterectomy of the small intestine (44202), mobilization of the splenic flexure with partial colectomy (44213), and closure of an enterostomy (44227), all performed via use of a laparoscope. These codes are intended to parallel many of the existing subsections in the CPT codebook for open procedures. As a result, a number of cross-references included within the open-approach codes refer users to alternative and/or related procedures for laparoscopic intestinal services. Additional parenthetical notes (such as those included after code 44188) are exclusionary notes, ie, identifying codes that should not be reported together or codes that should be used to replace other codes that have been deleted.

In addition, unlisted code 44239 has been deleted and renumbered to a more relevant location.

Clinical Example (44202)

A 23-year-old female with Crohn's disease has a severe sigmoid stenosis. Failing medical treatment, the operation includes laparoscopic assessment of the intestinal tract for active Crohn's disease. The sigmoid colon is mobilized through four laparoscopic ports. The mesenteric and intestinal resection is accomplished intra- and extracorporeally. The resected specimen is delivered through a suprapubic incision. Intestinal continuity is restored with an end-to-end anastomosis using a transanal stapling device. The incision and port sites are closed. Postoperative care manages the associated ileus, immunosuppressive medications, and wound care. Outpatient follow-up includes assessment for anastomotic complications.

Description of Procedure (44202)

Under general anesthesia, surgical laparoscopy is performed. A supraumbilical incision is made, and the peritoneum is grasped with sutures on the fascia. The peritoneum is opened under direct vision. A blunt trocar is inserted. Gas flow is initiated to distend the abdomen, and the laparoscope is introduced. Gas flow and intra-abdominal pressure are carefully monitored so as not to impair ventilation or venous return. The viscera are inspected. Three additional trocars are placed to expose the mobilized area and resect the pathologic segment of intestine (in this case, the sigmoid). The mesenteric vessels are identified, double clamped and ligated through the laparoscope. The specimen is delivered to the abdominal wall in the lower abdomen. A separate incision is placed in the abdomen to deliver the specimen from the wound. An extracorporeal anastomosis is performed through the incision. Intracorporeal anastomoses are performed through the laparoscope. A trans-anal circular stapling device is used to perform the anastomosis. Meticulous hemostasis is obtained and the trocar are removed. The trocar sites are individually closed as is the lower abdominal incision.

Clinical Example (44213)

After laparoscopic colon resection for middle to low rectal cancer, an end-to-end colorectal anastomosis between the splenic flexure and the rectum is performed, requiring mobilization of the entire splenic flexure.

Description of Procedure (44213)

Laparoscopic mobilization of the splenic flexure involves placement of additional operative trocar ports (one or possibly two) to attain proper traction tension for the tedious dissection. With medial traction to expose the lateral line of Toldt, dissection of the colon is carried out cephalad, along the line of Toldt, lateral to the descending colon. The transverse colon is retracted toward the pelvis, while the omentum is retracted cephalad, then the omentum is dissected from the transverse colon, in order to enter the lesser sac for access to the colon mesentery. This dissection is carried to the spleen and then the ligaments are taken down from the lower pole of the spleen and the splenic hilum. Next, the colonic mesentery is divided in one of two ways: (1) the transverse mesentery is divided through the lesser sac up to the splenic flexure and the proximal descending colon; or (2) the transverse colon is retracted in the cephalad direction and the descending colon is retracted laterally in order to isolate the ligament of Treitz as a landmark for the retroperitoneal dissection of splenic flexure mesentery. During the procedure, the operative table will be repositioned multiple times to allow gravity to assist in the retraction of the hollow organs. For example, the Trendelenburg position is used while the omentum is dissected off of the transverse colon and the reverse Trendelenburg position is used while the mesentery of the transverse colon is divided through the lesser sac.

Clinical Example (44227)

A 73-year-old man, 3 months status post Hartmann procedure for perforated diverticulitis presents for reversal of his colostomy.

Description of Procedure (44227)

Under general anesthesia, surgical laparoscopy is performed. A supraumbilical incision is made, and the peritoneum is grasped with sutures on the fascia. The peritoneum is opened under direct vision. A Hassan blunt trocar is inserted. Gas flow is initiated to distend the abdomen, and the laparoscope is introduced. Gas flow and intra-abdominal pressure are carefully monitored so as not to impair ventilation or venous return. Two 5-mm trocars are placed in the right lower quadrant and another 5-mm trocar is placed in the mid-epigastrium. The viscera are inspected. The previous operation typically involves pelvic sepsis and creates dense adhesions that maximally complicate the re-exploration; therefore, laparoscopic lysis of adhesions is oftentimes the first step performed. The rectal stump is identified after mobilizing any adherent small bowel off the top of the Hartmann pouch. The stoma is dissected free from the anterior abdominal wall fascia. The colon is mobilized from the transverse colon distally including the splenic flexure. The descending colon will serve as the segment for the anastomosis. The ureters are identified bilaterally with care to prevent injury. Once the colon is fully mobilized from inside the abdomen, the colostomy is freed up from the skin of the anterior abdominal wall using an elliptical incision, and carried down into the peritoneal cavity. With the transient loss of pneumoperitoneum, the colostomy is resected and the anvil of a circular stapler is placed in the proximal colon. After securing it with a purse-string suture, the proximal bowel is reduced into the abdominal cavity and the colostomy site is closed in two layers. Once pneumoperitoneum has been reinstituted, an anastomosis is performed using the circular stapling device. While the pelvis is filled with irrigation solution, a rigid proctoscopy is performed with insufflation of the rectum to assure that the anastomosis does not create an air leak and remains intact. Hemostasis is obtained. The trocars are removed, the fascial openings are closed as appropriate, and the individual wounds of the port sites are closed.

ENTEROSTOMY—EXTERNAL FISTULIZATION OF INTESTINES

▲44310 Ileostomy or jejunostomy, non-tube

►(For laparoscopic procedure, use 44187)◄

►(Do not report 44310 in conjunction with 44144, 44150-44153, 44155, 44156, 45113, 45119, 45136)◄

▲44320 Colostomy or skin level cecostomy;

►(For laparoscopic procedure, use 44188)◄

►(Do not report 44320 in conjunction with 44141, 44144, 44146, 44605, 45110, 45119, 45126, 45563, 45805, 45825, 50810, 51597, 57307, or 58240)◄

Rationale

The separate procedure designation has been removed from codes 44310 and 44320 in favor of inclusion of an exclusionary parenthetical note listed subsequent to each code that identifies the service codes that should not be reported together with the 44310 and 44320 services. Additional parenthetical notes have been added to the open approach ileostomy and colostomy codes to direct users to the laparoscopic "counterparts" for these services.

Clinical Example (44320)

A 67-year-old male presents with a history of rectal bleeding and a biopsy-proven sigmoid carcinoma at 35 cm from the anal verge. The lesion is completely obstructing the patient and, because of multiple medical problems, the decision is made to perform a diverting colostomy to decompress the colon and to allow time for proper medical stabilization of the patient prior to definitive resection. After the decision to operate has been made, the surgeon reviews laboratory and radiologic studies, and assesses the need for further diagnostic procedures prior to surgery. The surgeon discusses the procedure with the patient, and obtains informed consent. At operation, a dissection of the left colon is performed. The left colon is mobilized and brought out as a colostomy and drains placed as indicated. Postoperative care of the patient includes monitoring of ventilator settings, hemodynamics, intravenous nutrition, antibiotics, and fluid balance. Wound checks and dressing changes are made to assure an absence of infection, hematoma, and drainage. Communication occurs with the patient and family, as well as coordination of care with other physicians and health care providers. Drains are removed as indicated. Oral feeding is resumed after a return of bowel function. The patient's diet is advanced, intravenous feeding is discontinued, and the nutritional status of the patient is also monitored to ensure that adequate nutritional intake occurs. The medical status of the patient is reviewed with other consultants, discussed with the patient and family, and appropriate decisions are then made for further care of the patient. A decision is made to discharge the patient to allow further stabilization of his medical status, prior to definitive resection. The patient is followed in the office as needed to monitor for wound complications or infection until cleared for surgery by the medical consultants.

Description of Procedure (44320)

A skin incision is made, and the anterior abdominal wall is carefully divided. The peritoneum is entered and a thorough exploration of the abdomen is undertaken, including palpating and visualizing (where possible) the spleen, liver, stomach, duodenum, pancreas, small bowel, large bowel, kidneys, and pelvis, including bladder and rectum. Adhesions are lysed by sharp and blunt dissection. A self-retaining retractor is secured to the operating table, and rings and blades are selected and inserted to obtain adequate visualization of the operative site. The small bowel is mobilized and isolated with laparotomy packs. An incision of the muco-cutaneous junction of the previously constructed ileostomy is incised and the ileostomy is carefully separated from the subcutaneous fat and fascia or muscle of the abdominal wall, taking care to preserve the blood supply of the ileum. The distal bowel is measured for the appropriate length to create a pouch. A point chosen proximal to the distal end is isolated from its mesenteric blood supply for future use as an intussuscepted nipple valve. The pouch components are folded into the appropriate pouch configuration and held in place with sutures. The common wall anastomosis is performed. The valve component is intussuscepted and secured in place with suture or staples. The prior ileostomy site is assessed for suitability for placement of the pouch nipple and, if adequate, is prepared for a pouch nipple-mucocutaneous anastomosis. The pouch is delivered through the abdominal wall into the ileostomy site and carefully secured in place with sutures. The position of the nasogastric tube is adjusted and ascertained to be in the correct place for drainage. The abdominal cavity is irrigated with saline, and another inspection of the abdomen is made for other abnormalities. A closed-system suction drain may be inserted for drainage of a localized area.

The self-retaining retractor is removed and disassembled; sponge, needle, and instrument counts are obtained and confirmed, prior to closure of the abdomen. The anterior abdominal wall is closed with a standard technique, and subcutaneous tissue is irrigated and drained with a closed-suction drain when indicated. The skin is closed in a standard fashion. After the skin is closed and dressed, a special pouch intubation catheter is selected and placed into the nipple valve and the pouch.

REPAIR

44620 Closure of enterostomy, large or small intestine;

44625 with resection and anastomosis other than colorectal

44626 with resection and colorectal anastomosis (eg, closure of Hartmann type procedure)

►(For laparoscopic procedure, use 44188)◄

Rationale

In tandem with the establishment of a code to report performance of laparoscopic colostomy or skin level cecostomy, a cross-reference has been added to the open approach codes to refer the user to code 44188.

Rectum

EXCISION

45110 Proctectomy; complete, combined abdominoperineal, with colostomy

►(For laparoscopic procedure, use 45395)◄

▲**45119** Proctectomy, combined abdominoperineal pull-through procedure (eg, colo-anal anastomosis), with creation of colonic reservoir (eg, J-pouch), with diverting enterostomy when performed

►(For laparoscopic procedure, use 45397)◄

Rationale

In tandem with addition of codes to identify laparoscopic proctectomy, a cross-reference was added to the open approach codes to refer users to 45395 and 45397.

Clinical Example (45119)

A 53-year-old female requires radical extirpation of a 4-cm rectal cancer with a resection margin at the level of the levators. A total mesorectal resection with proctectomy is performed. The remaining colon is mobilized proximal to the splenic flexure. A colonic J-pouch is fashioned in the descending colon. The J-pouch anastomosis to the rectum is either through a transanal or abdominal approach. A diverting loop ilesotomy in the right lower quadrant protects the anastomosis. The abdominal incision is closed. Postoperative care manages the associated ileus and wound care. Outpatient follow-up includes assessment for anastomotic complications.

Description of Procedure (45119)

Through a midline incision, the abdomen is explored. The physician establishes the intraoperative staging of the rectal cancer assessing for extra pelvic extension of the tumor. The colon is mobilized from the midtransverse colon distally including the splenic flexure. The descending colon will serve as the segment for creation of the J-pouch. The sigmoid colon is resected enbloc with the rectum. A total mesorectal excision (TME) is included to provide adequate margins for a malignancy. The ureters are identified bilaterally with care to prevent injury. The rectosigmoid segment is resected and removed from the operative field. The specimen is forwarded to the pathologist where it is properly opened; thus, allowing the surgeon to establish the adequacy of the distal margin. The J-pouch is created using a linear gastrointestinal stapler. The anorectal junction is prepared by placing circumferential sutures transanally. The J-pouch is introduced into the pelvis and advanced to the anorectal junction. A hand-sewn, transanal anastomosis is performed. The previously marked ileostomy site is identified in the right lower quadrant. The ileostomy is prepared by incising the skin and opening the rectus fascia. The rectus muscles are split and the posterior fascia is incised. The terminal ileum is brought out through the ileostomy site. A stoma bar is placed beneath the ileostomy to prevent stoma retraction. Two active drains are placed within the pelvis and the abdominal incision is closed. The ileostomy is secured to the stoma.

ENDOSCOPY

⊙**45378** Colonoscopy, flexible, proximal to splenic flexure; diagnostic, with or without collection of specimen(s) by brushing or washing, with or without colon decompression (separate procedure)

⊙**45392** with transendoscopic ultrasound guided intramural or transmural fine needle aspiration/biopsy(s)

(Do not report 45392 in conjunction with 45330, 45341, 45342, 45378, 76872)

Rationale

The moderate sedation bull's-eye indicator has been added to denote that moderate sedation is inherent in these prcodures. Therefore, conscious sedation should not be reported separately.

▶LAPAROSCOPY◀

▶Surgical laparoscopy always includes diagnostic laparoscopy. To report a diagnostic laparoscopy (peritoneoscopy) (separate procedure), use 49320.◀

▶*Excision*◀

●**45395** Laparoscopy, surgical; proctectomy, complete, combined abdominoperineal, with colostomy

▶(For open procedure, use 45110)◀

●**45397** proctectomy, combined abdominoperineal pull-through procedure (eg, colo-anal anastomosis), with creation of colonic reservoir (eg, J-pouch), with diverting enterostomy, when performed

▶(For open procedure, use 45119)◀

Rationale

New codes have been added to the Intestines (Except Rectum) and Rectum subsections of the Digestive System to identify laparoscopic performance of various services. These laparoscopic subsections are further sub-divided into areas of (1) Excision, (2) Repair, and (3) Enterostomy-External Fistulization of Intestines. Addition of these new sections follows the pattern used throughout the Digestive System section. To accommodate these changes, the descriptors of some of the existing open approach codes have been revised to denote the specific procedures for which they are intended to be used (ie, the additions improve granularity of each of the codes for more specific usage). In tandem with the addition of laparoscopic protectomy codes, cross-references direct the user to the open approach proctectomy codes 45110 and 45119.

Clinical Example (45395)

A 65-year-old man presents with a low rectal lesion that is 1 cm proximal to the dentate line and a biopsy-proven moderately differentiated adenocarcinoma. The lesion is T2 on endorectal ultrasound and negative for metastatic disease based on a previous computed tomographic position emission tomography (CT PET) scan. He had received preoperative chemoradiation and is 1 month post-radiotherapy. At laparoscopic operation, he undergoes a complete proctectomy with colostomy.

Description of Procedure (45395)

Under general anesthesia, surgical laparoscopy is performed. A right lower quadrant and suprapubic trocar and right upper quadrant and left lower quadrant trocars are placed. After an exploratory laparoscopy, the sigmoid colon is retracted medially and dissection along the line of Toldt is performed to the level of the splenic flexure. Next, the sigmoid colon is retracted laterally in order to isolate and transect the inferior mesenteric artery (IMA). The left ureter is isolated in the retroperitoneal space of the sigmoid and mobilized. The mesentery of the sigmoid is opened at the level of the pelvic brim and sharp dissection is performed to isolate and divide the IMA (through the right lower quadrant port with an endovascular stapler). The dissection is continued along the medial mesentery to the level of the inferior mesenteric vein (IMV), which is divided with an endovascular stapler. Sharp dissection of the lateral ligaments to the pelvic floor is carried out. The rectum is mobilized posterior to Waldeyer's fascia to the level of the pelvic floor. At the level of the descending sigmoid junction, the colon is divided intracorporeally with an endogastrointestinal stapler. Perineal dissection is carried out with transperineal removal of the specimen, and the perineal skin is closed. The descending colon is brought out through a previously marked ostomy site. Hemostasis is obtained. The trocars are removed and the fascial openings closed as appropriate, and the individual wounds of the port sites closed.

Clinical Example **(45397)**

A 72-year-old woman presents with a low rectal lesion 6 cm proximal to the dentate line that is a biopsy-proven moderately differentiated adenocarcinoma. The lesion is T3 without adenopathy on endorectal ultrasound and negative for metastatic disease based on CT PET scan. She had received preoperative chemoradiation and is 1 month post-radiotherapy. At laparoscopic operation, a total mesorectal resection with proctectomy is performed. The remaining colon is mobilized proximal to the splenic flexure. A colonic J-pouch is fashioned in the descending colon and anastomosed to the rectal stump or anus. A diverting loop ileostomy is created in the right lower quadrant to protect the anastomosis.

Description of Procedure **(45397)**

Under general anesthesia, surgical laparoscopy is performed. A right lower quadrant and suprapubic trocar and right upper quadrant and left lower quadrant trocars are placed. After an exploratory laparoscopy, the sigmoid colon is retracted medially and dissection along the line of Toldt is performed to the level of the splenic flexure. The medial mobilization and dissection of the sigmoid mesentery with intracorporeal ligation of the IMA and IMV is performed using an endovascular stapler. The rectum is mobilized to below the mesorectum for eventual intracorporeal transection of the rectum with an endovascular stapler for total mesorectal excision (TMC) resection. After transection of the rectum, the suprapubic or the left lower quadrant trocar site is extended in order to remove the specimen. Construction of the colonic J-pouch is accomplished by transecting the proximal colon at or near the descending sigmoid junction and folding the distal end of the remaining colon onto itself, creating a pouch. A circular stapler is placed in the rectal stump and while the anvil of the staple is placed in the J portion of the pouch, a double-stapled anastomosis is performed. If the lesion is closer to the anus, a transanal mucosectomy is performed and a hand-sewn coloanal pouch anastomosis is performed. A proximal diverting loop ileostomy is created. Hemostasis is obtained. The trocars are removed and the fascial openings closed as appropriate and the individual wounds of the port sites closed.

▶*Repair*◀

●**45400** Laparoscopy, surgical; proctopexy (for prolapse)

▶(For open procedure, use 45540, 45541)◀

●45402 proctopexy (for prolapse), with sigmoid resection

►(For open procedure, use 45550)◄

●45499 Unlisted laparoscopy procedure, rectum

Rationale

New codes have been added to the Intestines (Except Rectum) and Rectum subsections of the Digestive System to identify laparoscopic performance of various services. These laparoscopic subsections are further subdivided into areas of (1) Excision, (2) Repair, and (3) Enterostomy-External Fistulization of Intestines. Addition of these new sections follows the pattern used throughout the Digestive System section. To accommodate these changes, the descriptors of some of the existing open approach codes have been revised to denote the specific procedures for which they are intended to be used (ie, the additions improve granularity of each of the codes for more specifc usage). Code 45499 has been established in tandem with the deletion of unlisted code 44239.

Clinical Example (45400)

A 75-year-old woman presents with full-thickness rectal prolapse. She has no history of constipation but has moderate symptoms of fecal incontinence. Laparoscopically, the rectum is mobilized, the prolapse is reduced, and the mobilized rectum is fixated to the sacrum.

Description of Procedure (45400)

Under general anesthesia, surgical laparoscopy is performed and a number of ports are inserted to permit adequate instrumentation. After an exploratory laparoscopy, the sigmoid colon and rectum are mobilized off the presacral fascia, with great care to protect the presacral autonomic nerves and ureters. The presacral space is entered and the rectum mobilized adequately to reduce any prolapse. An appropriate section of the rectum is chosen for attachment to the sacrum to maintain reduction of the prolapse. The mesorectum of this section of rectum is affixed to the sacrum or sacral promontory. Hemostasis is obtained. The trocars are removed; the fascial openings are closed as appropriate; and, the individual wounds of the port sites are closed.

Clinical Example (45402)

A 75-year-old woman presents with full-thickness rectal prolapse. She has a history of severe constipation and has no significant symptoms of fecal incontinence. Laparoscopically, the rectum is mobilized and the sigmoid colon is resected. The specimen is removed through a small incision. Laparoscopically, an anastomosis is fashioned using an end-to-end stapling device and the distal rectum is fixed to the sacrum.

Description of Procedure (45402)

Under general anesthesia, surgical laparoscopy is performed and a number of ports are inserted to permit adequate instrumentation. After an exploratory laparoscopy, the sigmoid colon and rectum are mobilized off the presacral fascia with great care to protect the presacral autonomic nerves and ureters. The presacral space is entered and the rectum mobilized adequately to reduce any prolapse. The sigmoid colon is resected, with or without an accompanying portion of the upper rectum. The vascular supply to this piece of bowel is ligated, either by dividing the inferior mesenteric artery at the proximal and distal ends or by dividing individual branches of the sigmoid arteries and preserving the inferior mesenteric artery. The bowel is divided at the distal point of transection, below the confluence of the taeniae coli, using a laparoscopic stapling device. The proximal bowel is extracted through a small muscle-splitting incision, and the anvil of a stapler inserted before returning the proximal end of the bowel to the abdomen and closing the fascia. The anastomosis is fashioned with a transanal circular stapling device. An appropriate section of the rectum is chosen for attachment to the sacrum to maintain reduction of the prolapse. The mesorectum of this section of the rectum is affixed to the sacrum or sacral promontory. Hemostasis is obtained. The trocars are removed and the fascial openings closed as appropriate and the individual wounds of the port sites closed.

REPAIR

▲45540 Proctopexy (eg, for prolapse); abdominal approach

▶(For laparoscopic procedure, use 45400)◀

▲45550 with sigmoid resection, abdominal approach

▶(For laparoscopic procedure, use 45402)◀

Rationale

New codes have been added to the Intestines (Except Rectum) and Rectum subsections of the Digestive System to identify laparoscopic performance of various services. These laparoscopic subsections are further subdivided into areas of (1) Excision, (2) Repair, and (3) Enterostomy-External Fistulization of Intestines. The addition of these new sections follows the pattern used throughout the Digestive System section. To accommodate these changes, the descriptors of some of the existing open approach codes have been revised to denote the specific procedures for which they are intended to be used (ie, the additions improve granularity of each of the codes for more specifc usage). In tandem with the revision of the open approach proctectomy codes, cross-references direct the user to the laparoscopic approach codes 45400 and 45402.

Clinical Example (45550)

A 75-year-old female presents with a long history of chronic constipation and recent onset of full-thickness rectal prolapse. After the decision to operate has been made, the surgeon reviews all laboratory and radiologic studies, and determines that no further evaluation is required. The surgeon reviews the intended procedure with the patient and her spouse and informed consent is obtained. A preoperative mechanical and antibiotic bowel preparation is performed. At operation, a complete rectosigmoid mobilization is performed down to the pelvic floor posteriorly. The redundant sigmoid colon is resected and a primary anastomosis is performed. The mobilized rectum is sutured fixated to the sacral promontory with four permanent sutures. The wound is closed in layers. Postoperative care includes all necessary hospital and office visits during the 90-day global period to assure normal recovery and the absence of any complications.

Description of Procedure (45550)

The patient is prepped and draped under anesthesia, placed in the supine position, and readied for the abdominal incision. The surgeon makes an abdominal incision of his or her choice. The incision is carried through the subcutaneous tissues and other layers of tissue, individually entering the peritoneal cavity. The peritoneal cavity is thoroughly explored for other abnormalities and is appropriately packed. The self-retaining retractor is secured to the operating table and the appropriate appendages are attached to provide visualization. The packs are repositioned as needed to mobilize the distal descending colon and the sigmoid colon. Once that is done, rectal mobilization must be accomplished to the level of the lateral stocks of the rectum. Rectopexy sutures are placed appropriately to the rectum at the upper level of the lateral stocks and the presacral fascia. The sutures are tagged and not tied at this time. An appropriate length of bowel for resection is determined. The mesentery is divided to that part of the bowel to devascularize it. The resection is carried out controlling the distal rectal stump and proximal colon site of resection to avoid leakage. Anastomosis is made in the fashion of choice by the operating surgeon. Rectopexy sutures are tied down, securing the rectum to the presacral fascia. The abdominal cavity is irrigated with a saline solution to ensure hemostasis and cleansing. Exploration for foreign bodies, such as sponges, instruments, and needles, is carried out. All are removed and counts are verified. The retractor is removed and disassembled. The anterior abdominal wall is closed in a standard technique, irrigating the subcutaneous tissue. The skin is closed in the surgeon's fashion of choice.

OTHER PROCEDURES

►Surgical diagnostic anorectal exam (45990) includes the following elements: external perineal exam, digital rectal exam, pelvic exam (when performed), diagnostic anoscopy, and diagnostic rigid proctoscopy.◄

●45990 Anorectal exam, surgical, requiring anesthesia (general, spinal, or epidural), diagnostic

►(Do not report 45990 in conjunction with 45300-45327, 46600, 57410, 99170)◄

Rationale

Code 45990 is intended to report performance of a diagnostic anorectal exam that requires anesthesia. As is noted in the descriptor language, this code may be used for anorectal exam performed under general, spinal, or epidural anesthesia. Parenthetical notes have been included to identify codes that should not be report concurrently with code 45990.

A surgical diagnostic anorectal exam includes the following elements: external perineal exam, digital rectal exam, pelvic exam (when performed), diagnostic anoscopy, and diagnostic rigid proctoscopy. If during the exam a procedure is initiated, then only that procedure code would be reported instead of 45990.

45999 Unlisted procedure, rectum

(For unlisted laparoscopic procedure, rectum, use ▶45499◀)

Rationale

In tandem with the deletion and renumbering of code 44239, the cross-reference following 45999 has been revised to reference the new unlisted code 45499.

Clinical Example (45990)

A 35-year-old man with severe rectal pain is referred for evaluation. Initial office evaluation revealed no external evidence or signs of anorectal pathology. Due to severe pain, further evaluation including DRE, anoscopy, and proctoscopy cannot be performed in the office and the patient is referred to a facility. Under anesthesia (general, spinal, or epidural), a complete examination of the perianal skin, anal verge, anal canal, and rectum is performed. This includes visual inspection of the perineal skin, digital rectal exam (DRE) of the anal canal and distal rectum, anoscopic examination, and proctoscopic examination. No anorectal source of pain is identified.

Description of Procedure (45990)

Under anesthesia (general, spinal, or epidural), a complete examination of the perianal skin, anal verge, anal canal, and rectum is performed. This includes visual inspection of the perineal skin, DRE of the anal canal and distal rectum (a sweep of the entire coccyx and at least half of the sacrum), anoscopic examination, and proctoscopic examination. No anorectal source of pain is identified.

Anus

INTRODUCTION

46500 Injection of sclerosing solution, hemorrhoids

(For excision of hemorrhoids, see 46250-46262; for destruction, see 46934-46936; for ligation, see 46945, 46946; for hemorrhoidopexy, use 46947)

●**46505** Chemodenervation of internal anal sphincter

▶(For chemodenervation of other muscles, see 64612-64614, 64640)◀

▶(Report the specific service in conjunction with the specific substance(s) or drug(s) provided)◀

Rationale

Code 46505 is used to report chemodenervation of the internal anal sphincter. The procedure code identifies the injection of botulinum toxin into the internal anal sphincter muscle tissue to allow loosening of the anal opening and accommodate healing of the fissure that has developed at that orifice site. Parenthetical notes include a cross-reference to the location of other chemodenervation procedures as well as a notation on the use of other codes to separately identify materials used for the procedure.

Initial medical management of anal fissures consists of keeping the stools soft to avoid tearing the anal skin; frequent sitz baths to increase local blood flow and relax the sphincter; topical steroid-anesthetic medications to decrease the inflammatory response and to provide local anesthesia; and topical application of dilute nitroglycerin paste to produce local relaxation of the exposed smooth muscle of the anus. The goal of medical therapy is to create the effect of a temporary or reversible sphincterotomy, reducing sphincter pressure only until the fissure has healed. If this fails after reasonable treatment duration, the next step has traditionally been surgical intervention with a lateral internal sphincterotomy, with or without removing the fissure itself.

Code 46505 is intended to report the injection of botulinum toxin into the internal anal sphincter area as another type of medical therapy before resorting to surgical intervention. Botulinum toxin causes denervation of the internal anal sphincter. The toxin acts rapidly and paralysis occurs within a few hours. Clinical visits are maintained during the "weakened" state of the muscle (for 3 to 4 months). This reduction in the resting pressure of the anal muscle produces the equivalent of a surgical lateral internal sphincterotomy and thus allows the fissure to heal.

Clinical Example (46505)

A 38-year-old woman presents with a history of bright red rectal bleeding and pain with every bowel movement. She has a posterior midline fissure that has failed treatment with topical creams and nitroglycerin ointment. Treatment of the fissure by injection of chemodenervation agent (eg, botulinum toxin) is performed to temporarily relax the internal anal sphincter, allow healing of the fissure, and minimize the complication of fecal incontinence associated with a surgical sphincterotomy.

Description of Procedure (46505)

Under anesthesia, a digital rectal exam and anoscopic evaluation are performed. Forty units of botulinum toxin are injected in divided doses at the posterior midline and both lateral quadrants of the intersphincteric area.

REPAIR

●46710 Repair of ileoanal pouch fistula/sinus (eg, perineal or vaginal), pouch advancement; transperineal approach

●46712 combined transperineal and transabdominal approach

Rationale

Two codes have been added to identify repair of an ileoanal fistula or sinus by a transperineal approach or via a combined transperineal and transabdominal approach. Development of these codes allows report of circumferential transanal pouch advancement to repair a pouch-vaginal or pouch-perineal fistula or a long exit conduit of an S-pouch.

Clinical Example (46710)

A 35-year-old woman presents with passage of stool through the vagina. Her history includes a prior proctocolectomy and ileal pouch-anal anastomosis for ulcerative colitis. Crohn's disease has been considered. At operation, she undergoes a transperineal mobilization of the pouch with advancement and re-anastomosis.

Description of Procedure (46710)

Under general anesthesia, the distal pouch is mobilized for 6 to 10 cm. If residual anal canal mucosa is present, a completion mucosectomy is performed. An operating anoscope is inserted, and the level of the anastomosis is defined. An epinephrine-containing solution is injected below the level of the previous anastomosis. Cautery is used to circumferentially dissect the pouch immediately proximal to the dentate line. This is deepened to the internal sphincter that is defined and protected with great care. Hemostasis is meticulous with cautery. Dissection proceeds proximally. The previous anastomosis is reached and dissection continues past this point, generally for a distance of 6 to 10 cm until the pouch has been circumferentially mobilized. For cases with a pouch-vaginal or anastomosis-vaginal fistula, this dissection has divided the fistula tract. Attention is turned to the vaginal or perineal end of the tract, which is excised and debrided, before being closed with one or more layers of meticulously placed absorbable sutures. The distal end of the mobilized pouch is trimmed, excising the anal transitional zone or fistula site. Great attention is made to avoid making the pouch too short or rendering it ischemic. The new distal margin of the pouch is sutured circumferentially to the dentate line as a new hand-sewn ileo-anal anastomosis. Hemostasis is assessed for, and obtained, at each stage of the procedure.

Clinical Example (46712)

A 35-year-old woman presents with passage of stool through the vagina. Her history includes a prior proctocolectomy and ileal pouch-anal anastomosis for ulcerative colitis. Crohn's disease has been considered. At operation, she undergoes a transperineal and transabdominal mobilization of the pouch with advancement and re-anastomosis.

Description of Procedure (46712)

The patient is placed under general anesthesia in the perineolithotomy position. The abdomen is opened through a lower midline incision and dissection is performed to mobilize the pelvic reservoir from the sacrum, the lateral pelvic walls, and then from the vagina. Complete mobilization of the pelvic pouch is performed to the level of the anastomosis. After this is completed, attention is turned to the perineal area. An epinephrine-containing solution is injected below the level of the previous anastomosis. Cautery is used to circumferentially dissect the pouch immediately proximal to the dentate line. This is deepened to the internal sphincter that is defined and protected with great care. Hemostasis is meticulous with cautery. Dissection proceeds proximally. This is carried up to the level of the abdominal dissection. This divides any fistula tracts. The old pouch is brought into the abdomen and assessed for viability. If the old pouch is viable, it is returned to the pelvis, ensuring it is not under too much tension, and sewn to the anal canal. If the old pouch was not salvaged, a new neo-pelvic reservoir is constructed and sewn to the anal canal. When this is completed, attention is returned to the abdominal incision and a temporary loop ileostomy is created. All wounds are closed as appropriate.

Abdomen, Peritoneum, and Omentum

EXCISION, DESTRUCTION

49200 Excision or destruction, open, intra-abdominal or retroperitoneal tumors or cysts or endometriomas;

49201 extensive

►(For open cryoablation of renal tumor, use 50250)◄

►(For percutaneous cryotherapy ablation of renal tumors, use Category III code 0135T)◄

Rationale

In tandem with the addition of codes to report performance of open and percutaneous renal tumor cryoablation of tumors, cross-references have been added following 49200-49201 to direct the user to codes 50250 and 0135T.

Urinary System

Kidney

EXCISION

50240 Nephrectomy, partial

(For laparoscopic partial nephrectomy, use 50543)

●50250 Ablation, open, one or more renal mass lesion(s), cryosurgical, including intraoperative ultrasound, if performed

►(For laparoscopic ablation of renal mass lesions, use 50542)◄

►(For percutaneous cryotherapy ablation of renal tumors, use 0135T)◄

Rationale

Code 50250 was added to describe open cryosurgical ablation of renal mass lesions. As indicated in the descriptor of code 50250, intraoperative ultrasound is considered to be an inherent component of the procedure and should not be reported separately.

A cross-reference was added after code 50250 to reference the laparoscopic procedure code 50542.

Open cryoablation of renal tumor(s) is an extension of this technology to treat renal cancers in a select group of patients that include those who have tumors 4 cm or smaller in size and may be poor surgical candidates; refuse a radical or a partial nephrectomy; or have multiple comorbid illnesses, a solitary kidney, or renal insufficiency, or for those patients for whom renal preservation is required. Open cryoablation is a viable treatment option that results in decreased morbidity and rapid recovery for renal cell carcinoma patients.

Existing codes describe laparoscopic surgical ablation of renal mass lesions (50542) and open cryoablation of liver tumor(s) (47381).

Clinical Example (50250)

A 59-year-old female with intermittent nausea and vomiting undergoes an abdominal computed tomography that reveals an incidental 2.5-cm solid mass of the anterior midpole of the right kidney. The patient has chronic renal failure with a baseline creatinine of 3.2. The patient is referred to a urologist and focal cryoablation of the mass is decided upon in order to preserve renal function. Since the patient has undergone multiple prior abdominal procedures, an open approach is selected. The patient receives usual follow-up care in the hospital and office during the 90-day global period.

Description of Procedure (50250)

A 16 F Foley catheter is placed in the bladder and the patient is placed in the flank position. A flank incision is made, the 11th or 12th rib is resected, and the mass is exposed. The kidney is mobilized, the ureter is identified, and fatty tissue is dissected from the kidney. A cryosurgical probe is inserted into the mass. Ultrasound may be used to monitor the freeze depth. A second freeze is performed. Meticulous hemostasis is carried out and drains are placed. The incision is closed in layers.

INTRODUCTION

▶*Renal Pelvis Catheter Procedures*◀

▶Internally Dwelling◀

⊙●**50382** Removal (via snare/capture) and replacement of internally dwelling ureteral stent via percutaneous approach, including radiological supervision and interpretation

▶(For bilateral procedure, use modifier 50)◀

⊙●**50384** Removal (via snare/capture) of internally dwelling ureteral stent via percutaneous approach, including radiological supervision and interpretation

▶(For bilateral procedure, use modifier 50)◀

▶(Do not report 50382, 50384 in conjunction with 50395)◀

▶Externally Accessible◀

⊙●**50387** Removal and replacement of externally accessible transnephric ureteral stent (eg, external/internal stent) requiring fluoroscopic guidance, including radiological supervision and interpretation

▶(For bilateral procedure, use modifier 50)◀

►(For removal and replacement of externally accessible ureteral stent via ureterostomy or ilieal conduit, use 50688)◄

►(For removal without replacement of an externally accessible ureteral stent not requiring fluoroscopic guidance, see **Evaluation and Management** services codes)◄

●**50389** Removal of nephrostomy tube, requiring fluoroscopic guidance (eg, with concurrent indwelling ureteral stent)

►(Removal of nephrostomy tube not requiring fluoroscopic guidance is considered inherent to E/M services. Report the appropriate level of E/M service provided)◄

Rationale

Four codes, two subsections, and related cross-references have been established to report removal of ureteral stents. These codes are differentiated by approach (percutaneous and transurethral) and type (internally dwelling and externally dwelling). The code families are further differentiated by reporting removal or removal-replacement. These procedures are commonly performed for the treatment of ureteral strictures and obstructions. Ureteral stents are thin catheters threaded into the ureter for diversion of the urine either internally into the bladder or externally into a collection system. These stents must be monitored while in place and removed when no longer needed; they are required to be periodically changed, especially when they are chronically indwelling.

Prior to the addition of these codes, reporting ureteral stent exchange was possible only with the existing endoscopic approach codes. As 50382, 50384, and 50387 are unilateral procedures, instructional cross-references have been added following these codes to instruct the use of modifier 50 for bilateral procedures.

Code 50382 is intended to report a percutaneous approach for the removal and replacement of an internally dwelling ureteral stent. This capture approach uses a thread-like element at the end that forms a loop and is used to snare and extract the stent from the bladder. Code 50384 is reported for only removal of ureteral stent via percutaneous approach. Code 50387 is reported for removal and replacement of an externally accessible ureteral stent via the transnephric approach. Code 50389 is reported for those instances in which a ureteral stent has been placed with the loops in the renal pelvis and urinary bladder. Following clearance of blood after the stent placement, the nephrostomy catheter removal is performed under fluoroscopic guidance. In the Externally Accessible Stent subsection, exclusionary cross-references following 50387 and 50389 indicate that stent removals that do not require fluoroscopic guidance are considered to be inherent in the Evaluation and Management procedures. A cross-reference following 50387 directs the user to 50688 to differentiate the transnephric removal of the ureteral stent reported with 50387 from ureterostomy or ilieal conduit approaches for ureteral stent exchange.

Clinical Example (50382)

An 80-year-old with a chronic indwelling double-J ureteral stent placed for ureteral obstruction is seen after a failed attempt to exchange the stent was made via cystoscopy. The stent was inadvertently fractured, with the distal end removed at cystoscopy, and is now inaccessible from a urethral approach. It is, therefore, elected to retrieve and exchange the stent percutaneously from a transnephric approach.

Description of Procedure (50382)

The physician orders medication for conscious sedation. A small skin incision is made after infiltration of the skin and subcutaneous tissues with 1% lidocaine of the selected entry site. A needle is introduced into the appropriate renal calyx with the help of imaging guidance to ensure appropriate needle positioning. The physician injects contrast once the needle is in place, and fluoroscopy is used to confirm position and to identify relevant anatomy. A guidewire is introduced into the renal pelvis, the needle is removed, and the tract is serially dilated to the appropriate diameter. A guidewire is introduced into the renal pelvis again, this time followed by a sheath placement over the wire into the renal pelvis. A safety guidewire is introduced into the bladder, traversing the ureter under fluoroscopic imaging guidance with periodic contrast injection. Under fluoroscopic guidance, a snare device is negotiated into the renal pelvis through the sheath and used to grasp the proximal end of the indwelling stent, and the stent is partially pulled out through the sheath. Once the proximal end of the indwelling stent has been externalized, it is cannulated with a guidewire, which is maneuvered past the side holes into the ureter. The old ureteral stent is removed completely over the guidewire, leaving the guidewire in place in the bladder. The physician confirms the length of the replacement stent. The replacement stent is advanced over the wire until the distal loop is in the bladder. (If balloon dilation of the ureter is necessary for stent passage, this is separately reportable.) The distal loop is deployed. Once the stent position is confirmed to be satisfactory, the wire is withdrawn, allowing the proximal loop to reform in the renal pelvis. The guide, sheath, and safety wire are removed. Images are obtained documenting the final stent position.

Clinical Example (50384)

A 75-year-old male with chronic ureteral obstruction has been maintained for 2 years with a chronic indwelling ureteral stent. However, the patient now has end-stage renal disease and no urine output, and it is elected to remove the ureteral stent. An attempt to remove the stent cystoscopically has failed, with removal of the distal portion of the catheter but retention of the proximal and ureteral portions after the stent was inadvertently fractured. The patient is referred, therefore, for percutaneous removal of the indwelling stent.

Description of Procedure (50384)

The physician orders medication for conscious sedation. A small skin incision is made after infiltration of the skin and subcutaneous tissues with 1% lidocaine of the selected entry site. The physician introduces a needle into the appropriate renal calyx, using imaging guidance to ensure appropriate needle positioning. He or she injects contrast once the needle is in place, and fluoroscopy is used to confirm the position and to identify relevant anatomy. A guidewire is introduced into the renal pelvis, the needle is removed, and the tract is serially dilated to the appropriate diameter. A guidewire is introduced into the renal pelvis again, this time followed by a sheath placement over the wire into the renal pelvis. A safety guidewire is introduced into the bladder, traversing the ureter under fluoroscopic imaging guidance with periodic contrast injection. Next, under fluoroscopic guidance, a snare device is negotiated into the renal pelvis through the sheath and used to grasp the proximal end of the indwelling stent, and the stent is pulled out through the sheath, maintaining wire position in the bladder. Once the proximal end of the indwelling stent has been externalized, it is cannulated with a guidewire, which is then maneuvered past the side holes into the ureter. The old ureteral stent is removed completely over the guidewire. The guidewire(s) and sheath are removed. A sterile dressing is applied.

Clinical Example (50387)

A 64-year-old male with a current right transnephric single-piece internal/external (tube hub accessible at the patient's flank) capped ureteral stent presents for routine fluoroscopically guided catheter exchange.

Description of Procedure (50387)

The physician infiltrates the skin and subcutaneous tissues with 1% lidocaine at the catheter entry site. Contrast may be injected into the catheter to assess anatomy and to help with subsequent positioning of both pigtails of the new stent. The suture fixing the proximal pigtail in position is cut, and a selective guidewire is introduced through the hub of the stent and advanced through the stent into the bladder. Fluoroscopy is used to help maneuver the wire through the catheter lumen; the guidewire often is difficult to position due to multiple side holes in the catheter. Once the guidewire has exited the distal end hole of the stent, the indwelling catheter is removed over the guidewire and discarded. A new nephroureteral stent is advanced over the wire with diameter and length chosen to fit the patient's anatomy. Once in the bladder, the guidewire is partially removed to allow formation of the distal loop within the bladder. Fluoroscopic assessment of the proximal portion of the catheter is done to be certain that the proximal pigtail will reform within the renal pelvis. Once the catheter is appropriately positioned, the guidewire is removed, and the suture is pulled to cinch the proximal pigtail in position. Minor adjustments to the catheter position are performed to decrease patient discomfort from the catheter tip poking into the wall of the bladder or renal collecting system. Contrast may be injected to ensure appropriate positioning and functioning of the new catheter. Once final adjustments are made, the catheter site is dressed appropriately. It may be sutured to the skin. The catheter may be capped to internal drainage or a drainage bag may be attached for partial external drainage. An image is obtained documenting final catheter position for the patient record.

Clinical Example (50389)

A 62-year-old male with bladder carcinoma had a left internal ureteral stent placed 5 days earlier via transnephric approach. A nephrostomy catheter had been left in place due to moderate bleeding at the time of the stent placement. He now presents for removal of the nephrostomy catheter under fluoroscopic guidance to avoid displacing the previously placed ureteral stent.

Description of Procedure (50389)

Contrast is injected through the indwelling nephrostomy catheter, confirming that the ureteral stent is in place and functioning. A note is made that no large thrombus is present in the collecting system. The skin site is anesthetized with local anesthetic. The suture fixing the nephrostomy pigtail in position is released, and a wire is carefully introduced through the indwelling nephrostomy catheter into the collecting system. This maneuver is watched fluoroscopically to be certain that the nephrostomy catheter pigtail and/or retention suture do not hook the proximal pigtail of the double-J stent. Adjustments are made with fluoroscopic guidance to ensure that the ureteral stent is not dislodged as the nephrostomy catheter is pulled out over the wire. Once the nephrostomy catheter is out, a permanent image of the final ureteral stent position is made for the patient's record. A thick sterile dressing is applied to the flank site.

LAPAROSCOPY

Surgical laparoscopy always includes diagnostic laparoscopy. . . .

50541 Laparoscopy, surgical; ablation of renal cysts

50542 ablation of renal mass lesion(s)

(For open procedure, see 50220-50240)

►(For open cryosurgical ablation, use 50250)◄

►(For percutaneous cryotherapy ablation of renal tumors, use 0135T)◄

Rationale

In tandem with the addition of codes to report performance of open and percutaneous renal tumor cryoablation of tumors, cross-references have been added following 50542 to direct the user to codes 50250 and 0135T.

OTHER PROCEDURES

50590 Lithotripsy, extracorporeal shock wave

⊙●**50592** Ablation, one or more renal tumor(s), percutaneous, unilateral, radiofrequency

►(50592 is a unilateral procedure. For bilateral procedure, report 50592 with modifier 50)◄

►(For imaging guidance and monitoring, see 76362, 76394, 76940)◄

►(For percutaneous cryotherapy ablation of renal tumors, use 0135T)◄

►(For imaging guidance and monitoring, see 76362, 76394, 76940)◄

Rationale

Code 50592 was established to report percutaneous radiofrequency ablation of renal tumors, with the addition of cross-references to indicate the unilateral nature of the procedure. This code differs by approach from the existing CPT codes that report radiofrequency ablation (RFA) of renal tumors from a laparoscopic (50542) or open (49200-49201) approach. This procedure is frequently performed for the treatment of renal masses as a palliative therapy for inoperative stage IV renal cell carcinoma. Inclusion of the moderate sedation bull's-eye indicator with this code denotes that moderate sedation is inherent and not separately reported.

As this procedure is considered to be unilateral, a cross-reference has been added to instruct bilateral reporting for this procedure.

Clinical Example (50592)

A 76-year-old man with poor cardiac function and history of previous open-heart surgery has a 3.0-cm enhancing solid renal mass that was incidentally found as a result of a computed tomography scan performed due to the patient's complaint of abdominal pain. The patient's comorbidities rule out open total or partial nephrectomy as too risky. The patient is referred for percutaneous renal tumor ablation.

Description of Procedure (50592)

The physician supervises the start of an IV and the administration of 0.625 mg intravenous droperidol. He or she oversees equipping of the room, positioning of the patient, and dispersing of electrodes (ground pads) and skin temperature sensors. The physician obtains and interprets the initial localization image (included in 76362, 76394, or 76940, separately reportable) for selection of the site for initial electrode placement. The physician supervises as the nurse administers a dose (or doses) of IV conscious sedation, which typically is 50 µgs fentanyl and 1 mg midazolam. A small incision is made to facilitate radio frequency (RF) needle electrode placement. A 17-gauge, internally cooled radiofrequency needle electrode is introduced into the center of the lesion under imaging guidance (imaging included in 76362, 76394, or 76940) to avoid organs and major blood vessels. Needle tip location is confirmed using the imaging guidance (imaging included in 76362, 76394, or 76940). The physician applies RF power as many times as needed until satisfactory core heating is achieved. Intratumoral temperature is monitored before and after each treatment (based on the type of radio frequency ablation device used) to confirm the completion of the treatment. The physician repeats the process for overlapping ablations as needed to ensure complete tumor necrosis and satisfactory margins. The RF electrode is withdrawn after satisfactory necrosis, and the physician cauterizes to achieve hemostasis along the needle tract. The incision sites are cleaned and sterile adhesive dressings are applied.

Ureter

INTRODUCTION

▲**50688** Change of ureterostomy tube or externally accessible ureteral stent via ileal conduit

(If imaging guidance is performed, use 75984)

Rationale

Consistent with the addition of 50387 to report a transnephric approach removal and replacement of an externally accessible ureteral stent, 50688 was revised to clarify the intent of this code for ureteral tube change via ileal conduit.

Bladder

LAPAROSCOPY

Surgical laparoscopy always includes diagnostic laparoscopy. . . .

51990 Laparoscopy, surgical; urethral suspension for stress incontinence

51992 sling operation for stress incontinence (eg, fascia or synthetic)

(For open sling operation for stress incontinence, use 57288)

(For reversal or removal of sling operation for stress incontinence, use 57287)

●**51999** Unlisted laparoscopy procedure, bladder

Rationale

For consistency purposes throughout the CPT codebook, 51999 was added to describe an unlisted laparoscopic procedure code for the bladder.

VESICAL NECK AND PROSTATE

▲**52647** Laser coagulation of prostate, including control of postoperative bleeding, complete (vasectomy, meatotomy, cystourethroscopy, urethral calibration and/or dilation, and internal urethrotomy are included if performed)

▲**52648** Laser vaporization of prostate, including control of postoperative bleeding, complete (vasectomy, meatotomy, cystourethroscopy, urethral calibration and/or dilation, internal urethrotomy and transurethral resection of prostate are included if performed)

Rationale

Codes 52647 and 52648 have been editorially revised to eliminate the word "contact" from the code's nomenclature and to reflect current clinical practice.

When first introduced 10 years ago, there were two approaches to the treatment of benign prostatic hyperplasia (BPH) with lasers. The first laser treatment option involves placing laser fibers close to, but not in direct contact with, prostatic tissue thereby coagulating underlying tissue. The second laser treatment option involves placing the laser fiber in direct contact with prostatic tissue thereby transmitting high energy to the tissue and vaporizing the tissue. The former technique created coagulation necrosis while the latter caused immediate cavitation.

Over the past 10 years, there have been advances in laser fiber technology and laser techniques. Diffuser tip laser technology allows urologists to insert the fiber directly into the gland and coagulate large volumes of tissue, while the newest high-energy fibers permit vaporization and cavitation without direct tissue contact. Because the important issue in clinical outcomes is whether prostate tissue was coagulated or vaporized, not which fiber was selected to accomplish the operative endpoint, codes 52647 and 52648 nomenclature have been updated to reflect these important advances in technology.

Clinical Example (52647)

A 70-year-old male has severe, obstructive symptoms secondary to BPH.

Description of Procedure (52647)

During cystoscopic examination under anesthesia, a 25-gram obstructive prostate is noted. A right-angle laser fiber is passed into the prostatic fossa through a continuous-flow resectoscope and laser energy is delivered for 90 seconds to each of four quadrants and to the median lobe. The procedure is approximately 30 minutes in duration. A suprapubic tube may be inserted prior to the procedure or a Foley catheter inserted following the procedure. The procedure is performed on an ambulatory basis or for a 1-day stay. The patient returns to the office on the fifth postoperative day and the Foley catheter is removed or the patient is instructed to turn the valve on the suprapubic tube to initiate a voiding trail. He may be placed on an intermittent catheter until successful voiding begins, a process that may take up to 2 weeks. Though not common for all, some patients may also require placement of a suprapubic tube.

Clinical Example (52648)

A 75-year-old male has severe, obstructive symptoms secondary to BPH.

Description of Procedure (52648)

During cystoscopic examination under anesthesia, a 65-gram obstructive prostate is noted. A right-angle laser fiber is passed into the prostate fossa through a continuous-flow resectoscope with the delivery of laser energy for 45 seconds at a time. Prostate tissue is vaporized at 20 different points within the prostatic fossa, ultimately creating a resected cavity similar to a transurethral resection of the prostate. After completion of the laser procedure, a resectoscope sheath may be inserted transurethrally to resect debris and remaining prostate tissue. The procedure is approximately an hour in duration. A catheter is placed and the patient is discharged on the second postoperative day. He returns to the office on the fifth postoperative day and his catheter is removed with a voiding trail. Though not common for all, some patients may also require placement of a suprapubic tube.

Male Genital System

Prostate

INCISION

55700 Biopsy, prostate; needle or punch, single or multiple, any approach

►(For prostate needle biopsy saturation sampling for prostate mapping, use Category III code 0137T)◄

(If imaging guidance is performed, use 76942)

Rationale

In tandem with the establishment of code 0137T, a cross-reference has been added to 55700 to direct the user to report 0137T for needle biopsy saturation sampling for prostate mapping.

Female Genital System

Vagina

REPAIR

57291 Construction of artificial vagina; without graft

57292 with graft

●**57295** Revision (including removal) of prosthetic vaginal graft, vaginal approach

Rationale

A code has been added to the Female Genital System/Vagina/Repair section, to report the revision or removal of a prosthetic graft using a vaginal approach. Revision of a vaginal graft is performed when a complication, such as an infection, occurs and the graft material needs to be dealt with surgically. Removal of a graft is included in this code, and, therefore, not separately reported.

Clinical Example (57295)

A 65-year-old Gravida 4 Para 4 female patient complains of vaginal discharge, discomfort, and painful intercourse. She underwent abdominal sacral colpopexy using mesh about 1 year ago, which was uncomplicated. Her past medical history is negative. Her pertinent physical examination reveals mesh eroding through the apex of the vagina. Vaginal apical support is adequate. The surgeon decides that excision is necessary and performs this via the vaginal route.

Description of Procedure (57295)

Access to the vaginal apex is achieved using deep vaginal retractors. Dissection around the eroding mesh is performed sharply. Care is taken not to disect too deeply to avoid entering the bladder or rectum. The vaginal epithelium is dissected sharply around the eroding mesh, creating a plane between the vaginal epithelium and the endopelvic fascia. This dissection is taken circumferentially about 2 cm. The eroding mesh is grasped placing tension outward. All of the eroding material is excised sharply, being careful to avoid the rectum, bladder, and small bowel. Once the excision is complete, the remaining edges of the endopelvic fascia are re-approximated with delayed absorbable sutures and the vaginal epithelium is also closed in layers. Irrigation is carried out and a urinary catheter and vaginal packing is placed to complete the procedure.

ENDOSCOPY

57420 Colposcopy of the entire vagina, with cervix if present;

▲57421 with biopsy(s) of vagina/cervix

(For colposcopic visualization of cervix and adjacent upper vagina, use 57452)

(When reporting colposcopies of multiple sites, use modifier 51 as appropriate. For colposcopic examinations/procedures involving the vulva, see 56820, 56821; cervix, see 57452-57461)

▶(For endometrial sampling (biopsy) performed in conjunction with colposcopy, use 58110)◀

(57450, 57451 have been deleted)

Rationale

In tandem with the establishment of 58110 to report endometrial sampling performed in conjunction with colposcopy, 57421 has been editorially revised to clarify that endometrial biopsies are not included in this code.

A cross-reference following 57421 has been added to direct users to the new code.

Clinical Example (57421)

A 42-year-old female has a Pap smear showing a high-grade squamous intraepithelial lesion. Three years ago, she had a radical hysterectomy for stage IB squamous cell carcinoma of the cervix. Acetic acid is applied to the vagina. Colposcopic examination of the entire vagina is performed. An area of aceto white changes is identified. The area is infiltrated with 1% lidocaine and a biopsy is obtained under colposcopic guidance. Hemostasis is obtained with silver nitrate or monsol solution.

Description of Procedure (57421)

Acetic acid is applied to the entire vagina. After adequate time for acetic acid effect, surfaces of the vagina are evaluated with the colposcope at several magnifications. Colposcopic evaluation reveals a suspicious lesion at the vaginal cuff and a second area in the mid-vagina. Both areas are injected with local anesthetic, biopsies are taken, and bleeding is controlled with Monsel's solution or silver nitrate.

Cervix Uteri

(For cervicography, see Category III code 0003T)

ENDOSCOPY

(For colposcopic examinations/procedures involving the vulva, see 56820, 56821; vagina, see 57420, 57421)

57452 Colposcopy of the cervix including upper/adjacent vagina;

57461 with loop electrode conization of the cervix

(Do not report 57456 in addition to 57461)

►(For endometrial sampling (biopsy) performed in conjunction with colposcopy, use 58110)◄

Corpus Uteri

EXCISION

58100 Endometrial sampling (biopsy) with or without endocervical sampling (biopsy), without cervical dilation, any method (separate procedure)

(For endocervical curettage only, use 57505)

►(For endometrial sampling (biopsy) performed in conjunction with colposcopy (57420, 57421, 57452-57461), use 58110)◄

Rationale

In tandem with the establishment of 58110 to report endometrial sampling performed in conjunction with colposcopy, an instructional note has been added following code 58100 instructing users to report 58110 in conjunction with 57420, 57421, 57452, 57454, 57455, 57456, 57460, and 57461 for endometrial sampling performed in conjunction with colposcopy.

✚●58110 Endometrial sampling (biopsy) performed in conjunction with colposcopy (List separately in addition to code for primary procedure)

►(Use 58110 in conjunction with 57420, 57421, 57452-57461)◄

Rationale

Add-on code 58110 was established to report endometrial sampling performed in conjunction with colposcopy. An instructional note has been added following 58110 to instruct users to report 58110 in conjunction with 57420, 57421, 57452, 57454, 57455, 57456, 57460, and 57461 for endometrial sampling performed in conjunction with colposcopy.

Clinical Example (58110)

A 48-year-old female presents for evaluation of an abnormal cervical cytology result that shows "atypical glandular cells." An interval history and physical

⊘=Modifier 51 Exempt ⊙=Conscious Sedation ✚=Add-on Code ⊬=FDA approval pending examination, including a pelvic exam, is performed. Colposcopy of the cervix is performed, and the exocervix appears normal. In order to evaluate the patient for a lesion in either the endocervix or endometrium, both an endocervical curettage and an endometrial biopsy are performed to determine the source of the atypical glandular cells in the lower genital tract.

Note: Survey results for 58100 were used to develop this recommendation.

Description of Procedure (58110)
Since the speculum has already been properly positioned, the physician work for this add-on begins by prepping the cervix with an antiseptic solution. The anterior lip of the cervix is grasped with a tenaculum and the uterus is sounded with a uterine sound to gauge the depth of the endometrial cavity. The endometrial curette is passed through the cervix to the fundus of the uterus. The endometrial biopsy is performed in four quadrants by applying suction with a syringe attached to the hollow curette. Three passes with the suction curette are typically performed. The curette is withdrawn and the tissue is placed in formalin. The tenaculum is removed. Pressure is applied to the cervix to control any postoperative bleeding. The speculum is removed and the patient is taken down from the lithotomy position.

Nervous System

Skull, Meninges, and Brain

ENDOVASCULAR THERAPY

61624 Transcatheter permanent occlusion or embolization (eg, for tumor destruction, to achieve hemostasis, to occlude a vascular malformation), percutaneous, any method; central nervous system (intracranial, spinal cord)

(See also 37204)

(For radiological supervision and interpretation, use 75894)

61626 non-central nervous system, head or neck (extracranial, brachiocephalic branch)

(See also 37204)

(For radiological supervision and interpretation, use 75894)

●61630 Balloon angioplasty, intracranial (eg, atherosclerotic stenosis), percutaneous

●61635 Transcatheter placement of intravascular stent(s), intracranial (eg, atherosclerotic stenosis), including balloon angioplasty, if performed

►(61630 and 61635 include all selective vascular catheterization of the target vascular family, all diagnostic imaging for arteriography of the target vascular family, and all related radiological supervision and interpretation. When diagnostic arteriogram (including imaging and selective catheterization) confirms the need for angioplasty or stent placement, 61630 and 61635 are inclusive of these services. If angioplasty or stenting are not indicated, then the appropriate codes for selective catheterization and imaging should be reported in lieu of 61630 and 61635)◀

●61640 Balloon dilatation of intracranial vasospasm, percutaneous; initial vessel

+●61641 each additional vessel in same vascular family (List separately in addition to code for primary procedure)

+●61642 each additional vessel in different vascular family (List separately in addition to code for primary procedure)

▶(Use 61641 and 61642 in conjunction with 61640)◀

▶(61640, 61641, 61642 include all selective vascular catheterization of the target vessel, contrast injection(s), vessel measurement, roadmapping, postdilatation angiography, and fluoroscopic guidance for the balloon dilatation)◀

Rationale

Five codes and related cross-references were established to report intracranial angioplasty, stent placement, and balloon dilatation for initial and additional vessels. Intracranial angioplasty and stenting are intended to treat impaired cerebral circulation due to arterial narrowing that may result in symptoms of ischemia, such as repeated transient neurological deficits, ischemic attacks, cerebral infarction, or death. These codes are separated into two families differentiated by balloon angioplasty and stenting for the treatment of intracranial atherosclerotic stenosis and balloon dilatation for the treatment of vasospasm.

Code 61630 is reported for intracranial percutaneous endovascular balloon angioplasty. Code 61635 is reported for intracranial percutaneous endovascular stent placement. As indicated in the cross-reference guideline following these codes, all selective vascular catheterization and diagnostic imaging for arteriography of the target vascular family and all related radiological supervision and interpretation are included in 61630 and 61635 and are not separately reported. Codes 61630 and 61635 also include the confirmation of the need for angioplasty or stent placement via diagnostic arteriogram (including imaging and selective catheterization). The instructional cross-reference also indicates that these codes are not appropriately reported when angioplasty or stenting are not performed, instructing the user to report the appropriate codes for selective catheterization and imaging. Unless performed in separate vessels, codes 61630 and 61635 would not be reported together because 61630 is a component procedure of 61635.

Codes 61640-61642 are reported for intracranial endovascular balloon dilatation for the treatment of the smooth muscle lining of the intracranial vessel. This is most frequently necessary following subarachnoid hemorrhage, in which changes in the intima lining are detected, ultimately resulting in luminal narrowing and rigidity of the vessel wall. This code family is differentiated by the dilatation of the initial vessel (61640); and two add-on codes for dilatation of each additional vessel in the same vascular family (61641); and each additional vessel in a different vascular family from the initial dilatation (61642). The cross-reference following 61642 instructs that 61641 and 61642 are reported with 61640. As instructed in the cross-reference guideline following 61642, all selective vascular catheterization of the target vessel, contrast injections, vessel measurement, roadmapping, post-dilatation angiography, and fluoroscopic guidance for the balloon dilatation are included in codes 61640, 61641, and 61642 and would not be separately reported.

Clinical Example (61630)

A 66-year-old male presents with a history of left hemisphere transient ischemic attacks that persist on medical therapy. A carotid duplex exam demonstrated no significant stenosis of the left carotid bifurcation. Magnetic resonance angiography of the head is suspicious for significant stenosis of the M1 segment of the left middle cerebral artery. The patient is referred for possible intracranial angioplasty.

Note: The proposed new code includes all selective vascular catheterization of the target vascular family, all diagnostic imaging for arteriography of the target vascular family, and all related radiological supervision and interpretation. Additionally, when the diagnostic arteriogram (including imaging and selective catheterization) confirms the need for angioplasty or stent placement, 61630 is inclusive of these services. If angioplasty or stenting are not indicated, then the appropriate codes for selective catheterization and imaging should be reported in lieu of code 61635.

Description of Procedure (61630)

The common femoral artery is accessed and a sheath is placed under sterile conditions. A bolus dose of intravenous heparin is administered. The activated coagulation time (ACT) is checked. Additional heparin is given as necessary throughout the procedure, and the ACTs are monitored at appropriate intervals. Pressurized, continuous heparin-saline flush systems are prepared. Meticulous examination of these systems is performed by the physician to exclude the possibility of residual air bubbles. The left common carotid artery is selectively catheterized with a 5 Fr catheter. Biplane anteroposterior (AP) and lateral angiograms of the cervical common carotid artery are obtained. If necessary, oblique views are obtained to profile the carotid bifurcation. Biplane AP and lateral (and possibly oblique) angiograms of the intracranial vessels are also obtained to determine that no interval change has occurred since the original diagnostic angiogram. The catheter is advanced into the external carotid artery over a steerable guidewire. Utilizing an exchange wire placed into the external carotid artery, a neuroguide catheter is placed into the common carotid artery.

A common carotid artery angiogram is obtained to confirm the appropriate positioning of the guide catheter below the carotid bifurcation and to exclude the possibility of arterial spasm, dissection, or thromboembolus during the guide catheter placement. The guide catheter is advanced into the internal carotid artery over a steerable guidewire. A cervical internal carotid artery angiogram is obtained to confirm the appropriate positioning of the guide catheter and to exclude the possibility of arterial spasm, dissection, or thromboembolus. The guide catheter is placed on a continuous heparin flush using a flow control Y-connector. Biplane AP, lateral, and oblique angiograms of the cerebral vessels are obtained.

High-magnification biplane angiograms are obtained, centered upon the arterial stenosis. The target lesion must be carefully reassessed for subtle changes that indicate the development of subacute intraluminal thrombus, which is a contraindication to the performance of an angioplasty. Precise, quantitative measurements of the stenotic artery are obtained to determine the proper diameter and length of the angioplasty balloon to be used. External reference markers may be placed on the skin in order to calculate the precise dimensions. The physician prepares the appropriate size angioplasty balloon. Meticulous preparation is done by the physician to eliminate the air within the balloon. A steerable micro-guidewire and a low-profile microcatheter are advanced through the guide catheter into the intracranial arteries using an angiographic roadmap. The micro-guidewire and microcatheter are advanced gently across the arterial stenosis. The guidewire is removed and replaced with an exchange length wire, leaving the wire tip beyond the stenotic area. The physician removes the microcatheter. The micro-angioplasty balloon is advanced over the exchange wire and across the stenosis. Slowly the balloon is inflated to dilate the lesion under fluoroscopic control while monitoring the balloon pressure. The physician deflates the balloon and withdraws it into the internal carotid artery, leaving the guidewire across the stenosis. Post-angioplasty angiograms are obtained by injecting contrast through the guide catheter to confirm satisfactory dilation of vessel lumen and antegrade filling of distal blood vessels. Fifteen minutes pass before the angiogram is repeated so as to exclude the possibility of hyperacute thrombotic occlusion or rebound stenosois. If evidence of rebound stenosis arises, the balloon is placed again to re-dilate the lesion or exchanged for a larger angioplasty balloon, if needed. Again, the physician waits 15 minutes and repeats the angiogram to exclude the possibility of hyperacute thrombotic occlusion or rebound stenosois. After a 15-minute period of observation with no further evidence of restenosis or acute arterial occlusion, the balloon and wire are removed and final angiograms are obtained of the regional circulation to check for possible embolic complications. The physician removes the guide catheter. All fluoroscopy, contrast injection, angiography, and image interpretation associated with the arterial stenosis treated is included in the procedure up to this point

Clinical Example (61635)

A 66-year-old male presents with a history of left hemisphere transient ischemic attacks that persist on medical therapy. A carotid duplex exam demonstrated no significant stenosis of the left carotid bifurcation. Magnetic resonance angiography of the head is suspicious for significant stenosis of the M1 segment of the left middle cerebral artery. The patient is referred for possible intracranial stent.

Note: The proposed new code includes all selective vascular catheterization of the target vascular family, all diagnostic imaging for arteriography of the target vascular family, and all related radiological supervision and interpretation. Additionally, when the diagnostic arteriogram (including imaging and selective catheterization) confirms the need for angioplasty or stent placement, 61635 is inclusive of these services. If angioplasty or stenting are not indicated, then the appropriate codes for selective catheterization and imaging should be reported in lieu of code 61635.

Description of Procedure (61635)

The common femoral artery is accessed and a 5 Fr sheath is placed under sterile conditions. A bolus dose of intravenous heparin is administered. The right common carotid artery is selectively catheterized with a 5 Fr catheter. The physician advances the catheter into the internal carotid artery over a guidewire. Using a neuro exchange wire, a neuroguide catheter is placed into the internal carotid artery. Biplane anteroposterior (AP) and lateral angiograms of the cerebral vessels are obtained. High-magnification biplane angiograms are obtained centered upon the arterial stenosis. Precise, quantitative measurements of the stenotic artery are obtained to determine the proper diameter and length of the angioplasty balloon to be used. External reference markers may be placed on the skin to calculate the precise dimensions. Injection of a contrast in the AP and lateral images and placement of an external marker help to measure the diameter and length of stenotic segment and assess local flow dynamics.

The physician prepares the appropriate size of angioplasty balloon and stent systems. A hydrophilic guidewire and a low profile microcatheter are advanced through the guide catheter using an angiographic roadmap into the stenotic vessel. The microcatheter is passed across the middle cerebral artery stenosis. The physician removes the guidewire and replaces it with an exchange wire, leaving the tip beyond the stenotic area. The micro-angioplasty balloon is advanced over the exchange wire and across the stenosis. Slowly, the physician inflates the balloon to pre-dilate the lesion under fluoroscopic control while monitoring the balloon's pressure. The balloon is deflated and withdrawn into the internal carotid artery, leaving the guidewire across the stenosis. Postangioplasty angiograms are obtained by injecting contrast through the guide catheter to confirm satisfactory pre-dilation of the vessel lumen such that a subsequent passage of the stent will be possible. If pre-dilation appears to be insufficient to allow subsequent stent placement, then the balloon is placed again to re-dilate the region or it is exchanged with a larger angioplasty balloon and the angioplasty is repeated as necessary. The angioplasty balloon is removed, leaving the micro-exchange wire across the lesion.

The physician advances the stent delivery system across the stenosis and deploys the stent. The stent delivery catheter is withdrawn into the internal carotid artery, leaving the micro-guidewire across the stenosis. Post-stent placement angiograms are obtained by injecting contrast through the guide catheter to confirm satisfactory dilation of the vessel lumen and antegrade filling of the distal blood vessels. After a 15-minute wait, the angiogram is repeated to exclude the possibility of hyperacute thrombotic occlusion. The guidewire is removed. Final angiograms of the entire vascular circulation are obtained to check for possible embolic complications. The guide catheter is removed.

Clinical Example (61640)

A 42-year-old female with recent subarachnoid hemorrhage deteriorates clinically. She undergoes complete cerebral angiography (separately reportable even if performed on the same day), which demonstrates significant spasm of the supraclinoid segment of the right internal carotid artery. After receiving the report of this finding, the attending neurosurgeon requests balloon dilatation of the spastic segment.

Note: The proposed new code includes all selective vascular catheterization of the target vessel, contrast injection(s), vessel measurement, roadmapping, postdilatation angiography, and fluoroscopic guidance for balloon dilatation.

Description of Procedure (61640)

The common femoral artery is accessed and a sheath is placed under sterile conditions. A bolus dose of intravenous heparin is administered. The activated coagulation time (ACT) is checked. Additional heparin is given as necessary throughout the procedure, and the ACTs are monitored at appropriate intervals. Pressurized, continuous heparin-saline flush systems are prepared. Meticulous examination of these systems is performed by the physician to exclude the possibility of residual air bubbles. The left common carotid artery is selectively catheterized with a 5 Fr catheter. Biplane anteroposterior (AP) and lateral angiograms of the cervical common carotid artery are obtained. If necessary, oblique views are obtained to profile the carotid bifurcation. Biplane AP and lateral (and possibly oblique) angiograms of the intracranial vessels are also obtained to determine that no interval change has occurred since the original diagnostic angiogram. The catheter is advanced into the external carotid artery over a steerable guidewire. Using an exchange wire placed into the external carotid artery, a neuroguide catheter is placed into the common carotid artery.

A common carotid artery angiogram is obtained to confirm the appropriate positioning of the guide catheter below the carotid bifurcation and to exclude the possibility of arterial spasm, dissection, or thromboembolus during guide catheter placement. The guide catheter is advanced into the internal carotid artery over a steerable guidewire. A cervical internal carotid artery angiogram is obtained to confirm appropriate positioning of the guide catheter and to exclude the possibility of arterial spasm, dissection, or thromboembolus. The guide catheter is placed on a continuous heparin flush using a flow-control Y-connector. Biplane AP, lateral, and oblique angiograms of the cerebral vessels are obtained. High-magnification biplane angiograms are obtained, centered upon the arterial stenosis. The target lesion must be carefully reassessed for subtle changes that indicate the development of subacute intraluminal thrombus, which is a contraindication to performance of angioplasty.

Precise, quantitative measurements of the stenotic artery are obtained to determine the proper diameter and length of the angioplasty balloon to be used. External reference markers may be placed on the skin in order to calculate the precise dimensions. The appropriate size angioplasty balloon is prepared. Meticulous preparation is done by the physician to eliminate the air within the balloon. A steerable micro-guidewire and a low-profile microcatheter are advanced through the guide catheter into the intracranial arteries using an angiographic roadmap. The micro-guidewire and microcatheter are advanced gently across the arterial stenosis. The guidewire is removed and replaced with an exchange length wire, leaving the wire tip beyond the stenotic area. The microcatheter is removed. The micro-angioplasty balloon is advanced over the exchange wire and across the stenosis. Slowly the physician inflates the balloon to dilate the lesion under fluoroscopic control while monitoring the balloon's pressure. The balloon is deflated and withdrawn into the internal carotid artery, leaving the guidewire across the stenosis. Post-angioplasty angiograms are obtained by injecting contrast through the guide catheter to confirm satisfactory dilation of the vessel lumen and antegrade filling of the distal blood vessels. After a 15-minute wait, the physician repeats the angiogram to exclude the possibility of hyperacute thrombotic occlusion or rebound stenosois. If evidence of rebound stenosis arises, the balloon is placed again to re-dilate the lesion or it is exchanged for a larger angioplasty balloon if needed. Again the physician waits 15 minutes and repeats the angiogram to exclude the possibility of hyperacute thrombotic occlusion or rebound stenosois. After a 15-minute period of observation with no further evidence of re-stenosis or acute arterial occlusion, the balloon and wire are removed; final angiograms are obtained of the regional circulation to check for possible embolic complications. The guide catheter is removed. All fluoroscopy, contrast injection, angiography, and image interpretation associated with the arterial stenosis treated is included in the procedure up to this point.

Clinical Example (61641)

A 55-year-old male presents with a recent subarachnoid hemorrhage. Complete cerebral angiography (separately reportable even if performed on the same day) demonstrated significant vasospasm in the supraclinoid left internal carotid artery and the M1 segment of the left middle cerebral artery. After receiving the report of this finding, the attending neurosurgeon requests balloon dilatation of the spastic segments. The internal carotid spasm balloon dilatation is completed (separately reportable) and the M1 segment spasm is now to be balloon dilated.

Note: Code 61641 is considered an add-on procedure code that should be reported in conjunction with 61640. Additionally, the proposed new code includes all selective vascular catheterization of the target vessel, contrast injection(s), vessel measurement, roadmapping, post-dilatation angiography, and fluoroscopic guidance for balloon dilatation.

Description of Procedure (61641)

A second bolus dose of intravenous heparin may be administered. The activated coagulation time (ACT) is checked. Additional heparin is given as necessary throughout the procedure, and the ACTs are monitored at appropriate intervals. Biplane anteroposterior (AP), lateral, and oblique angiograms of the cerebral vessels are obtained. High-magnification biplane angiograms are obtained, centered upon the arterial stenosis. The target lesion must be carefully reassessed for subtle changes that indicate the development of subacute intraluminal thrombus, which is a contraindication to the performance of an angioplasty. Precise, quantitative measurements of the stenotic artery are obtained to determine the proper diameter and length of the angioplasty balloon to be used. External reference markers may be placed on the skin in order to calculate the precise dimensions. The physician prepares the appropriate size angioplasty balloon. Meticulous preparation is done by the physician to eliminate the air within the balloon. A steerable micro-guidewire and a low-profile microcatheter are advanced through the guide catheter into the second target intracranial arterie(s) (additional vessel, same vascular family) using an angiographic roadmap. The micro-guidewire and microcatheter are advanced gently across the arterial stenosis. The physician removes the guidewire and replaces it with an exchange length wire, leaving the wire tip beyond the stenotic area. The microcatheter is removed. The micro-angioplasty balloon is advanced over the exchange wire and across the stenosis. Slowly the physician inflates the balloon to dilate the lesion under fluoroscopic control while monitoring the balloon's pressure. The balloon is deflated and withdrawn into the internal carotid artery, leaving the guidewire across the stenosis.

Post-angioplasty angiograms are obtained by injecting contrast through the guide catheter to confirm satisfactory dilation of the vessel lumen and antegrade filling of the distal blood vessels. After a 15-minute wait, the physician repeats the angiogram to exclude the possibility of hyperacute thrombotic occlusion or rebound stenosois. If evidence of rebound stenosis arises, the balloon is placed again to re-dilate the lesion or it is exchanged for a larger angioplasty balloon if needed. Again 15 minutes is allowed to pass and the angiogram is repeated to exclude the possibility of hyperacute thrombotic occlusion or rebound stenosois. After a 15-minute period of observation with no further evidence of re-stenosis or acute arterial occlusion, the balloon and wire are removed and final angiograms of the regional circulation are obtained to check for possible embolic complications. The guide catheter is removed. All fluoroscopy, contrast injection, angiography, and image interpretation associated with the arterial stenosis treated is included in the procedure up to this point.

Clinical Example (61642)

A 55-year-old male presents with a recent subarachnoid hemorrhage. A complete cerebral angiography (separately reportable even if performed on the same day) demonstrated significant vasospasm in the supraclinoid left internal carotid artery and the M1 segment of the right middle cerebral artery. After receiving the report of this finding, the attending neurosurgeon requests balloon dilatation of the spastic segments. The left internal carotid spasm balloon dilatation is completed (separately reportable) and the right M1 segment spasm is now to be dilated.

Note: Code 61642 is considered an add-on procedure code that should be reported in conjunction with 61640. Additionally, the proposed new code includes all selective vascular catheterization of the target vessel, contrast injection(s), vessel measurement, roadmapping, post-dilatation angiography, and fluoroscopic guidance for balloon dilatation.

Description of Procedure (61642)

A second bolus dose of intravenous heparin may be administered. The activated coagulation time (ACT) is checked. Additional heparin is given as necessary throughout the procedure, and the ACTs are monitored at appropriate intervals. Pressurized, continuous heparin-saline flush systems are prepared. Meticulous examination of these systems is performed by the physician to exclude the possibility of residual air bubbles. The left common carotid artery is selectively catheterized with a 5 Fr catheter. Biplane anteroposterior (AP) and lateral angiograms of the cervical common carotid artery are obtained. If necessary, oblique views are obtained to profile the carotid bifurcation. Biplane AP and lateral (and possibly oblique) angiograms of the intracranial vessels are also obtained to determine that no interval change has occurred since the original diagnostic angiogram. A catheter is advanced into the external carotid artery over a steerable guidewire. Using an exchange wire placed into the external carotid artery, a neuroguide catheter is placed into the common carotid artery.

A common carotid artery angiogram is obtained to confirm appropriate positioning of the guide catheter below the carotid bifurcation and to exclude the possibility of arterial spasm, dissection, or thromboembolus during guide catheter placement. The guide catheter is advanced into the internal carotid artery over a steerable guidewire. A cervical internal carotid artery angiogram is obtained to confirm appropriate positioning of the guide catheter and to exclude the possibility of arterial spasm, dissection, or thromboembolus. The guide catheter is placed on continuous heparin flush using a flow-control Y-connector. Biplane AP, lateral, and oblique angiograms of the cerebral vessels are obtained. High magnification biplane angiograms are obtained, centered upon the arterial stenosis. The target lesion must be carefully reassessed for subtle changes that indicate the development of subacute intraluminal thrombus, which is a contraindication to the performance of an angioplasty.

Precise, quantitative measurements of the stenotic artery are obtained to determine the proper diameter and length of the angioplasty balloon to be used. External reference markers may be placed on the skin in order to calculate the precise dimensions. The physician prepares the appropriate size angioplasty balloon. Meticulous preparation is done by the physician to eliminate the air within the balloon. A steerable micro-guidewire and a low-profile microcatheter are advanced through the guide catheter into the additional vessel (in a vascular family different from the vessel coded in 61640). The micro-guidewire and microcatheter are advanced gently across the arterial stenosis. The physician removes the guidewire and replaces it with an exchange length wire, leaving the wire tip beyond the stenotic area. The microcatheter is removed. The micro-angioplasty balloon is advanced over the exchange wire and across the stenosis. Slowly the physician inflates the balloon to dilate the lesion under fluoroscopic control while monitoring the balloon's pressure. The balloon is deflated and withdrawn into the internal carotid artery, leaving the guidewire across the stenosis. Post-angioplasty angiograms are obtained by injecting contrast through the guide catheter to confirm satisfactory dilation of the vessel lumen and antegrade filling of the distal blood vessels. After a 15-minute wait, the physician repeats the angiogram to exclude the possibility of hyperacute thrombotic occlusion or rebound stenosois. If evidence of rebound stenosis arises, the balloon is placed again to re-dilate the lesion or it is exchanged for a larger angioplasty balloon if needed. Again, 15-minutes is allowed to pass and the angiogram is repeated to exclude the possibility of hyperacute thrombotic occlusion or rebound stenosis. After a 15-minute period of observation with no further evidence of re-stenosis or acute arterial occlusion, the balloon and wire are removed and final angiograms of the regional circulation are obtained to check for possible embolic complications. The guide catheter is removed. All fluoroscopy, contrast injection, angiography, and image interpretation associated with the arterial stenosis treated is included in the procedure up to this point.

Extracranial Nerves, Peripheral Nerves, and Autonomic Nervous System

DESTRUCTION BY NEUROLYTIC AGENT (EG, CHEMICAL, THERMAL, ELECTRICAL OR RADIOFREQUENCY)

(Codes 64600-64681 include the injection of other therapeutic agents (eg, corticosteroids).

Somatic Nerves

64612 Chemodenervation of muscle(s); muscle(s) innervated by facial nerve (eg, for blepharospasm, hemifacial spasm)

▲64613 neck muscle(s) (eg, for spasmodic torticollis, spasmodic dysphonia)

64614 extremity(s) and/or trunk muscle(s) (eg, for dystonia, cerebral palsy, multiple sclerosis)

▶(For chemodenervation guided by needle electromyography or muscle electrical stimulation, see 95873, 95874)◀

(For chemodenervation for strabismus involving the extraocular muscles, use 67345)

▶(For chemodenervation of internal anal sphincter, use 46505)◀

Rationale

Code 64613 was revised in order to avoid limiting the muscle groups that this code describes. As the code descriptor indicates, chemodenervation can be performed on cervical spinal muscles to treat spasmodic torticollis. However, chemodenervation may also be performed to treat spasmodic dysphonia, which affects a different group of muscles in the neck region. The descriptor of code 64613 was revised to specify neck muscle(s) rather than cervical spinal muscle(s).

A parenthetical note has been added as a cross-reference to direct users to the correct code for chemodenervation of the internal anal sphincter, 46505.

Clinical Example (64613)

Physician time is recorded only for practice expense purposes.

Sympathetic Nerves

●64650 Chemodenervation of eccrine glands; both axillae

●64653 other area(s) (eg, scalp, face, neck), per day

▶(Report the specific service in conjunction with code(s) for the specific substance(s) or drug(s) provided)◀

▶(For chemodenervation of extremities (eg, hands or feet), use 64999)◀

64680 Destruction by neurolytic agent, with or without radiologic monitoring; celiac plexus

⊘=Modifier 51 Exempt ⊙=Conscious Sedation ✚=Add-on Code ⁄⁄=FDA approval pending

Rationale

Two codes (64650 and 64653) were added to describe chemodernervation of the eccrine glands and other areas including scalp, face, and neck. Existing chemodenervation codes do not adequately describe structures like eccrine sweat glands, which are innervated by sympathetic nerves. Code 64650 is intended to be reported for chemodenervation of the eccrine glands. Code 64653 is intended to be reported per day for chemodenervation of other areas, including the scalp, face, and neck, regardless of the number of injections provided per session.

An instructional parenthetical note has been added to instruct the user that the specific substance(s) or drug(s) is separately reported. Chemodenervation aids in the treatment of severe focal hyperhidrosis. An additional parenthetical instructs the use of unlisted code 64999.

Clinical Example (64650)

A 26-year-old female patient presents with profuse sweating under the arms since puberty. She reports interference in performing her duties in the workplace, interference with interactions with others in the workplace and elsewhere, and multiple daily changes of clothes. She has not responded to over-the-counter or prescription-strength antiperspirants. A decision was made to perform botulinum toxin injections in both axillae.

Description of Procedure (64650)

The patient is positioned and draped. Prior to administering botulinum toxin type A, the locations of excessive sweating are mapped to maximize treatment effectiveness. The physician paints the prepared axillae areas with an iodine solution and, when dry, dusts the areas with starch powder. Within a 10- to 15-minute period, the presence of sweat will cause the prepped areas to turn a dark purple. The physician outlines the reactive area of excessive sweating with a surgical marking pen and removes the starch-iodine compound. With the surgical marking pen, the physician marks a nonlinear staggered pattern of sites 1.5 cm apart because botulinum toxin type A diffuses under the skin to a diameter of approximately 2 cm and this ensures uninterrupted coverage of the entire treatment area. The physician preps the area with antimicrobial solution.

The physician reconstitutes the vacuum-dried botulinum toxin type A (100 U per vial) with 4 ml sterile saline solution and draws four separate 1-ml syringes. The physician administers a series of 12 to 15 intradermal injections per axilla to distribute 50 U evenly among the injection sites. At a 10° to 30° angle, the physician slowly injects an aliquot of botulinum toxin type A into the dermis to obtain a visible wheal that confirms placement and avoids puncturing the skin at the mapping marks so as not to carry any ink into the skin. Compression is held to facilitate hemostasis. The physician discusses the follow-up assessment. He also addresses pain management, dressings if required, and care of the treated skin area. The physician monitors for pain as well as skin surface reaction throughout the process.

Clinical Example (64653)

A 66-year-old male patient undergoes a surgical excision of a mixed-cell tumor of the left parotid gland. Following surgery, he develops a complication of gustatory hyperhidrosis where he has excessive sweating when he smells or eats certain foods. He is referred for evaluation and treatment of excessive sweating on the left cheek. A decision was made to perform botulinum toxin injections in the affected area.

Description of Procedure (64653)

The patient is positioned and draped. Prior to administering botulinum toxin type A, the locations of excessive sweating are mapped to maximize treatment effectiveness. The physician paints the area(s) with an iodine solution and, when dry, dusts the area(s) with starch powder. Within a 10- to 15-minute period, the presence of sweat will cause the prepped areas to turn a dark purple. The physician outlines the reactive area of excessive sweating with a surgical marking pen, and removes the starch-iodine compound. With the surgical marking pen, the physician marks a nonlinear staggered pattern of sites 1.5 cm apart because botulinum toxin type A diffuses under the skin to a diameter of approximately 2 cm and this ensures uninterrupted coverage of the entire treatment area. The physician preps the area(s) with antimicrobial solution.

The physician reconstitutes the vacuum-dried botulinum toxin type A (100 U per vial) with 4 ml sterile saline solution and draws four separate 1-ml syringes. The physician administers a series of 12 to 15 intradermal injections per area to distribute 50 U evenly among the injection sites. At a 10° to 30° angle, the physician slowly injects an aliquot of botulinum toxin type A into the dermis to obtain a visible wheal that confirms placement and avoids puncturing the skin at mapping marks so as not to carry any ink into the skin. Compression is held to facilitate hemostasis. The physician monitors for pain as well as skin surface reaction throughout the process.

Eye and Ocular Adnexa

Anterior Segment

ANTERIOR SCLERA

Excision

66150 Fistulization of sclera for glaucoma; trephination with iridectomy

66172 trabeculectomy ab externo with scarring from previous ocular surgery or trauma (includes injection of antifibrotic agents)

►(For transciliary body sclera fistulization, use Category III code 0123T)◄

Rationale

In tandem with the establishment of code 0123T to report tranciliary sclera fistulization, a cross-reference has been added following fistulization code 66172 to direct the user to the new code.

⊘=Modifier 51 Exempt ⊙=Conscious Sedation ✚=Add-on Code ⁄⁄=FDA approval pending

Ocular Adnexa

EYELIDS

Repair (Brow Ptosis, Blepharoptosis, Lid Retraction, Ectropion, Entropion)

▲67901 Repair of blepharoptosis; frontalis muscle technique with suture or other material (eg, banked fascia)

▲67902 frontalis muscle technique with autologous fascial sling (includes obtaining fascia)

Rationale

The codes for eyelid surgical repair, 67901 and 67902, have been revised to reflect the current practice of using banked fascial strips that is similar to the work described in 67901 and not 67902, which requires the physician to harvest the fascia with a fascial stripper from the same patient (autologous) who will be receiving this autogenous fascia to repair an eyelid defect (eg, brow ptosis, blepharoptosis).

Description of Procedure (67901)

The correct surgical site is confirmed. A marking pen is used to delineate the planned six incisions in the eyelid and above the brow. Antibiotic ointment and a protective device (eg, protective shell) are placed on the cornea. Lidocaine with epinephrine is infiltrated for hemostasis and for anesthesia. Five minutes are allowed to pass.

A traction suture is placed through the upper eyelid margin and clamped inferiorly. The eyelid incisions are made just above the lash line through skin and orbicularis oculi muscle. The suprabrow incisions are made to the level of periosteum. A superiorly directed pocket is created at each suprabrow incision.

A fascia needle is used to thread the banked fascia between the incisions in the eyelids and brow forming two rectangles with two pieces of fascia. The eyelid incisions are closed with absorbable 7-0 suture. The upper eyelid traction suture is removed. The protective device is removed. Tension on the two fascia ends that finally exit the suprabrow incision is adjusted until optimal eyelid height and contour are obtained. Square knots are tied in the fascia, secured with suture, and buried deep in the suprabrow wounds.

The suprabrow incisions are closed in layers with 7-0 absorbable suture. The eyelid incisions may be closed according to the surgeon's preference. Antibiotic ointment is placed on the wounds and in the conjunctival cul-de-sac. A traction suture is placed in the lower lid margin and taped to the brow with adhesive strips.

Description of Procedure (67902)

The correct surgical site and the site for harvesting the fascia autograft are confirmed. The thigh is positioned. An incision is made in the thigh approximately 2.5 in above the knee joint. The incision is carried through skin and subcutaneous tissue until the fascia lata is identified. Three cuts in the fascia are made to create a U shape. The fascia is separated from the underlying muscle. A ligature is placed on the free end of the fascia. The free end of the fascia is threaded into the fascia stripper. The stripper is directed superiorly beneath the skin for about 20 cm in a line from the head of the fibula to the iliac crest. The fascia is cut superiorly by activating the cutting mechanism of the stripper. The fascia and stripper are removed. The skin wound is closed in layers and the thigh is dressed with a pressure dressing.

The fascia is cleaned of subcutaneous tissue and fat and cut to produce two strips of appropriate size.

A marking pen is used to delineate the planned six incisions in the eyelid and above the brow. Antibiotic ointment and a protective device (eg, protective shell) are placed on the cornea. Lidocaine with epinephrine is infiltrated for hemostasis. Five minutes are allowed to pass. A traction suture is placed through the upper eyelid margin and clamped inferiorly. The three eyelid incisions are made just above the lash line through skin and orbicularis oculi muscle. The three suprabrow incisions are made to the level of periosteum. A superiorly directed pocket is created above each suprabrow incision.

A fascia needle is used to thread the two pieces of fascia between the incisions in the eyelids and brow, forming two rectangles. The eyelid incisions are closed with absorbable 7-0 suture. The upper eyelid traction suture is removed. The protective device is removed. Tension on the two fascia ends that exit two of the suprabrow incisions is adjusted until optimal eyelid height and contour are obtained. Square knots are tied in the fascia, secured with suture, and buried deep in the suprabrow wounds.

The suprabrow incisions are closed in layers with 7-0 absorbable sutures. Antibiotic ointment is placed on wounds and in the conjunctival cul-de-sac. A traction suture is placed in the lower lid margin and taped to the brow with adhesive strips.

Auditory System

Middle Ear

INTRODUCTION

▶(69410 has been deleted)◀

Rationale

Code 69410 has been deleted because the baffle technique is no longer performed. No other code is recommended for reporting this service.

Operating Microscope

The surgical microscope is employed when the surgical services are performed using the techniques of microsurgery. Code 69990 should be reported (without modifier 51 appended) in addition to the code for the primary procedure performed. Do not use 69990 for visualization with magnifying loupes or corrected vision. Do not report code 69990 in addition to procedures where use of the operating microscope is an inclusive component (15756-15758, 15842, 19364, 19368, 20955-20962, 20969-20973, 26551-26554, 26556, 31526, 31531, 31536, 31541, ►31545, 31546, ◄31561, 31571, 43116, 43496, 49906, 61548, 63075-63078, 64727, 64820-64823, 65091-68850).

+69990 Microsurgical techniques, requiring use of operating microscope (List separately in addition to code for primary procedure)

Radiology

Most notable of the revisions to the Radiology section is the deletion of code 76375 and addition of codes 76376 and 76377, with the addition of cross-references to the applicable codes and deletion of the existing cross-references to 76375 for 3-dimensional rendering. Also significant are changes in the Radiation Oncology section and deletion of the nuclear medicine supply codes.

Radiology

Diagnostic Radiology (Diagnostic Imaging)

Head and Neck

70450 Computed tomography, head or brain; without contrast material

70470 without contrast material, followed by contrast material(s) and further sections

►(To report 3D rendering, see 76376, 76377)◄

70480 Computed tomography, orbit, sella, or posterior fossa or outer, middle, or inner ear; without contrast material

70482 without contrast material, followed by contrast material(s) and further sections

►(To report 3D rendering, see 76376, 76377)◄

70486 Computed tomography, maxillofacial area; without contrast material

70488 without contrast material, followed by contrast material(s) and further sections

►(To report 3D rendering, see 76376, 76377)◄

70490 Computed tomography, soft tissue neck; without contrast material

70492 without contrast material followed by contrast material(s) and further sections

►(To report 3D rendering, see 76376, 76377)◄

Chest

71250 Computed tomography, thorax; without contrast material

71270 without contrast material, followed by contrast material(s) and further sections

►(To report 3D rendering, see 76376, 76377)◄

Spine and Pelvis

72131 Computed tomography, lumbar spine; without contrast material

72133 without contrast material, followed by contrast material(s) and further sections

►(To report 3D rendering, see 76376, 76377)◄

72192 Computed tomography, pelvis; without contrast material

72194 without contrast material, followed by contrast material(s) and further sections

►(To report 3D rendering, see 76376, 76377)◄

Upper Extremities

73200 Computed tomography, upper extremity; without contrast material

73202 without contrast material, followed by contrast material(s) and further sections

►(To report 3D rendering, see 76376, 76377)◄

Lower Extremities

73700 Computed tomography, lower extremity; without contrast material

73702 without contrast material, followed by contrast material(s) and further sections

►(To report 3D rendering, see 76376, 76377)◄

Abdomen

74150 Computed tomography, abdomen; without contrast material

74170 without contrast material, followed by contrast material(s) and further sections

►(To report 3D rendering, see 76376, 76377)◄

(For computed tomographic colonography, see Category III codes 0066T, 0067T. Do not report 74150-74170 in conjunction with 0066T, 0067T)

Rationale

Cross-references have been added to report 3-dimensional rendering (76376, 76377) after the following codes: 70470, 70482, 70488, 70492, 71270, 72133, 72194, 73202, 73702, and 74170.

Vascular Procedures

AORTA AND ARTERIES

Selective vascular catheterizations should be coded . . .

Additional second and/or third order arterial . . .

For angiography performed in conjunction with . . .

Diagnostic angiography (radiological supervision and interpretation) . . .

1. Contrast injections, angiography, roadmapping, and/or fluoroscopic guidance for the intervention,
2. Vessel measurement, and
3. Post-angioplasty/stent angiography,

Diagnostic angiography performed at the time . . .

1. No prior catheter-based angiographic study is available and a full diagnostic study is performed, and the decision to intervene is based on the diagnostic study, OR

2. A prior study is available, but as documented in the medical record:

   b. There is inadequate visualization of the anatomy and/or pathology, OR

   c. There is a clinical change during the procedure that requires new evaluation outside the target area of intervention.

Diagnostic angiography performed at a separate . . .

Diagnostic angiography performed at the time . . .

(For intravenous procedure, see 36000-36013, 36400-36425 and 36100-36248 for intra-arterial procedure)

(For radiological supervision and interpretation, see 75600-75978)

75600 Aortography, thoracic, without serialography, radiological supervision and interpretation

Rationale

For *CPT 2005*, introductory guidelines were added to the Aorta and Arteries and the Veins and Lymphatics subsections of the Diagnostic Radiology Vascular Procedure section to instruct appropriate reporting for the CPT subsections related to selective vascular catheterization imaging. These revisions were intended to clarify the circumstances under which a provider should report both a diagnostic angiogram or venogram radiological supervision and interpretation service and an interventional therapeutic vascular radiological supervision and interpretation service. For *CPT 2006*, these guidelines have been revised to clarify that diagnostic angiography codes should not be used to report radiological supervision and interpretation services such as contrast injections, vessel measurement, and post-angioplasty imaging that have already been captured through the reporting of the radiological supervision and interpretation code(s) for the therapeutic intervention(s). This does not preclude the separate reporting of diagnostic angiography/venography performed at the time of transcatheter therapeutic radiological and interpretation service(s). Such services are separately reportable, unless these services are specifically included in the therapeutic code descriptor. Additionally, for those uses permitted by 75898, completion angiography for the therapeutic intervention is separately reportable.

VEINS AND LYMPHATICS

For venography performed in conjunction with . . .

Diagnostic venography (radiological supervision and interpretation) . . .

1. Contrast injections, venography, roadmapping, and/or fluoroscopic guidance for the intervention,
2. Vessel measurement, and
3. Post-angioplasty/stent venography,

Diagnostic venography performed at the time . . .

1. No prior catheter-based venographic study is available and a full diagnostic study is performed, and decision to intervene is based on the diagnostic study, OR
2. A prior study is available, but as documented in the medical record:
   a. The patient's condition with respect to the clinical indication has changed since the prior study, OR
   b. There is inadequate visualization of the anatomy and/or pathology, OR
   c. There is a clinical change during the procedure that requires new evaluation outside the target area of intervention.

Diagnostic venography performed at a separate . . .

Diagnostic venography performed at the time . . .

(For injection procedure for venous system, see 36000-36015, 36400-36510)

(For injection procedure for lymphatic system, use 38790)

75801 Lymphangiography, extremity only, unilateral, radiological supervision and interpretation

✍ Rationale

For *CPT 2005*, introductory guidelines were added to the Aorta and Arteries and Veins and Lymphatics subsections of the Diagnostic Radiology Vascular Procedure section to instruct appropriate reporting for the CPT subsections related to selective vascular catheterization imaging. These revisions were intended to clarify the circumstances under which a provider should report both a diagnostic angiogram/venogram radiological supervision and interpretation service and an interventional therapeutic vascular radiological supervision and interpretation service. For *CPT 2006*, these guidelines have been revised to clarify that diagnostic angiography codes should not be used to report radiological supervision and interpretation services such as contrast injections, vessel measurement, and post-angioplasty imaging that have already been captured through the reporting of the radiological supervision and interpretation code(s) for the therapeutic intervention(s). This does not preclude the separate reporting of diagnostic angiography/venography performed at the time of transcatheter therapeutic radiological and interpretation service(s). Such services are separately reportable, unless these services are specifically included in the therapeutic code descriptor. Additionally, for those uses permitted by 75898, completion angiography for the therapeutic intervention is separately reportable.

TRANSCATHETER PROCEDURES

Therapeutic transcatheter radiological supervision and interpretation . . .

1. Contrast injections, angiography/venography, roadmapping, and fluoroscopic guidance for the intervention,

2. Vessel measurement, and

3. Completion angiography/venography (except for those uses permitted by 75898).

Unless specifically included in the code descriptor, diagnostic angiography/venography performed at the time of transcatheter therapeutic radiological and interpretation service(s) is separately reportable (eg, no prior catheter based diagnostic angiography/venography study of the target vessel is available, prior diagnostic study is inadequate, patient's condition with respect to the clinical indication has changed since the prior study or during the intervention). See 75600-75893.

►Codes 75956 and 75957 include all angiography of the thoracic aorta and its branches for diagnostic imaging prior to deployment of the primary endovascular devices (including all routine components of modular devices), fluoroscopic guidance in the delivery of the endovascular components, and intraprocedural arterial angiography (eg, confirm position, detect endoleak, evaluate runoff).◄

►Code 75958 includes the analogous services for placement of each proximal thoracic endovascular extension. Code 75959 includes the analogous services for placement of a distal thoracic endovascular extension(s) placed during a procedure after the primary repair.◄

▲75900 Exchange of a previously placed intravascular catheter during thrombolytic therapy with contrast monitoring, radiological supervision and interpretation

(For procedure, use 37209)

Rationale

Consistent with the revision of code 37209 to expand the use of the code for arterial and venous catheter exchange with the addition of the word "intravascular," code 75900, the component imaging code, has been similarly revised with the addition of "intravascular."

Clinical Example (75900)

A 58-year-old man is undergoing thrombolytic therapy for a thrombosed left femoral-popliteal graft. Urokinase has been infusing into the proximal portion of the graft for 14 hours, via a catheter placed from the right groin. There has been some clinical improvement. A routine follow-up angiogram has shown clearing of the clot in the graft but there has been embolization of the thrombus to the tibial trifurcation.

Description of Procedure (75900)

In order to treat the distal occlusion, a guidewire is manipulated into the distal popliteal artery and the infusion catheter is exchanged for a new catheter, which has its tip positioned within the distal thrombus. The catheter is secured in the right groin and covered with a sterile dressing, and the infusion is continued.

75954 Endovascular repair of iliac artery aneurysm, pseudoaneurysm, arteriovenous malformation, or trauma, radiological supervision and interpretation

●75956 Endovascular repair of descending thoracic aorta (eg, aneurysm, pseudoaneurysm, dissection, penetrating ulcer, intramural hematoma, or traumatic disruption); involving coverage of left subclavian artery origin, initial endoprosthesis plus descending thoracic aortic extension(s), if required, to level of celiac artery origin, radiological supervision and interpretation

►(For implantation of endovascular graft, use 33880)◄

●75957 not involving coverage of left subclavian artery origin, initial endoprosthesis plus descending thoracic aortic extension(s), if required, to level of celiac artery origin, radiological supervision and interpretation

▶(For implantation of endovascular graft, use 33881)◀

●75958 Placement of proximal extension prosthesis for endovascular repair of descending thoracic aorta (eg, aneurysm, pseudoaneurysm, dissection, penetrating ulcer, intramural hematoma, or traumatic disruption), radiological supervision and interpretation

▶(Report 75958 for each proximal extension)◀

▶(For implantation of proximal endovascular extension, see 33883, 33884)◀

●75959 Placement of distal extension prosthesis(s) (delayed) after endovascular repair of descending thoracic aorta, as needed, to level of celiac origin, radiological supervision and interpretation

▶(Do not report 75959 in conjunction with 75956, 75957)◀

▶(Report 75959 once, regardless of number of modules deployed)◀

▶(For implantation of distal endovascular extension, use 33886)◀

Rationale

In concert with the conversion of Category III codes 0033T-0040T to Category I codes, four imaging codes and guidelines have been added to report imaging for endovascular thoracic aorta prosthesis placement. As indicated in the guidelines, codes 75956 and 75957 include all angiography of the thoracic aorta and its branches for diagnostic imaging prior to deployment of the primary endovascular devices (including all routine components of modular devices), fluoroscopic guidance in the delivery of the endovascular components, and intraprocedural arterial angiography (eg, confirm position, detect endoleak, evaluate runoff). Code 75959 includes the analogous services for placement of each proximal thoracic endovascular extension. Code 75958 includes the analogous services for placement of a distal thoracic endovascular extension(s) placed during a procedure after the primary repair.

Cross-references following codes 75956-75959 refer the user to the appropriate component surgical codes, 33880-33886, for endovascular thoracic aorta prosthesis placement. A cross-reference following the proximal extension placement code 75958 instructs that this imaging code is appropriately reported one time for the placement of each proximal extension. In contrast, cross-references following the distal extension placement imaging code 75959 instruct that this code is reported one time, regardless of the number of extensions placed during a session, and that this code is not reported in addition to 75956 and 75957.

Clinical Example (75956)

A 68-year-old male with hypertension, a 50-pack-per-year smoking habit, and previous myocardial infarction is found to have a 7.0-cm diameter descending thoracic aortic aneurysm that begins immediately beyond the origin of the left subclavian artery. Risks and benefits of open surgical repair, endovascular repair, and watchful waiting have been discussed, and the patient has chosen endovascular repair. Perioperative risk evaluation, including cardiac workup, indicated suitability for the endovascular approach. Imaging studies (typically a combination of computed tomography scan, magnetic resonance imaging, and/or angiography) demonstrate that the aneurysm is within acceptable parameters for endovascular repair if the left subclavian artery origin is covered by the endoprosthesis. Endovascular repair of the descending thoracic aortic aneurysm is performed. The proximal extent of the endoprosthesis covers the left subclavian artery origin.

Description of Procedure (75956)

The physician directs the technical personnel throughout the procedure. He or she interprets imaging of the vessel being treated, including complete views of the target vessel in all projections necessary. Accurate radiological views, exposures, shielding, image size, and injection sequences are ensured, and radiation protection for the patient and staff are managed. Real-time analysis of all imaging occurs during the procedure, including pretreatment imaging, fluoroscopic and angiographic imaging throughout the procedure as required to perform the procedure, and postprocedure fluoroscopic and angiographic imaging. This includes all imaging to manipulate the wires, catheters, and devices into position as well as to correct positioning and deployment, open balloons, and assess postoperative success and complications. Quantitative measurements of the lesion, target vessel, and landing zones are obtained to confirm appropriate prosthesis and balloon sizes. Continuous fluoroscopic imaging is provided during all catheter or stent manipulations to assess proper position.

Clinical Example (75957)

A 68-year-old male with hypertension, a 50-pack-per-year smoking habit, and previous myocardial infarction is found to have a 7.0-cm diameter descending thoracic aortic aneurysm that begins several centimeters beyond the left subclavian artery origin. Risks and benefits of open surgical repair, endovascular repair, and watchful waiting have been discussed, and the patient opted for endovascular repair. Perioperative risk evaluation including cardiac workup indicated suitability for an endovascular approach. Imaging studies (typically a combination of computed tomography scan, magnetic resonance imaging, and/or angiography) demonstrate that the aneurysm is within acceptable parameters for endovascular repair. Endovascular repair of his descending thoracic aortic aneurysm is performed. The proximal portion of the endoprosthesis does not cover the left subclavian artery origin.

Description of Procedure (75957)

The physician directs the technical personnel throughout the procedure. He or she interprets imaging of the vessel being treated, including complete views of the target vessel in all projections necessary. Accurate radiological views, exposures, shielding, image size, and injection sequences are ensured, and radiation protection for the patient and staff are managed. Real-time analysis of all imaging occurs during the procedure, including pretreatment imaging, fluoroscopic and angiographic imaging throughout the procedure as required to perform the procedure, and postprocedure fluoroscopic and angiographic imaging. This includes all imaging to manipulate the wires, catheters, and devices into position as well as to correct positioning and deployment, open balloons, and assess postoperative success and complications. Quantitative measurements of the lesion, target vessel, and landing zones are obtained to confirm appropriate prosthesis and balloon sizes. Continuous fluoroscopic imaging is provided during all catheter or stent manipulations to assess proper position.

Clinical Example (75958)

A 68-year-old male with hypertension, a 50-pack-per-year smoking habit, and previous myocardial infarction underwent endovascular repair of the descending thoracic aortic aneurysm 1 year ago. On the follow-up computed tomography (CT) scan, he is found to have a proximal endoleak. Risks and benefits of endovascular endoleak repair have been discussed, and he opted to proceed. Perioperative risk evaluation, including cardiac workup, indicated suitability for endovascular repair. Imaging studies (typically a combination of CT scan, magnetic resonance imaging, and/or angiography) demonstrate that the endoleak is suitable for an endovascular approach. A proximal endovascular extension is deployed.

Description of Procedure (75958)

The physician directs the technical personnel throughout the procedure. He or she interprets imaging of the vessel being treated, including complete views of the target vessel in all projections necessary. Accurate radiological views, exposures, shielding, image size, and injection sequences are ensured, and radiation protection for the patient and staff are managed. Real-time analysis of all imaging occurs during the procedure, including pretreatment imaging, fluoroscopic and angiographic imaging throughout the procedure as required to perform the procedure, and postprocedure fluoroscopic and angiographic imaging. This includes all imaging to manipulate the wires, catheters, and devices into position as well as to correct positioning and deployment, open balloons, and assess postoperative success and complications. Quantitative measurements of the lesion, target vessel, and landing zones are obtained to confirm appropriate prosthesis and balloon sizes. Continuous fluoroscopic imaging is provided during all catheter or stent manipulations to assess proper position.

Clinical Example (75959)

A 68-year-old male with hypertension, a 50-pack-per-year smoking habit, and previous myocardial infarction underwent endovascular repair of the descending thoracic aortic aneurysm 1 year ago. On the follow-up computed tomography scan, he is found to have a distal endoleak. Placement of a distal extension is undertaken to seal the leak.

Description of Procedure (75959)

The physician directs the technical personnel throughout the procedure. He or she interprets imaging of the vessel being treated, including complete views of the target vessel in all projections necessary. Accurate radiological views, exposures, shielding, image size, and injection sequences are ensured, and radiation protection for the patient and staff are managed. Real-time analysis of all imaging occurs during the procedure, including pretreatment imaging, fluoroscopic and angiographic imaging throughout the procedure as required to perform the procedure, and postprocedure fluoroscopic and angiographic imaging. This includes all imaging to manipulate the wires, catheters, and devices into position as well as to correct positioning and deployment, open balloons, and assess postoperative success and complications. Quantitative measurements of the lesion, target vessel, and landing zones are obtained to confirm appropriate prosthesis and balloon sizes. Continuous fluoroscopic imaging is provided during all catheter or stent manipulations to assess proper position.

Other Procedures

▲76012 Radiological supervision and interpretation, percutaneous vertebroplasty or vertebral augmentation including cavity creation, per vertebral body; under fluoroscopic guidance

76013 under CT guidance

(For procedure, see 22520-22522►, 22523-22525◄)

Rationale

In tandem with the establishment of the percutaneous vertebral augmentation codes 22523-22525, code 76012 has been revised to allow reporting this imaging code to report imaging services required in the performance of percutaneous vertebral augmentation. The cross-reference following 76013 has been revised to refer the user to the percutaneous vertebral augmentation procedure codes in addition to codes 22520-22522 for percutaneous vertebroplasty.

Clinical Example (76012)

A 75-year-old white female who had been living independently develops sudden, severe low back pain after bending over to retrieve a laundry item. Her family physician orders a plain film spine series that reveals an acute compression fracture of L2. He prescribes bedrest and narcotic analgesic to be taken as needed. The pain is unrelieved with medication, and immobilization provides minimal relief. The medication is increased to 4 to 6 times daily, with no significant change. After 2 weeks of immobilization and narcotic analgesics, the patient remains bed-ridden with a clouded sense of sensorium from narcotics. No improvement in pain or mobility is seen.

Description of Procedure (76012)

The patient is placed in the prone position on the angiography-fluoroscopy table. The left L2 pedicle is fluoroscopically localized. Needle placement is monitored fluroscopically to confirm needle position within the trabecular space. Injection of contrast is monitored fluoroscopically to obtain the epidural venogram. Injection of polymethyl-methacrylate (PMMA) is monitored to ensure no migration occurs into or towards the outlined venous plexus. This procedure is repeated if bilateral pedicular injections are required. Radiologist review of final anterior-posterior and lateral images of the lumbar spine show PMMA within the vertebral body with no migration into the surrounding veins.

76362 Computed tomography guidance for, and monitoring of, visceral tissue ablation

▶(For percutaneous cryotherapy ablation of renal tumors, use 0135T)◀

(For percutaneous radiofrequency ablation, ▶see◀ 47382▶, 50592◀)

Rationale

In tandem with the establishment of the percutaneous renal tumor cryotherapy ablation code 0135T, a cross-reference has been added following the computed tomography (CT) visceral tissue ablation imaging code 76362 to direct the user to this new ablation code. The modality of imaging used to guide percutaneous cryotherapy ablation of renal tumor(s) is dependent on patient-specific clinical considerations and physician preference. The imaging guidance codes (76362, 76394, 76940) are appropriate for reporting visceral tissue ablation imaging services in addition to the percutaneous cryotherapy ablation of renal tumor code 0135T.

76370 Computed tomography guidance for placement of radiation therapy fields

▶(76375 has been deleted)◀

▶(2D reformatting is no longer separately reported. To report 3D rendering, see 76376, 76377)◀

▶(Codes 76376, 76377 require concurrent physician supervision of image postprocessing 3D manipulation of volumetric data set and image rendering)◀

●**76376** 3D rendering with interpretation and reporting of computed tomography, magnetic resonance imaging, ultrasound, or other tomographic modality; not requiring image postprocessing on an independent workstation

▶(Use 76376 in conjunction with code(s) for base imaging procedure(s))◀

▶(Do not report 76376 in conjunction with 70496, 70498, 70544-70549, 71275, 71555, 72159, 72191, 72198, 73206, 73225, 73706, 73725, 74175, 74185, 75635, 78814-78816, 0066T, 0067T)◀

●**76377** requiring image postprocessing on an independent workstation

▶(Use 76377 in conjunction with code(s) for base imaging procedure(s))◀

▶(Do not report 76377 in conjunction with 70496, 70498, 70544-70549, 71275, 71555, 72159, 72191, 72198, 73206, 73225, 73706, 73725, 74175, 74185, 75635, 78814, 78815, 78816, 0066T, 0067T)◀

Rationale

Two codes were added to report 3-dimensional (3D) image rendering. Code 76376 was added to report 3D rendering with interpretation and reporting of computed tomography (CT), magnetic resonance imaging (MRI), ultrasound, or other tomographic modality, not requiring image post-processing on an independent workstation. Code 76377 was added to report 3D rendering with interpretation and reporting of CT, MRI, ultrasound, or other tomographic modality; requiring image post processing on an independent workstation. The current 2-dimensional (2D) reformatting-3D rendering code 76375 has been deleted because it no longer describes current technology. To report CT colonography, see Catagory III codes 0066T and 0067T.

Parenthetical notes were added to indicate that 76375 was deleted and that 2D reformatting is no longer separately reported. The cross-reference directs the user to the 3D image rendering codes 76376 and 76377.

An instructional parenthetical note was added to indicate that 3D image rendering codes 76376 or 76377 require concurrent physician supervision of image post-processing 3D manipulation of volumetric data set and image rendering.

Another instructional parenthetical note directs the user to report codes 76376 and 76377 in conjunction with the code for the base imaging procedure(s).

Two exclusionary parenthetical notes have been added to preclude reporting 76376 and 76377 in addition to procedures inherent in image rendering.

The 3D image rendering codes were added to accurately reflect the levels of complexity of image post-processing and rendering currently being performed. Advances in technology have, in many situations, expedited 2D image reformatting so that it can now be performed rapidly by a technologist without a separate workstation or the need to take a scanner off-line for image processing. On the other hand, complex 3D image rendering often requires extensive independent workstation processing by a supervising physician and specially trained technologist. A few applications can be performed on the scanner using optional and expensive hardware and software. Additionally, with the evolution of scanner capabilities to produce 2D reformatting virtually in real time, it is felt that the 2D reformats should be included in the base procedure code and not separately reported. The new 3D rendering codes will address complex renderings such as shaded surface rendering, volumetric rendering, maximum intensity projections (MIPs), fusion imaging, and quantitative analysis (segmental volumes and surgical planning).

Clinical Example (76376)

A 27-year-old female patient Grava 2 Para 1 has previously delivered an infant with a cleft lip and palate. The obstetrician performs a pelvic exam and concludes that the uterine size appears consistent with a 20- to 22-weeks gestation. The patient is scheduled for a 2-dimensional (2D) ultrasound examination to confirm fetal dating of the pregnancy and to evaluate for possible fetal abnormalities including a possible facial cleft malformation.

An ultrasound technologist scans the patient in a conventional ultrasound unit that has 2D ultrasound capabilities. Sagittal and transverse images of the pregnant uterus are obtained in 2D ultrasound (coded separately). The attending physician evaluates the images and concludes that the images generated from the 2D ultrasound are not able to confidently exclude or identify a facial cleft anomaly. A 3-dimensional (3D) ultrasound is ordered to better visualize the facial structures in 3D shaded surface rendering.

Description of Procedure (76376)

The physician supervises the technologist in creating the 3D images, interprets the images, and dictates a report for the medical record.

Clinical Example (76377)

A 50-year-old male presented to his physician with hematuria. Renal ultrasound (coded separately) identified a 3-cm lower pole, right renal mass consistent with renal cell carcinoma, previously diagnosed with ultrasound. The patient is a possible candidate for nephron-sparing partial nephrectomy, and a computerized tomographic (CT) scan of the abdomen is ordered by the patient's urologist. Three-dimensional (3D) rendering is requested for further evaluation.

A CT examination of the abdomen, both before and after the use of contrast media, is performed (coded separately). Subsequent postprocessing and 3D reconstruction is performed demonstrating the patient is a candidate for partial nephrectomy.

Description of Procedure (76377)

The physician supervises and/or creates 3D reconstructions of the organs of interest using an independent workstation. He or she adjusts the projection of the 3D reconstructions to optimize visualization of the anatomy or pathology. The physician interprets the 3D reformatted images resulting from the study, typically including cine review. The images are compared to all pertinent available prior studies and a report is dictated for the medical record.

76394 Magnetic resonance guidance for, and monitoring of, visceral tissue ablation

(For percutaneous radiofrequency ablation, ►see◄ 47382►, 50592◄)

(For focused ultrasound ablation treatment of uterine leiomyomata, see Category III codes 0071T, 0072T)

►(For percutaneous cryotherapy ablation of renal tumors, use 0135T)◄

Rationale

An instructional parenthetical note has been added after 76394 to direct the user to percutaneous radiofrequency ablation, 50592.

In tandem with the establishment of the percutaneous renal tumor cryotherapy ablation code 0135T, a cross-reference has been added following the magnetic resonance (MR) visceral tissue ablation imaging code 76394 to direct the user to this new ablation code. The modality of imaging used to guide percutaneous cryotherapy ablation of renal tumor(s) is dependent on patient-specific clinical considerations and physician preference. The imaging guidance codes (76362, 76394, 76940) are appropriate for reporting visceral tissue ablation imaging services in addition to the percutaneous renal tumor cryotherapy ablation code 0135T.

Diagnostic Ultrasound

Ultrasonic Guidance Procedures

76940 Ultrasound guidance for, and monitoring of, visceral tissue ablation

(Do not report 76940 in conjunction with 76986)

(For ablation, see 47370-47382►, 50592◄)

►(For percutaneous cryotherapy ablation of renal tumors, use 0135T)◄

Rationale

An instructional parenthetical has been added after 76940 to direct the user to percutaneous radiofrequency ablation, 50592.

In tandem with the establishment of the percutaneous renal tumor cryotherapy ablation code 0135T, a cross-reference has been added following the ultrasound (U/S) visceral tissue ablation imaging code 76940 to direct the user to this new ablation code. The modality of imaging used to guide percutaneous cryotherapy ablation of renal tumor(s) is dependent on patient-specific clinical considerations and physician preference. The imaging guidance codes (76362, 76394, 76940) are appropriate for reporting visceral tissue ablation imaging services in addition to the percutaneous renal tumor cryotherapy ablation code 0135T.

Radiation Oncology

Radiation Treatment Delivery

▲77412 Radiation treatment delivery, three or more separate treatment areas, custom blocking, tangential ports, wedges, rotational beam, compensators, electron beam; up to 5 MeV

77413 6-10 MeV

77414 11-19 MeV

77416 20 MeV or greater

Rationale

In tandem with the establishment of 77422 and 77423 for neutron beam therapy delivery, 77412 has been editorially revised to exclude the series of codes 77412-77416 from use for reporting neutron therapy delivery.

●77421 Stereoscopic X-ray guidance for localization of target volume for the delivery of radiation therapy

►(Do not report 77421 in conjunction with 77432, 0083T)◄

Rationale

Code 77421 was added to report stereoscopic X-ray guidance. Stereoscopic X-ray guidance is used for imaging and localizing target volumes in certain anatomical sites immediately prior to 3D or intensity-modulated radiation therapy (IMRT) .

The tumor target volume mapped for 3D or IMRT may vary on a daily basis depending on errors in setup and internal motion of the target volume or surrounding tissues. This technology detects any 3D deviations between actual and planned target position. Locating the target volume on orthogonal X rays with (when target volumes cannot be well seen on X rays) or without (if the target volume can be seen on X rays) the help of implanted markers ensures accurate treatment of the target and spares normal tissues. This process is not described by 77417, which describes taking a port film once a week for setup corrections alone.

Using stereoscopic X-ray guidance, physicians can more accurately ensure that the target volume is treated to the planned dose of radiation.

Clinical Example (77421)

A 60-year-old male presented with prostate cancer. The patient opted for external beam radiotherapy, and the plan is to deliver 78 Gy at 2 Gy per fraction to the prostate and seminal vesicles using highly conformal radiotherapy. Service includes acquisition and review of positioning X rays and physician-directed repositioning as necessary.

Description of Procedure (77421)

A radiation oncologist oversees the patient preparation, including placement of infrared markers. The infrared markers are placed either on the patient to monitor the patient's position or on the treatment couch to localize the position of the couch. Two sets of X rays are acquired to visualize internal anatomy or implanted marker positions immediately prior to treatment. This is done using kV or MV X-ray units that may be a combination of two kV X-ray units and two amorphous silicon flat panel detectors or an X-ray unit attached to the gantry or MV X rays with an electronic portal imaging device (EPID), which takes two orthogonal images. These two high-resolution X rays are acquired prior to treatment delivery in order to visualize the internal anatomy or implanted markers.

The stereoscopic X-ray images are compared with the imported digital reconstructed radiographs (DRRs) from the treatment planning system or generated DRRs from the stored computed tomography treatment planning scan data, which are in the same plane as the X rays taken. The DRRs serve as a reference for identifying rotational or movement discrepancies, positioning, and guidance for the delivery of radiation and enable real-time analysis of the targeted area.

Alignment, registration, and fusion of the two images are done manually or automatically using previously implanted markers, direct visualization of the target volume, or surrounding bony anatomy. These procedures are done under the supervision of the radiation oncologist.

The rotational errors of the patient setup and the table movement necessary to optimally align the patient's target volume at the isocenter in longitudinal, lateral, and vertical directions are calculated. The deviations, if present, are determined and corrected by adjusting the patient's treatment position to the treatment target volume isocenter. This is performed by applying the required translational shifts to the treatment couch performed by the therapist and done under physician supervision.

The radiation oncologist reviews the images daily and compares with previous shifts. Feedback by the physician is given to the therapists about the adequacy of registrations and, if necessary, about the steps necessary to improve future registrations as well as for required treatment modifications.

▸Neutron Beam Treatment Delivery◂

●**77422** High energy neutron radiation treatment delivery; single treatment area using a single port or parallel-opposed ports with no blocks or simple blocking

●**77423** 1 or more isocenter(s) with coplanar or non-coplanar geometry with blocking and/or wedge, and/or compensator(s)

Rationale

Codes 77422 and 77423 for reporting neutron therapy and a new subheading titled Neutron Beam Treatment Delivery have been established to report neutron beam therapy delivery to allow tracking and monitoring of neutron therapy and the ability to differentiate the type of radiation therapy reported.

Code 77422 is intended to describe high-energy neutron radiation treatment delivery to a single treatment area using a single port or parallel-opposed ports with no blocks or simple blocking.

Code 77423 is intended to describe high-energy neutron radiation treatment delivery to one or more isocenter(s) with coplanar or noncoplanar geometry with simple or complex blocking and/or wedge, and/or compensator(s).

High-energy neutron therapy treats radioresistant tumors and especially advanced, unresectable tumors. Its largest application is in salivary gland tumors, paranasal sinuses, locally extended head and neck disease, advanced prostate cancer, and sarcoma of bone, soft tissue, or cartilage. Radioresistant tumors are tumors known not to respond well to conventional photon or electron therapy.

Nuclear Medicine

Listed procedures may be performed independently . . .

Radioimmunoassay tests are found in the . . .

The services listed do not include the ▶radiopharmaceutical or drug◀. Diagnostic and therapeutic radiopharmaceuticals ▶and drugs◀ supplied by the physician should be reported separately ▶using the appropriate supply code(s), in addition to the procedure code◀.

✍ Rationale

The introductory statement to the Nuclear Medicine section has been editorially revised. The editorial revision in the guideline indicates that supplies should be separately reported for the use of the codes. Also the word *provision* has been deleted because it has erroneously led providers to interpret the meaning as the introduction of or administration of a radiopharmaceutical or drug. In addition, the phase "radium and other radioelements" has been outdated and replaced with the word *radiopharmaceutical*, which is intended to be all-inclusive, ie, encompassing other words such as *radionuclide*, *radioelement*, etc.

Diagnostic

HEMATOPOIETIC, RETICULOENDOTHELIAL AND LYMPHATIC SYSTEM

▶(78160, 78162, 78170, 78172 have been deleted)◀

CARDIOVASCULAR SYSTEM

▶(78455 has been deleted)◀

✍ Rationale

Nuclear medicine codes 78160, 78162, 78170, 78172, and 78455 have been deleted. These codes were reported for procedures and provision of radiopharmaceuticals, which are obsolete or inappropriately reported with CPT codes.

78472 Cardiac blood pool imaging, gated equilibrium; planar, single study at rest or stress (exercise and/or pharmacologic), wall motion study plus ejection fraction, with or without additional quantitative processing

(For assessment of ▶right ventricular ejection fraction◀ by first pass technique, use 78496)

✍ Rationale

The parenthetical note following 78472 has been revised in order to clarify the appropriate use of 78496.

The current language has led to misinterpretation of the use of add-on code 78496. Code 78496 was developed as an add-on code specifically for right ventricle ejection fraction and to be used only in conjunction with 78472 primarily in the evaluation of patients with known or suspected pulmonary disease.

OTHER PROCEDURES

78805 Radiopharmaceutical localization of inflammatory process; limited area

78807 tomographic (SPECT)

(For imaging bone infectious or inflammatory disease with a bone imaging radiopharmaceutical, see 78300, 78305, 78306)

(78810 has been deleted. To report, see 78811-78813)

(For PET of brain, see 78608, 78609)

(For PET myocardial imaging, see ►78459, ◄78491, 78492)

Rationale

The cross-reference following 78807 has been updated to include a reference to position emission tomography (PET) myocardial imaging code 78459.

Therapeutic

79101 Radiopharmaceutical therapy, by intravenous administration

(Do not report 79101 in conjunction with 36400, 36410, 79403, 90760, 90774 or 90775, 96409)

Rationale

In tandem with the revisions of the Hydration and Therapeutic, Prophylactic, and Diagnostic Injections and Infusions subsections, the cross-reference following 79101 has been revised to include the new codes.

Pathology and Laboratory

For 2006, a new therapeutic drug assay code has been added to the CPT codebook for the first time since 2001. In the Chemistry subsection, a series of occult blood test codes has been added. Also, significant changes have been made to the molecular diagnostics and lipoprotein test codes. In the Immunology subsection, the B cell, natural killer cell, and stem cell codes added for *CPT 2005* have been deleted and renumbered. Other important changes include the revision of the cytopathology guidelines and the addition of new codes to the Surgical Pathology subsection.

Pathology and Laboratory

Therapeutic Drug Assays

●**80195** Sirolimus

Rationale

Code 80195 has been established to report a new immunoassay test to monitor drug levels of sirolimus in blood. Sirolimus is an immunosuppressive therapy medication for solid organ transplant recipients. Monitoring of this therapy is recommended due to potential toxic effects associated with high levels of sirolimus.

Clinical Example (80195)

The service provided is to measure the concentration of sirolimus in the patient's blood following sirolimus immunosuppressive therapy. The sirolimus measurements must be made on a regular basis to monitor blood levels of the drug for as long as the patient is being administered the drug. This is done to adjust and optimize the dosage of the drug for each individual and to minimize toxic side effects.

Chemistry

▲**82270** Blood, occult, by peroxidase activity (eg, guaiac), qualitative; feces, consecutive collected specimens with single determination, for colorectal neoplasm screening (ie, patient was provided three cards or single triple card for consecutive collection)

●**82271** other sources

●**82272** Blood, occult, by peroxidase activity (eg, guaiac), qualitative, feces, single specimen (eg, from digital rectal exam)

▶(82273 has been deleted. To report, use 82271)◀

Rationale

Chemistry code 82270 has been revised to expand the intent of this code to report evaluation of triple sample specimens with single determination for colorectal neoplasm screening. Code 82273 has been deleted and renumbered 82271. The intent of code 82273 has not changed. A cross-reference has been added to instruct the user to the appropriate code. Code 82272 has been added to this series in order to provide a mechanism for reporting tests performed on a single specimen. These changes allow a more accurate description of the physician-patient role in the service that is furnished and reported.

Previously code 82270 failed to distinguish between a single specimen fecal occult blood test (FOBT) that is primarily done in the office setting, eg, after a digital rectal exam, and a three-specimen FOBT that the patient typically collects at home. While a physician may furnish a single-specimen FOBT for diagnostic purposes, three-specimen determination is essential for proper screening.

Code 82270 is constructed to permit the laboratory (eg, reference laboratory, hospital laboratory, physician office laboratory) to use this code for analysis of peroxidase activity, irrespective of the number of samples received, when the patient is asked to collect and return three consecutive samples. There may be times where the laboratory receives only two samples when the patient was specifically asked to collect three. Under this scenario, the laboratory should perform analysis of the two collected specimens, report the results accordingly, and record one unit of 82270.

These changes permit more accurate reporting of the FOBT service, and encourage appropriate use of FOBT as a screening test for colorectal cancer.

Clinical Example (82270)

A 72-year-old patient is seen for a follow-up visit for her hypertension and diabetes. During the visit, the physician discusses the importance of colorectal cancer screening with the patient, including all recommended screening options. The patient agrees that screening for colorectal cancer with a set of three fecal occult blood cards is appropriate, and the physician supplies the kit and instructions.

Clinical Example (82272)

A 57-year-old female is seen for fatigue and mentions that she has had dark stools. During the visit, the physician performs a digital rectal exam and obtains a fecal specimen for guaiac-based occult blood test.

82726 Very long chain fatty acids

►(For long-chain (C20-22) omega-3 fatty acids in red blood cell (RBC) membranes, use Category III code 0111T)◄

Rationale

A cross-reference was added following 82726 to direct the user to Category III code 0111T, which has been added to report long-chain omega-3 fatty acid testing.

83026 Hemoglobin; by copper sulfate method, non-automated

▲83036 glycosylated (A1C)

●83037 glycosylated (A1C) by device cleared by FDA for home use

Rationale

Code 83036 was revised to replace the word *glycated* with *glycosylated (A1C)* to better reflect current nomenclature. Code 83037 was established for reporting a glycosylated hemoglobin (A1C) test that is obtained in the patient's home with a Food and Drug Administration (FDA) cleared device. This testing platform may be used in a clinical setting to provide rapid turnaround Hg A1C levels as a means to enable physicians and other health care providers to manage glycemic control in people with diabetes. The purpose of this device is to provide a self-contained A1C system used by physicians and other health care providers to provide test results for use in their face-to-face interaction with patients.

Clinical Example (83037)

A 45-year-old patient with a history of type II diabetes and demonstrated capability of maintaining long-term, stable glycemic control arrives for a chronic care medical visit. It is determined that an A1C test has not been performed within the last 3 months.

Description of Procedure (83037)

After consent, a large drop of capillary blood or venous blood is obtained from the patient by standard techniques. The blood sample is deposited into a buffer solution and shaken in order to lyse red blood cells. The sample is then transferred to a self-contained, internally controlled system that automatically generates an A1C result. The A1C result is used to monitor the patient's overall diabetes therapy within the context of a systematic glycemic control plan.

▲83630 Lactoferrin, fecal; qualitative

●83631 quantitative

Rationale

Code 83631 was added to describe quantitative determination of lactoferrin in feces. Additionally, code 83630 was revised to clarify the intent of this code for qualitative determinations of lactoferrin in feces.

The quantitative test described in 83631 is used to determine the presence of intestinal inflammation, differentiate inflammatory from non-inflammatory gastrointestinal disease, monitor patient response to therapy, and predict inflammatory bowel disease recurrence.

Clinical Example (83631)

A 56-year-old male patient presented with diarrhea (of a 2-week duration) containing a significant amount of blood and mucus. A test for Clostridium difficile was ordered and a sigmoidoscopy performed. The sigmoidoscopy revealed little or no ulceration extending beyond the rectal area. Due to the acute onset of the diarrhea and age of the patient, there was no strong indication of inflammatory bowel disease. Fecal lactoferrin levels were elevated (2500 micrograms/ml), indicating significant intestinal inflammation. Test results for Clostridium difficile toxin were negative.

The patient was placed on oral steroids and enemas containing non-steroidal anti-inflammatories.

The patient did not respond to treatment and returned to the physician after 1 week complaining of continued diarrhea with blood loss and subsequent weakness. The patient was admitted immediately to the hospital where a colonoscopy was performed. This showed ulceration far into the colon beyond the small section initially observed during sigmoidoscopy. Lactoferrin levels were recorded at 9000 micrograms/ml.

The patient's drug therapy was revised. After 5 days, the symptoms resolved and lactoferrin levels had dropped significantly to 400 micrograms/ml. The patient was discharged with further drug therapy adjustments.

One week later lactoferrin levels, which were being monitored on a daily basis, rose to 7000 micrograms/ml. The medication was changed before any diarrheal symptoms reappeared. After 1 week, fecal lactoferrin levels had dropped to less than 7 micrograms/ml.

●83695 Lipoprotein (a)

Rationale

Code 83695 was established to report direct quantitative measurement of Lipoprotein a [Lp(a)] in serum, an indicator for increased risk for myocardial infarction, stroke, coronary artery disease, vein graft restenosis, and retinal arterial occlusions when present in elevated blood concentrations.

Lp(a) measurements evaluate disorders of lipid metabolism, are genetically determined, and show wide intrapopulation and interpopulation variability.

Lp(a) is a distinct class of lipoprotein and is considered a risk factor determinant for coronary heart disease (CHD) and cerebrovascular disease. Lp(a) is a cholesterol and kringle-containing plasma lipoprotein with a lipid composition similar to low-density lipoprotein (LDL). It has low apoprotein constituents, apo B-100 and apo(a). Lp(a) can be measured using several methods.

The test can be run using ELISA and immunoturbidometric platforms with monoclonal antibodies against unique apo(a) epitopes used in the determination for Lp(a) being performed on a venipuncture serum sample.

Clinical Example (83695)

A 55-year-old black female visits her physician for cholesterol, triglyceride, and HDL testing. She is concerned by her family's long history of coronary heart disease (CHD). Her lipid profile is normal. In light of the strong family history, her physician additionally performs a Lipoprotein(a) test to obtain additional information on the patient's risk of developing heart disease. Her Lp(a) result is elevated. The physician can make lifestyle changes and monitor the patient for changes.

●83700 Lipoprotein, blood; electrophoretic separation and quantitation

●83701 high resolution fractionation and quantitation of lipoproteins including lipoprotein subclasses when performed (eg, electrophoresis, ultracentrifugation)

●83704 quantitation of lipoprotein particle numbers and lipoprotein particle subclasses (eg, by nuclear magnetic resonance spectroscopy)

►(83715, 83716 have been deleted. To report, use 83700, 83701)◄

83718 Lipoprotein, direct measurement; high density cholesterol (HDL cholesterol)

83719 VLDL cholesterol

83721 LDL cholesterol

(For fractionation by high resolution electrophoresis ►or ultracentrifugation◄, use ►83701◄)

►(For lipoprotein particle numbers and subclasses analysis by nuclear magnetic resonance spectroscopy, use 83695)◄

(To report direct measurement, intermediate density lipoproteins (remnant lipoproteins), use Category III code 0026T)

Rationale

Lipoprotein analysis codes 83715 and 83716 have been deleted and renumbered to 83700 and 83701 to accommodate the addition of a third code (83704) to this series. Code 83704 has been added to allow a separate reporting mechanism for lipoprotein analysis by nuclear magnetic resonance (NMR) spectroscopy. Deleted code 83716 grouped analysis of lipoproteins by nuclear magnetic resonance (NMR) with two other technologies (electrophoresis and ultracentrifugation). The cross-reference following code 83721 was revised to direct users to the appropriate codes for ultracentrifugation (83701). Also, a second cross-reference was added to direct users to the appropriate codes for nuclear magnetic spectroscopy (83704).

NMR provides high-resolution direct lipoprotein particle quantification to measure lipoproteins and lipoprotein subclasses directly by exploiting natural pre-existing spectroscopic differences that exist among particles of different size. The distinct spectroscopic signal emitted by each of the lipoprotein subclasses indicates the presence of that particular subclass in a patient's plasma, and also provides from its measured amplitude a direct means of quantifying the number of subclass particles giving rise to the signal. By achieving simultaneous absolute quantification of 10 lipoprotein subclasses, the NMR analysis test provides physicians with absolute quantitative lipoprotein particle information.

Subclass particle quantification is particularly useful in assessing and managing the CVD risk of patients with elevated triglyceride levels and the metabolic abnormalities associated with insulin resistance and diabetes.

Clinical Example (83704)

The patient is a 48-year-old male, status post four vessel coronary artery bypass graft surgery 1 year prior to presentation, who returns to the cardiologist for a follow-up evaluation. Post bypass surgery, the patient completed cardiac rehabilitation, maintained daily aerobic exercise, and adopted a strict vegetarian diet (10% of calories from fat). He tolerates diet and activity as indicated without cardiovascular symptoms. His current medications include ASA 81 mg q day and pravastatin 20 mg q day. On physical examination, vital signs are normal and no objective abnormalities are noted: blood pressure 117/75; pulse 72, height 6'2"; weight 203 lb; waist circumference 38"; fasting glucose 105 mg/dL. A fasting lipid profile measured by standard chemical methods gave the following values:

Total cholesterol	156 mg/dL
LDL cholesterol	94 mg/dL
HDL cholesterol	34 mg/dL
Triglycerides	142 mg/dL

Description of Procedure (83704)

A fasting blood sample (greater than or equal to 3 cc) is obtained from the patient by venipuncture using an EDTA blood collection tube. Following centrifugation, the plasma is drawn off and transferred to a bar code-labeled collection vial and refrigerated for up to 4 days. The specimen is placed into its own specimen bag along with a completed requisition form and shipped by overnight express to the laboratory using a polystyrene plastic box kept cool with a frozen ice brick.

Upon receipt by the laboratory, the bar-coded plasma source tube is accessioned into the laboratory information system (LIS) and a bar-coded daughter vial is generated. A sampling of 300 ml of plasma is transferred to the daughter vial, diluted by two times with 300 ml of buffer, placed in a defined position in the nuclear magnetic resonance (NMR) analysis rack, and refrigerated prior to placement on the NMR analyzer.

The NMR analyzer is a 400 MHz proton NMR spectrometer consisting of a 9.4 Tesla-shielded superconducting magnet, digital radiofrequency transmitter-receiver with proton detection and deuterium lock, temperature-controlled flow probe detector with pulsed magnetic field gradient coil for water suppression, Windows NT host workstation, and XYZ robot for automated plasma aspiration and transport to the flow probe detector. The daily set-up procedure is performed using a standard sample of trimethylacetate. This procedure includes adjusting the current in the correction coils to optimize the homogeneity of the magnetic field across the sample; adjusting and verifying the sample temperature; and determining the normalization factor used to ensure day-to-day equivalence of detection sensitivity. NMR spectra of two different freshly-thawed quality control (QC) plasma samples are acquired automatically under prescribed conditions, and the data are processed and checked to verify that values for each lipoprotein parameter fall within previously established QC ranges.

The NMR analysis rack containing the patient's plasma sample is removed from the refrigerator and loaded onto the NMR analyzer. Each plasma specimen is sequentially aspirated, transported by flow injection to the detection probe, and heated to the measurement temperature. Spectra are acquired in triplicate, deconvoluted by software, and results transmitted to the LIS. The sample is removed from the detector and the transfer lines and detector cell cleaned and dried before injection of the succeeding sample. The patient's results are reviewed according to QC guidelines by the clinical analyst and approved for reporting to the physician. The report is transmitted to the physician by fax and a color hard copy sent by overnight express. Electronic access to the patient's results is also available via the Internet.

During the post-test patient management, the patient's results indicate that, despite having achieved the National Cholesterol Education Program (NCEP)-recommended LDL cholesterol goal of less than 100 mg/dL (less than the 20th percentile) on a regimen of diet, exercise, and a relatively low dose of a moderately potent statin (pravastatin 20 mg), risk of a recurrent cardiovascular event remains high owing to the presence of high numbers of LDL particles (1802 nmol/L; greater than the 80th percentile). Furthermore, the great majority of these LDL particles are small in size and, therefore, particularly atherogenic. The physician communicates her concern to the patient about the seriousness of the risk of having such high numbers of small LDL particles, and stresses the importance of complying with her diet and lifestyle recommendations. In addition, to achieve lower concentrations of LDL particles, a higher dose of a more potent statin (atorvastatin 40 mg) is prescribed. The primary goal of this more intensive LDL lowering therapy is to reduce the LDL particle number to less than 1100 nmol/L (less than the 20th percentile). Although secondary in importance, another source of clinical concern communicated to the patient is a desire to raise his very low level of protective large HDL subclass.

Codes 83890-►83914◄ are intended for use with molecular diagnostic techniques for analysis of nucleic acids.

Codes 83890-►83914◄ are coded by procedure rather than analyte.

Code separately for each procedure used . . .

When molecular diagnostic procedures are performed to test for oncology, hematology, neurology or inherited disorder, use the appropriate modifier to specify probe type or condition tested. (See **Appendix I** for a listing of appropriate modifiers to report with molecular diagnostic and cytogenetic procedures.)

(For microbial identification, see 87797, 87798)

►(For array technology using more than 10 probes, see 88384-88386)◄

83890 Molecular diagnostics; molecular isolation or extraction

▲83898 amplification of patient nucleic acid, each nucleic acid sequence

●83900 amplification of patient nucleic acid, multiplex, first two nucleic acid sequences

+▲83901 amplification of patient nucleic acid, multiplex, each additional nucleic acid sequence (List separately in addition to code for primary procedure)

►(Use 83901 in conjunction with 83900)◄

●83907 lysis of cells prior to nucleic acid extraction (eg, stool specimens, paraffin embedded tissue)

●83908 signal amplification of patient nucleic acid, each nucleic acid sequence

►(For multiplex amplification, see 83900, 83901)◄

●83909 separation and identification by high resolution technique (eg, capillary electrophoresis)

83912 interpretation and report

Rationale

In addition to numerous revisions to Appendix I of the CPT codebook, the molecular diagnostic procedure guidelines have been revised to reflect correct code ranges and to clarify that these tests are not performed for infectious diseases.

The genetic testing modifiers are appended to the molecular diagnostic code(s) 83890-83914 when the molecular diagnostic procedures are performed to test for oncology, hematology, neurology, or inherited disorder to specify the probe type or condition tested. The genetic testing modifiers may also be appended to the cytogenetic studies code(s) 88245-88291 when molecular diagnostic procedures are performed to test for oncologic or inherited disorders to specify the probe type or condition tested.

For a complete listing of the genetic testing modifiers, see Appendix I in *CPT 2006*. For more information on how to use CPT genetic testing modifiers, see the July 2005 *CPT Assistant* article titled Coding Commentary: Genetic Modifiers.

Four codes were established to report component procedures for molecular diagnostic testing. In addition, codes 83898 and 83901 were revised. Also, an instructional parenthetical note has been added to revised code 83901. A cross-reference was added to direct users to the appropriate codes for multiplex amplification (83900, 83901).

Code 83898 was revised to report amplification of each nucleic acid sequence rather than reporting each or single primer pair to better clarify the appropriate units of service. Code 83900 was established to report multiplex amplification of nucleic acid by each first two nucleic acid sequences again to alleviate confusion regarding the definition of the units of service. In the same light, indented code 83901 was revised to add-on code status to report multiplex amplification of nucleic acid by each additional nucleic acid sequence. Code 83901 must be listed separately in addition to the primary procedure code.

Lysis of the cell membrane, inactivation of the cellular nucleases, and separation of the desired nucleic acids require the extraction and purification of nucleic acids (RNA, DNA) from biological material. Code 83907 was established to report lysis of cells prior to nucleic acid extraction.

Code 83908 was established to report each nucleic acid sequence in signal amplification.

Code 83909 was established to report the high-resolution technique for separation and identification of nucleic acids currently performed via capillary electrophoresis. Post-amplification is used to yield precise separation of nucleic acids so that minor variations such as base variations may be identified.

The new and revised codes are used in a wide variety of clinical diagnostic tests for infectious agents, DNA-based disease markers, therapy selection in oncology, and predictors of inherited genetic disorders.

●**83914** Mutation identification by enzymatic ligation or primer extension, single segment, each segment (eg, oligonucleotide ligation assay (OLA), single base chain extension (SBCE), or allele-specific primer extension (ASPE))

Rationale

Code 83914 was established to report mutation identification of different alleles at the polymorphic sites within genomic DNA segments via enzymatic ligation or identification of primer extensions. The methods used for ligation or primer extension detections include those tests listed in the example (eg, statement in the code descriptor, oligonucleotide ligation assay [OLA], single base chain extension [SBCE], or allele-specific primer extension [ASPE]).

Prior to establishment of code 83914, the existing codes in the CPT codebook described only mutation detection methods using DNA sequencing and gel-electrophoresis methodologies to interrogate or identify variations in the DNA sequence.

Similar to all codes in the molecular diagnostic section, this code is intended to be reported in addition to other molecular diagnostic codes when identification of the presence of a mutation is necessary. These additional molecular diagnostic codes include 83890 (molecular isolation or extraction), 83901 (amplification of patient nucleic acid, multiplex, each multiplex reaction), and 83912 (interpretation and report).

Clinical Example (83914)

A 2-year-old female child presents with frequent respiratory infections, is frequently out of breath, and has abnormally salty sweat. Her medical records at birth indicate that the passing of meconium occurred 72 hours after birth. Additionally, her mother's sister had a 6-month-old infant that had presented with chronic respiratory infections. Her symptoms are not adequately controlled with medications and her level of disability is not improving.

Description of Procedure (83914)

Because her symptoms are suggestive for cystic fibrosis, the physician orders a series of tests to confirm the diagnosis and determine the prognosis. She undergoes a sweat test on two separate occasions to measure the amount of sodium chloride. The results of the sweat test are negative. A CF genetic test for the 25 recommended mutations is ordered to confirm CF and determine the mutations involved. To avoid the risk of a mismatch in the mutation detection, the physician has specified that a ligation or primer extension identification procedure be used for all 25 mutations. Additional tests are performed to measure how well the lungs, pancreas, and liver are functioning.

84233 Receptor assay; estrogen

84234 progesterone

84235 endocrine, other than estrogen or progesterone (specify hormone)

▲**84238** non-endocrine (specify receptor)

Rationale

Code 84238 has been revised with the deletion of the example (eg, statement in the descriptor) to clarify reporting for antibody assays.

Immunology

(Acetylcholine receptor antibody, see ►83519,◄ 86255, 86256)

(Actinomyces, antibodies to, use 86602)

(Adrenal cortex antibodies, see 86255, 86256)

86000 Agglutinins, febrile (eg, Brucella, Francisella, Murine typhus, Q fever, Rocky Mountain spotted fever, scrub typhus), each antigen

Rationale

The cross-reference following the Immunology subheading has been revised to include 83519 in addition to the other methods listed because many laboratories use the radioimmunoassay technique for acetylcholine receptor antibody assays.

86060 Antistreptolysin O; titer

(For antibodies to infectious agents, see 86602-86804)

86063 screen

(For antibodies to infectious agents, see 86602-86804)

(Blastomyces, antibodies to, use 86612)

►(86064 has been deleted. For B cells, total count, use 86355)◄

Rationale

In order to allay confusion, the flow cytometry quantitation B cells code 86064 has been deleted and relocated from its current alpha-order location in the Immunology subsection of Pathology and Laboratory to a location adjacent to the lymphocyte T-cell series of codes and renumbered to 86355 to report this service. The flow cytometric cross-reference has also been relocated after 86355.

●**86200** Cyclic citrullinated peptide (CCP), antibody

Rationale

Code 86200 was established to provide a mechanism for reporting testing for cyclic citrullinated peptide (CCP). This is a semi-quantitative/qualitative enzyme-linked immunosorbent assay (ELISA) for the detection of the IgG class of auto-antibodies specific to cyclic citrullinated peptide (CCP) in human serum or plasma. It is intended to aid in the diagnosis of rheumatoid arthritis (RA).

Anti-CCP is used to detect early RA. The sensitivity of the RA test allows detection before clinical manifestation of the disease, and due to its high specificity, may be used to differentiate RA from other forms of polyarthritidies. Additionally, anti-CCP antibodies can be detected in patients with seronegative RA (negative rheumatoid factor [RF]).

Clinical Example 1 (86200)

A 55-year-old woman presented with a 6-month history of pain and swelling of her hand joints and knees. This was associated with marked early morning stiffness and fatigue. Physical examination reveals swelling and tenderness of her proximal interphalangeal and metacarpophalangeal joints bilaterally as well as her left wrist joint. A blood sample is drawn for full blood count, biochemical indices, erythrocyte sedimentation rate (ESR), C-reactive protein (CRP), RF, anti-nuclear antibodies (ANA), and antibodies to cyclic citrullinated peptide (CCP). X rays of the hands are taken.

Results:

Hemoglobin = 10.2 g/dl

MCV = 88 fl

Chemistry panel = Normal

ESR = 45 mm/hr

CRP = 26 mg/dl (ref. < 20 mg/dl)

RF = < 22 IU/ml (ref. 0-22 IU/ml)

ANA = 1:40 (speckled pattern)

Anti-CCP = 15 units/ml (ref. 0-5 units/ml)

X ray of hands = soft tissue swelling, periarticular osteopenia

This patient had seronegative rheumatoid arthritis (clinical presentation, high anti-CCP, and X-ray features), and the disease is active (normocytic anemia, high ESR, and CRP).

Clinical Example 2 (86200)

A 38-year-old housewife presented with a 9-month history of pain and stiffness of the small joints of the hands, wrists, and ankles. She also complained of cold, white hands that have troubled her over the past year. Physical examination reveals swelling of her right wrist, ankle, and metacarpophalangeal joints bilaterally. A blood sample is drawn for a full blood count, biochemical indices, ESR, CRP, RF, and ANA anti-CCP. X rays of the hands are taken.

Results:

Hemoglobin = 11.8 g/dl

MCV = 86 fl

Chemistry panel = Normal

ESR = 30 mm/hr

CRP = 8 mg/dl (ref. < 20 mg/dl)

RF = < 22 IU/ml (ref. 0-22 IU/ml)

ANA = 1:80 (homogenous pattern)

Anti-CCP = < 5 units/ml (ref. 0-5 units/ml)

X ray of hands = soft tissue swelling

The patient is unlikely to have rheumatoid arthritis (negative RF and CCP). She may have a connective tissue disease (Raynaud's disease, borderline high ESR, and raised ANA titre) or an undifferentiated inflammatory polyarthritis.

86353 Lymphocyte transformation, mitogen (phytomitogen) or antigen induced blastogenesis

(Malaria antibodies, use 86750)

●**86355** B cells, total count

●**86357** Natural killer (NK) cells, total count

86359 T cells; total count

86360 absolute CD4 and CD8 count, including ratio

86361 absolute CD4 count

●**86367** Stem cells (ie, CD34), total count

►(For flow cytometric immunophenotyping for the assessment of potential hematolymphoid neoplasia, see 88184-88189)◄

86378 Migration inhibitory factor test (MIF)

(Mitochondrial antibody, liver, see 86255, 86256)

(Mononucleosis, see 86308-86310)

►(86379 has been deleted. For natural killer cells, total count, use 86357)◄

Rationale

A cross-references has been added after 86367 instructing users to 88184-88189 for reporting flow cytometric immunophenotyping for the assessment of potential hematolymphoid neoplasia.

Natural killer (NK) cell code 86379 has been deleted and renumbered to 86357 to report this service. Stem cell code 86587 has been deleted and renumbered to 86367. The flow cytometric cross-reference has also been relocated after code 86355. This relocation is an effort to allay confusion by putting the NK cell code and stem cell code in a location adjacent to the lymphocyte T-cell series of codes.

86430 Rheumatoid factor; qualitative

86431 quantitative

(Serologic test for syphilis, see 86592, 86593)

●**86480** Tuberculosis test, cell mediated immunity measurement of gamma interferon antigen response

Rationale

Code 86480 was established with the conversion of Category III code 0010T to Category I status. The language from the previous descriptor has been retained because the necessary effort and specific work required to perform this service has not changed. Code 86480 is intended to describe tuberculosis (TB) testing by cell-mediated immunity measurement of gamma interferon antigen response.

This in vitro blood test is an ELISA-based analysis that involves stimulation of a whole blood sample with TB-specific proteins and controls, and measurement of a single cytokine: Interferon gamma, using single-step sandwich ELISA technique. It measures cell-mediated immune (CMI) response (ie, specific T cell response) to determine TB infection with patient results compared to a universal cut-off value independent of risk stratification. A positive test result does not necessarily indicate the presence or absence of active TB disease. Other diagnostic procedures, such as X-ray examination of the chest and microbiological examination of sputum, should be used when active TB disease is suspected. The treatment options for a patient considered to have latent TB infection are at the discretion of the physician.

Clinical Example (86480)

An individual presents with an associated risk of having Mycobacterium tuberculosis (TB) infection or with suspected active TB. The disease is known to occur in individuals from countries with high TB prevalence, inmates and staff from correctional facilities, homeless persons, injection drug users, TB contacts, and patients with immunosuppressive conditions (eg, HIV disease). This test is most useful for determination of M. tuberculosis infection for those persons who have had prior Bacillus Calmette Guerin (BCG) vaccination or are exposed to non-tuberculous mycobacteria.

Tuberculosis testing is routinely performed for persons who are: (1) suspected as having active TB; (2) at increased risk for progression to active TB; (3) at increased risk for latent TB infection; or (4) at low risk for latent TB infection, but whose future activity may place them at increased risk for exposure (eg, military personnel and health care workers).

The test is based on the measurement of a CMI response in TB-infected individuals. The T cells of these individuals are sensitized to M. tuberculosis, and respond to stimulation with TB-specific proteins by secreting a cytokine called Interferon-gamma. The TB-specific proteins used in the test are ESAT-6 and CFP-10. Both are absent from all BCG strains and from most non-tuberculous mycobacteria, with the exception of M. kansasii, M. szulgai, and M. marinum. The ESAT-6 and CFP proteins stimulate Interferon-gamma responses in T cells from TB-infected individuals but not from uninfected or BCG-vaccinated persons.

86485 Skin test; candida

86580 tuberculosis, intradermal

(For tuberculosis test, cell mediated immunity measurement of gamma interferon antigen response, use ►86480◄)

►(86585 has been deleted. To report tuberculosis testing by intradermal (Mantoux) test, use 86580)◄

Rationale

In tandem with the conversion of Category III code 0010T to a Category I code, the cross-reference following code 86580 has been revised to refer the user to the new code. A cross-reference has also been added to note deletion of code 86580. Intradermal (Mantoux) tuberculosis testing is now reported with 86580.

86586 Unlisted antigen, each

▶(86587 has been deleted. For stem cells, total count, use 86367)◀

Rationale

A cross-reference has been added to note the deletion and renumbering of stem cell code 86587 from its previous alpha-order location in the Immunology subsection of Pathology and Laboratory to a location adjacent to the lymphocyte T-cell series of codes.

Stem cell code 86587 has been deleted and renumbered to 86367 to report this service.

Transfusion Medicine

86920 Compatibility test each unit; immediate spin technique

86922 antiglobulin technique

●**86923** electronic

▶(Do not use 86923 in conjunction with 86920-86922 for same unit crossmatch)◀

Rationale

Code 86923 was established to report a pretransfusion electronic crossmatch test. Additionally, an exclusionary parenthetical has been added to restrict reporting a manual test (86920-86922) with an electronic test (86923).

The electronic crossmatch code (86923) provides a third code to report crossmatching in addition to the immediate spin crossmatch (86920) and antiglobulin techniques (86922). This form of crossmatch does not include these techniques, hence a new code was necessary to report the service when the laboratory information system verifies ABO compatibility of the unit of blood with the intended recipient.

Clinical Example (86923)

An 80-year-old patient presenting with acute gastrointestinal bleeding secondary to an esophageal varix malformation presents with anemia. The patient has an ABO, Rh, and antibody screen performed. Because the patient has a negative antibody screen and no history of clinically significant antibodies, an electronic crossmatch may be performed. Since a prior ABO/Rh type is on file for the patient, a second patient ABO/Rh test is not required. An electronic crossmatch is then performed for each unit prepared for the patient.

Description of Procedure (86923)

The technologist verifies that the patient qualifies for an electronic crossmatch by reviewing the ABO/Rh and antibody screening data; he also reviews the antibody history and assesses whether any of the antibodies identified are clinically significant.

The technologist selects ABO/Rh compatible units from the inventory and performs an electronic verification of compatibility. The units are labeled for the patient and may then be issued for immediate transfusion or stored for future release.

●**86960** Volume reduction of blood or blood product (eg, red blood cells or platelets), each unit

Rationale

Code 86960 was established to report volume reduction of red blood cells or platelets.

Hospital transfusion services use "volume reduction" routinely to reduce the amount of ABO incompatible plasma from the platelets (or rarely a red blood cell component) that are to be transfused. Because apheresis-collected platelets contain a plasma volume of approximately 200 ml, and if that component contains an "incompatible" ABO plasma antibody, hemolysis of the recipient's red cells could occur. This shortage is alleviated by reducing the amount of plasma in the component prior to issue. This manual process requires centrifugation, sterile docking (connecting) another bag, expression off the residual plasma, and disconnection of the plasma-containing bag from the platelet component. The same type of process can be performed for whole blood-derived platelets (plasma volume of approximately 30 ml) when the recipient is a neonate. Volume reduction may also be required for the recipient with cardiac or renal problems that would restrict the amount of fluids (such as in a full plasma containing unit) that the patient should receive.

Clinical Example (86960)

A female pediatric patient whose blood type is B negative requires a platelet transfusion due to a low platelet count. The hospital transfusion service has no ABO type-specific (B) platelets, but does have an O negative component. This component contains antibodies (anti-A, B) in the plasma. By reducing the plasma content of the available unit, this platelet pheresis component is transfused without clinical sequelae.

Microbiology

87177 Ova and parasites, direct smears, concentration and identification

(Do not report 87177 in conjunction with 87015)

(For direct smears from a primary source, use 87207)

(For coccidia or microsporidia exam, use 87207)

►(For complex special stain (trichrome, iron hematoxylin), use 87209)◄

(For nucleic acid probes in cytologic material, use 88365)

(For molecular diagnostics, see 83890-83898, 87470-87799)

87205 Smear, primary source with interpretation; Gram or Giemsa stain for bacteria, fungi, or cell types

87207 special stain for inclusion bodies or parasites (eg, malaria, coccidia, microsporidia, trypanosomes, herpes viruses)

(For direct smears with concentration and identification, use 87177)

(For thick smear preparation, use 87015)

(For fat, meat, fibers, nasal eosinophils, and starch, see miscellaneous section)

●**87209** complex special stain (eg, trichrome, iron hemotoxylin) for ova and parasites

Rationale

Two microbiology cross-references regarding anatomic pathology special stains or complex stains codes (88312 and 88313) have been deleted because these are distinctly different analyses. These cross-references were previously located after codes 87177 and 87207. Instead, a separate microbiology code (87209) was added to describe complex special stains for ova and parasites, thus eliminating the need for a cross-reference.

Clinical Example (87209)

A 35-year-old man presents with severe diarrhea following a prolonged hiking expedition. Fecal analysis for parasites is requested, including trichrome stains to assess for intestinal parasite infestation.

Description of Procedure (87209)

The patient submits a fecal sample in PVA transport fluid and in Formalin transport fluid. A portion of the PVA specimen is processed, stained with the trichrome procedure, and microscopically analyzed for protozoa (88313). The Formalin sample is concentrated and microscopically examined for ova and parasites (87177).

●**87900** Infectious agent drug susceptibility phenotype prediction using regularly updated genotypic bioinformatics

87901 Infectious agent genotype analysis by nucleic acid (DNA or RNA); HIV 1, reverse transcriptase and protease

(For infectious agent drug susceptibility phenotype prediction for HIV-1, use ►87900◄)

Rationale

Category III code 0023T has been converted to Category I code 87900. Code 87900 is intended to describe infectious agent drug susceptibility phenotype prediction using regularly updated genotypic bioinformatics.

This service is widely used in the management of HIV patients on antiretroviral therapy. This service provides a quantitative prediction of drug susceptibility phenotype for each antiretroviral drug and provides the clinician with a numeric measure of susceptibility or resistance on which to base the selection of multi-drug regimens necessary for effective HIV disease management.

The prediction of phenotypic behavior derives from comparison of the genotypic patterns of the patient with a large relational database of actual phenotypic and genotypic information that is continuously updated with recent clinical isolates representing the changing nature of the pandemic.

Clinical Example (87900)

The patient is a 33-year-old male who has been treated for 2 years with three types of HIV medication. His viral load has generally been less than 50 copies during this time, with occasional blips greater than 200 copies. The patient admits to short periods of non-adherence. Today's visit to the clinic revealed a viral load of 5600 copies.

A plasma sample is drawn for HIV drug resistance testing (genotype and virtual phenotype).

The patient is instructed to continue the current course of therapy and return in 2 weeks when results of the virtual phenotype will be available.

The patient returns in 2 weeks. Results of the HIV drug resistance tests demonstrate a number of HIV gene mutations that suggest emerging resistance to drugs in the current treatment regimen. The virtual phenotype report shows that within the NRTI drug category, a number of agents demonstrate high levels of resistance.

The remaining drugs within the NRTI class show different levels of sensitivity (approximately 60-65% of matched samples were within the normal susceptibility range).

The virtual phenotype analysis also demonstrates levels of resistance or sensitivity to drugs within the other available drug classes including a high level of resistance to one of the drugs included in the current regimen and high sensitivity to drugs in the NRTI class.

87903 Infectious agent phenotype analysis by nucleic acid (DNA or RNA) with drug resistance tissue culture analysis, HIV 1; first through 10 drugs tested

+▲87904 each additional drug tested (List separately in addition to code for primary procedure)

(Use 87904 in conjunction with 87903)

Rationale

Add-on code 87904 has been revised to eliminate reference to the range of the number of drugs being tested to more accurately reflect the reporting for these procedures. The revised descriptor more appropriately describes the test process and resources required to analyze each additional drug that must be included in the phenotype test.

Taking into account the patient's clinical history, findings from the current physical examination, laboratory test results, and the HIV drug resistance data (including virtual phenotype), the clinician and patient agree to discontinue the current drug regimen and to institute a new regimen.

Clinical Example (87904)

The typical patient is a 36-year-old, white female. She has been HIV-1 positive for 7 years. For the past 9 months she has been taking a three-drug regimen. On this therapy, the HIV-1 RNA has been less then 50 copies/ml and the CD4 count has been greater than 500 cells/mm^3.

On periodic follow-up, the viral load has increased to 2200 copies/ml. This result is confirmed on repeat testing. The CD4 count has decreased to 450 cells/mm^3. The physician confirms by patient interview that she is taking her medicine as prescribed. The physician concludes his patient has failed highly active anti-retroviral therapy (HAART) for the first time. He orders an HIV phenotype resistance test. The physician expects the phenotype resistance test will test the patient's virus against all of the Food and Drug Administration approved and commonly prescribed anti-HIV drugs, including recently approved drugs. The patient is instructed to return in 4 weeks to adjust the antiretroviral therapy based on the results of the phenotype resistance test. Based on the HIV resistance phenotype test, the physician chooses four drugs as the new regimen to treat the patient.

Cytopathology

Codes 88141-88155, 88164-88167, 88174-88175 are used to report cervical or vaginal screening by various methods and to report physician interpretation services. Use codes 88150-88154 to report ►conventional◄ Pap smears that are examined using non-Bethesda reporting. Use codes 88164-88167 to report ►conventional◄ Pap smears that are examined using the Bethesda System of reporting. Use codes 88142-88143 to report ►liquid-based◄ specimens ►processed as◄ thin-layer preparations that are examined using any system of reporting (Bethesda or non-Bethesda). Use codes 88174-88175 to report automated screening of ►liquid-based◄ specimens that are examined using any system of reporting (Bethesda or non-Bethesda). Within each of these three code families choose the one code that describes the screening method(s) used. Codes 88141 and 88155 should be reported in addition to the screening code chosen when the additional services are provided. ►Manual rescreening requires a complete visual reassessment of the entire slide initially screened by either an automated or manual process. Manual review represents an assessment of selected cells or regions of a slide identified by initial automated review.◄

88141 Cytopathology, cervical or vaginal (any reporting system), requiring interpretation by physician

(Use 88141 in conjunction with 88142-88154, 88164-88167, 88174-88175)

88172 Cytopathology, evaluation of fine needle aspirate; immediate cytohistologic study to determine adequacy of specimen(s)

88173 interpretation and report

►(For fine needle aspirate, see 10021, 10022)◄

►(Do not report 88172, 88173 in conjunction with 88333 and 88334 for the same specimen)◄

88174 Cytopathology, cervical or vaginal (any reporting system), collected in preservative fluid, automated thin layer preparation; screening by automated system, under physician supervision

▲88175 with screening by automated system and manual rescreening or review, under physician supervision

(For manual screening, see 88142, 88143)

(88180 has been deleted. To report, see 88184-88189)

(For DNA ploidy analysis by morphometric technique, use 88358)

Rationale

The CPT add-on symbol (✚) and add-on status were eliminated from code 88141. The elimination of the add-on code status for code 88141 will allow reporting for professional interpretation by a physician or pathologist who is not associated with the laboratory providing the technical component.

Code 88175 was revised to broaden the intent of the code with the inclusion of review. The guidelines following 88140 in the Cytopathology subsection of the Pathology and Laboratory section were editorially revised for clarity and to provide instructions regarding manual rescreening and manual review.

Code 88175 previously described a complete visual re-assessment of the entire slide initially screened by either an automated or manual process. With the expansion of the language, code 88175 will also describe an assessment of selected cells or regions of a slide identified by initial automated review.

The introductory explanatory notes have been revised for three reasons. First, appropriate reporting instructions for conventional Pap smears using non-Bethesda (88150-88154) and the Bethesda system (88164-88167) have been added. Second, since a recent advance in technology for evaluation of liquid-based cervical or vaginal cytologies is available, the notes include appropriate reporting instructions for these services (88142-88143). Finally, and consistent with revised code 88175, the requirements for manual rescreening and manual review are clarified.

Additionally, two parenthetical notes were added following code 88173 clarifying the appropriate fine needle aspirate codes to report and restricting the reporting of codes 88172, 88173 in conjunction with 88333 and 88334 for the same specimen.

Clinical Example (88175)

An 18-year-old nulliparous sexually active female presents for annual exam desiring contraception. A cervical brush and scrape is submitted in a preservative fluid for preparation at a central laboratory of a liquid-based slide. The slide is mounted on an imager and scanned and followed by visualization of the 22 most significant fields by the cytotechnologist. No abnormalities are noted. It is filed as negative for atypical or malignant cells.

Cytogenetic Studies

When molecular diagnostic procedures are performed to test for oncologic or inherited disorder, use the appropriate modifier to specify probe type or condition tested. (See **Appendix I** ▶for a listing of appropriate modifiers to report with molecular diagnostic and cytogenetic procedures.◀)

(For acetylcholinesterase, use 82013)

(For alpha-fetoprotein, serum or amniotic fluid, see 82105, 82106)

(For laser microdissection of cells from tissue sample, see 88380)

88230 Tissue culture for non-neoplastic disorders; lymphocyte

Rationale

The guidelines that instruct the use of modifiers with the molecular laboratory testing code related to genetic testing have been revised to clarify the circumstances of use.

Surgical Pathology

88329 Pathology consultation during surgery;

88331 first tissue block, with frozen section(s), single specimen

88332 each additional tissue block with frozen section(s)

●**88333** cytologic examination (eg, touch prep, squash prep), initial site

●**88334** cytologic examination (eg, touch prep, squash prep), each additional site

▶(For intraoperative consultation on a specimen requiring both frozen section and cytologic evaluation, use 88331 and 88334)◀

▶(For percutaneous needle biopsy requiring intraprocedural cytologic examination, use 88333)◀

▶(Do not report 88333 and 88334 for non-intraoperative cytologic examination, see 88160-88162)◀

▶(Do not report 88333 and 88334 for intraprocedural cytologic evaluation of fine needle aspirate, see 88172)◀

Rationale

Two codes, 88333 and 88334, were established to report intraoperative cytologic examination (via touch or squash preparation) and consultation to provide immediate diagnoses during an intraoperative consultation without the involvement of frozen section. These codes are distinguished by the initial site examination (88333) and examination of each additional specimen (88334). Code 88334 is intended to be reported one time for each additional specimen in addition to the initial site examination (88333), and the frozen section evaluation (88331), as indicated in the cross-reference following code 88334.

Clinical Example (88333)

A 45-year-old woman with a mammary carcinoma previously diagnosed by needle biopsy presents for sentinel lymph node biopsy with possible axillary dissection. Following radioisotopic and methylene blue injection around the tumor, the surgeon performs an axillary lymph node biopsy guided by the tracers and methylene blue staining. The surgeon then requests an intraoperative pathology consultation. The pathologist performs an intraoperative touch prep examination on the sentinel lymph node. As the pathologist does not identify malignant cells, the surgeon elects not to proceed with the axillary lymph node dissection.

Description of Procedure (88333)

The pathologist comes to the operating room and reviews the pertinent clinical information with the surgeon. The pathologist takes the biopsy to the intraoperative pathology suite where the patient's original diagnosis is confirmed by a query into the anatomic pathology computer system. The specimen is dissected and grossly examined, and multiple cross sections are made and evaluated for macroscopic tumor involvement. A glass slide is labeled with the patient's name and another slide-specific identifier. The tissue is prepared and arranged for the cell transfer. A slide is carefully touched to the tissue and immediately fixed. It is stained by hematoxylin and eosin and coverslipped by the pathologist. The pathologist screens and evaluates the entire slide for evidence of malignant cells. Following this, the pathologist presents a verbal report intraoperatively to the surgeon and records a written confirmation of this report in the patient's medical record.

Clinical Example (88334)

A 45-year-old woman with a mammary carcinoma presents with a mammographically suspicious breast mass, treated with surgical mass excision. After an intraoperative diagnosis of malignancy is made by the pathologist on a lumpectomy specimen, the surgeon requests a pathology intraoperative assessment of the margins of the same specimen for the presence or absence of a tumor. As the pathologist identifies malignant cells at the anterosuperior surgical margin of resection, the surgeon elects to re-excise this margin.

Description of Procedure (88334)

Following the intraoperative frozen section or cytologic diagnosis of carcinoma rendered by the pathologist, whereby the tumor grossly approximates the anterosuperior surgical margin of resection, an additional glass slide is labeled with the patient's name and another slide-specific identifier. A touch preparation is performed from this margin of resection. The tissue is prepared and arranged for the cell transfer. A slide is touched carefully to the tissue and immediately fixed. The slide is stained by hematoxylin and eosin and coverslipped by the pathologist. The pathologist screens and evaluates the slide preparation for evidence of malignant cells, rendering a diagnosis of "Malignant cells present at the anterosuperior surgical margin of resection." Following this, the pathologist presents the verbal report and records a written confirmation of this report in the patient's medical record.

88380 Microdissection (eg, mechanical, laser capture)

●**88384** Array-based evaluation of multiple molecular probes; 11 through 50 probes

●**88385** 51 through 250 probes

●**88386** 251 through 500 probes

►(For preparation of array-based evaluation, see 83890-83892, 83898-83901)◄

►(For preparation and analyses of less than 11 probes, see 83890-83914)◄

Rationale

Three new codes were established to report array-based evaluation of multiple molecular probes with the inclusion of two parenthetical statements to instruct the user to report codes 83696 and 83912 for services that use less than 11 probes and to use codes 83890-83892, 83898-83901 for specimen preparation.

Code 88384 was established to report array-based evaluation of multiple probes, 11 through 50 probes. Code 88385 was established to report array-based evaluation of multiple probes, 51 through 250 probes. Code 88386 was established to report array-based evaluation of multiple probes, 251 through 500 probes.

The National Institutes of Health (NIH) defines microarray, sometimes called a gene chip or a DNA chip, as consisting of large numbers of molecules (often, but not always, DNA) distributed in rows in a very small space. It is a tool used to sift through and analyze the information contained within a genome. A microarray consists of different nucleic acid probes that are chemically attached to a substrate, which can be a microchip, a glass slide, or a microsphere-sized bead. Microarrays permit scientists to study gene expression by providing a snapshot of a variable multitude of genes that are present in a particular cell type.

In contrast to the CPT codes in the molecular diagnostics section of the 80000 series, these codes contain both the technical component to capture the actual performance of the array and the professional component to accommodate the professional interpretation of the data provided by the analysis. These codes do not include the technical components required to prepare the specimen or amplification of the genetic material for analysis, nor do they include the professional management and administrative oversight of these later components.

These codes were added to the Anatomic Pathology subsection because they were primarily intended to be used in the processing of specimens typically analyzed by traditional surgical and cytopathology techniques.

Clinical Example (88386)

A 48-year-old male patient is evaluated by an oncologist for myeloma. To aid in clarifying the patient's prognosis and treatment options, the clinician orders comparative genomic hybridization (CGH) array on the marrow. Anticoagulated marrow aspirate is submitted to the laboratory for gene dosage testing at 300 different chromosomal loci using commercial reagents that have been previously analytically validated in the clinical laboratory. A pathologist reviews a Wright's stained aspirate smear to determine whether the proportion of plasma cells is sufficient to warrant gene dosage testing. The marrow differential count reveals 30% plasma cells, which the pathologist determines is sufficient to proceed with gene dosage testing. A technologist performs the gene dosage test, along with controls. The pathologist assesses the gene dosage assay performance, including the examination of the positive and negative controls samples, interprets the finding in the patient, and assigns results (analytic interpretation), as well as the significance of the results for this patient (clinical interpretation). The analytic results in this patient were monosomy for chromosomes 13 and 22, monosomy for 17p13 (the TP53 locus), and partial monosomy of chromosome 14. The pathologist synthesizes these data, along with correlation of morphologic and clinical information. A report is composed, describing the patient's allelotype and the clinical implications of this result, including the clinical interpretation of the patient's increased risk of progression and relapse following standard therapy.

Description of Procedure (88386)

Discussion of the potential service is held with the technologist or referring pathologist or clinician prior to the receipt of the specimen. This discussion ensures that the patient is an appropriate candidate for the diagnostic evaluation and clarifies the necessity of referral of clinical history, tumor blocks, routine slides from biopsy and/or resection(s), and additional data (eg, immunostains, immunophenotyping, cytogenetics, as appropriate). A pathologist reviews a Wright's stained aspirate smear to determine whether the proportion of plasma cells is sufficient to warrant gene dosage testing. The marrow differential count reveals 30% plasma cells, which the pathologist determines is sufficient. Following the extraction, isolation, and purification of the sample by the technologist along with controls, the pathologist assesses the gene dosage assay performance, including the examination of the positive and negative control samples. He or she then analytically interprets the findings in the patient and assesses the significance of the results for this patient by correlating the analysis with clinical and morphologic data. The analytic results in this patient included monosomy for chromosomes 13 and 22, monosomy for 17p13 (the TP53 locus), and partial monosomy of chromosome 14. The pathologist analyzes the computer findings. The pathologist prepares the report, describing the patient's allelotype and the clinical implications of this result including the clinical interpretation that the patient is at increased risk of progression and relapse following a standardized chemotherapy regimen. The pathologist verbally communicates the results of the profile with the referring pathologist and/or clinician providing him or her with overall results and additional information regarding statistical data and limitations of the predictive value of the recurrence score. The pathologist also answers any questions specific to that clinical circumstance.

Other Procedures

●**89049** Caffeine halothane contracture test (CHCT) for malignant hyperthermia susceptibility, including interpretation and report

Rationale

Code 89049 was established to report performance of the caffeine halothane contracture test (CHCT) for identification of individuals who are susceptible to malignant hyperthermia (MH). MH becomes evident upon exposure to certain common anesthetic agents during surgery. The MH-susceptible patient will develop an extremely high metabolic rate, resulting in symptoms such as muscular rigidity and hyperthermia in excess of 110°F. When the anesthetized patient exhibits these symptoms, swift measures must be taken by the anesthesiologist to reverse the symptoms to prevent organ damage and death. Susceptibility to MH is inherited. The CHCT is performed on patients with a family history of MH or a past medical history indicating susceptibility. Upon confirmation of susceptibility, anesthetics can be planned to avoid triggering MH.

Prior to performance of the CHCT test, a sample of muscle tissue is required for the test. The work involved in excising the muscle tissue for the test is separately reported. Typically, a separate physician (ie, someone other than the individual performing the CHCT) will harvest the muscle from the patient. The physician who performs the harvest of the tissue should report a code that identifies the effort necessary to obtain the tissue needed for testing (eg, 27324, Biopsy, soft tissue of thigh or knee area; deep [subfascial or intramuscular]).

Clinical Example (89049)

A patient with a previous adverse reaction to anesthesia requires CHCT performed on freshly biopsied muscle for definitive diagnosis prior to further anesthesia exposure.

Note: Any work associated with obtaining the muscle specimen itself is separately reportable and should **not** be considered when evaluating the work of the CHCT.

Description of Procedure (89049)

The technician will prepare fresh Krebs-Ringer solution and the apparatus required to perform the test and confirm quality control. As part of the separately reported muscle biopsy procedure, muscle is obtained, preferably from the vastus group of the lower extremity. The muscle sample is placed on a tongue depressor and secured and placed in a Krebs-Ringer solution and maintained at room temperature. The muscle is promptly transported to the anesthesia testing laboratory. All caffeine contracture testing must be performed within 5 hours. The muscle is grossly inspected by the technician to ensure that the specimen is not stretched, distorted, or otherwise injured. The muscle sample is dissected to achieve a fascicle size of 1-2 cm in length and 0.1-0.5 cm in width.

The specimen is inspected under magnification to ensure the muscle fascicles are not nicked or otherwise injured. During this process, the muscle is not manually handled and is placed in a carbogenated Krebs-Ringer solution (95% oxygen and

5% carbon dioxide). Some of the testing components include a force transducer, glass chambers for exposure to testing solutions, a muscle twitch stimulator preferably made of platinum to allow twitch stimulation of 0.1-0.2 Hz every 5-10 seconds with a pulse duration up to 5 msec, ventilation hood to scavenge vapors, and a multi-channel electrophysiologic recorder. A technician mounts the muscle to the force transducer in the presence of the Krebs-Ringer solution and the muscle is allowed to equilibrate at 37°C for a minimum of 30 minutes until stable twitch height is attained upon stimulation. To attain adequate diagnostic criteria, a minimum of three muscle strips should be tested in each of the solutions. The solutions will include halothane and caffeine. The primary solution will again be carbogenated Krebs-Ringer with a pH of 7.4 and a temperature of 37°C. Halothane will be administered via a calibrated vaporizer to maintain a concentration of 3% (19-24 mm Hg partial pressure). Caffeine will be used in increasing concentrations from 0.5 mM to 32 mM. Positive results (the patient is susceptible to malignant hyperthermia) are considered with the following responses: contracture of muscle as greater than or equal to 0.5 g as measured by the force transducer in the presence of 3% halothane by 10 minutes duration; greater than or equal to 0.3 g increase in tension on exposure to 2 mM caffeine. The combined results of testing six strips gives statistical validation with the thresholds determined by the North American Malignant Hyperthermia consultants with a 98% sensitivity and 78% specificity of the test results. Each result is interpreted to review the characteristics of the testing, the validity of the testing in regards to the muscle specimen that was obtained, and the suitability of the testing conditions. The technician obtains and records measurements for physician review. The physician must remain on site throughout the procedure for consultation with the laboratory technician.

Medicine

Revisions to the Medicine section of the CPT codebook include complete and near complete revision of the Therapeutic or Diagnostic Infusions, Therapeutic, Prophylactic, or Diagnostic Injections and Chemotherapy Administration subsections, with the addition, revision, and deletion of many codes and guidelines. New codes and guidelines have been added to report moderate (conscious) sedation. Use of the new FDA approval pending indicator is evident in the Vaccines, Toxoids subsection. Also, important revisions have been made to the Ophthalmology subsection, with the deletion of the supply codes, and to the Acupuncture subsection.

Medicine

Immune Globulins

Codes 90281-90399 identify the immune globulin product only and must be reported in addition to the administration codes 90765-90768, 90772, 90774, 90775 as appropriate. Immune globulin products listed here include broad-spectrum and anti-infective immune globulins, antitoxins, and various isoantibodies.

Rationale

To correlate with the revisions of the Therapeutic, Prophylactic, and Diagnostic Infusion and Injections section, the injection codes listed in the explanatory text for immune globulins have been modified to list new codes 90765, 90768, 90772, 90774, and 90775.

Immunization Administration for Vaccines/Toxoids

Codes 90465-90474 must be reported in . . .

Report codes 90465-90468 only when the . . .

If a significant separately identifiable Evaluation . . .

(For allergy testing, see 95004 et seq)

(For skin testing of bacterial, viral, fungal extracts, see 86485-86586)

(For therapeutic or diagnostic injections, see ▶90772◀-90779)

Rationale

To correlate with the revisions of the Therapeutic, Prophylactic, and Diagnostic Infusion and Injections section, the injection codes listed in the explanatory parenthetical note have been revised to include the new codes.

Vaccines, Toxoids

▶To assist users to report the most recent new or revised vaccine product codes, the American Medical Association currently uses the CPT Web site, which features updates of CPT Editorial Panel actions regarding these products. Once approved by the CPT Editorial Panel, these codes will be made available for release on a semi-annual (twice a year—July 1 and January 1) basis. As part of the electronic distribution, there is a 6-month implementation period from the initial release date (ie, codes released on January 1 are eligible for use on July 1 and codes released on July 1 are eligible for use January 1).◀

▶The CPT Editorial Panel, in recognition of the public health interest in vaccine products, has chosen to publish new vaccine product codes prior to FDA approval. These codes are indicated with the ✗ symbol and will be tracked by the AMA to monitor FDA approval status. Once the FDA status changes to approval, the ⁄⁄ symbol will be removed. CPT users should refer to the AMA Internet site for the most up-to-date information on codes with the ⁄⁄ symbol. (www.ama-assn.org/ama/pub/category/10902.html)◄

Codes 90476-90748 identify the vaccine product . . .

(For immune globulins, see codes 90281-90399, 90765-90768, 90772-90775 for administration of immune globulins)

Rationale

The guidelines for the Vaccines, Toxoids section of the CPT codebook have been updated to explain the use of a new CPT symbol (⁄⁄) created to identify vaccine or toxoid products that have not yet received, at the time of their code assignment, FDA approval. Since it is anticipated that these vaccines will receive FDA approval, the American Medical Association (AMA) will update the status of these codes once the vaccine is approved by omitting the symbol assigned to these codes. News of these updates can be found on the AMA CPT Web site under Category I Vaccine Codes (www.ama-assn.org/ama/pub/category/10902.html) and in subsequent publications of the CPT codebook. The guidelines also have been updated to explain the "early release" of Category I vaccine product codes, which enables codes to be released electronically (www.ama-assn.org/ama/pub/category/10902.html) on a semi-annual basis (July 1 and January 1). As part of the electronic distribution, there is a 6-month implementation period from the initial release date (ie, codes released on January 1 are eligible for use on July 1 and codes released on July 1 are eligible for use January 1).

⊘ ⁄⁄ ●**90649** Human Papilloma virus (HPV) vaccine, types 6, 11, 16, 18 (quadrivalent), 3 dose schedule, for intramuscular use

Rationale

Code 90649 has been added for a vaccine product that is intended for use in individuals 9 through 26 years of age and developed to offer protection against the common types of the human papilloma virus (HPV) (Types 6, 11, 16, 18). Human papilloma virus, which may appear in the form of genital warts, is often a precursor to cervical dysplasia and cancer. This vaccine is currently pending FDA approval, as indicated by the newly created CPT symbol (⁄⁄). CPT users will be instructed to refer to the AMA Web site for updated information relating to the FDA status of this vaccine (www.ama-assn.org/ama/pub/category/10902.html). Once the FDA status changes to approval, the pending FDA approval symbol will be removed from the affected CPT codes and this update will be reflected on the AMA Web site posting and in subsequent CPT publications.

⊘ ⁄⁄ ▲**90680** Rotavirus vaccine, pentavalent, 3 dose schedule, live, for oral use

Rationale

A new vaccine product has been developed to offer protection from rotavirus, a cause of severe gastroenteritis in children. Code 90680 has been revised to describe the new rotavirus vaccine product, which contains five serotypes (G1, G2, G3, G4, and P1). This vaccine is currently pending FDA approval as indicated in the newly created CPT symbol (⁄⁄). CPT users are instructed to refer to the AMA CPT Web site for updated information related to the FDA status of this vaccine (www.ama-assn.org/ama/pub/-category/10902.html). Once the vaccine receives FDA approval, the symbol will be removed from code 90680 on the AMA CPT Web site and in subsequent CPT publications.

⊘▲**90713** Poliovirus vaccine, inactivated, (IPV), for subcutaneous or intramuscular use

Rationale

Code 90713 was revised to include reference to the intramuscular route of administration in addition to the subcutaneous route previously described for inactivated polio virus vaccine.

⊘●**90714** Tetanus and diphtheria toxoids (Td) adsorbed, preservative free, for use in individuals 7 years or older, for intramuscular use

Rationale

Code 90714 has been added to describe a preservative-free diphtheria (Td) vaccine that will be used as a routine vaccine in early adolescent and is recommended in individuals 7 years or older.

Code number 90714 was previously assigned to a vaccine that was deleted in *CPT 1999*. Code 90714 was reused to maintain proximal sequencing for vaccine codes for similar products (eg, influenza, Hepatitis A, Hemophilus influenza b, Hepatitis B).

⊘⁄⁄▲**90715** Tetanus, diphtheria toxoids and acellular pertussis vaccine (Tdap), for use in individuals 7 years or older, for intramuscular use

Rationale

Code 90715, first appearing in *CPT 2004*, has been revised to reflect the reduced amount of pertussis antigen contained in the tetanus, diphtheria, and pertussis combination vaccine products. In order to adequately identify and facilitate correct coding, the convention of using upper and lower case letters to distinguish between varying amounts of antigen components in related vaccine products is used. For example, in code 90702, the DT is used to reflect the increased diphtheria component for children younger than age 7, and in code 90718, Td is used to indicate the reduced antigen concentration of diphtheria for children age 7 and older. This vaccine is currently pending FDA approval, as indicated by the newly created CPT symbol (⁄⁄). CPT users should refer to the AMA Web site for updated information regarding FDA status of this vaccine (www.ama-assn.org/ ama/pub/category/10902.html). Once the vaccine receives FDA approval, the pending FDA approval symbol will be removed from the designated CPT codes. This update will also be posted on the AMA Web site and in subsequent publications.

This product is anticipated to be developed separately by two different vaccine manufacturers. Currently, it is recommended that adolescents receive a Td booster (90718). However, it is likely that new recommendations will be made that will include routine vaccination against pertussis as well as Td in the adolescent population.

⊘ ⁄⁄ ●90736 Zoster (shingles) vaccine, live, for subcutaneous injection

Rationale

Code 90736 has been established to report the administration of zoster vaccine. This vaccine is provided to reduce the occurrence, severity, and duration of shingles pain. The zoster vaccine is expected to be administered to older adults. CPT users will be instructed to refer to the AMA Web site for updated information related to the FDA status of this vaccine (www.ama-assn.org/ama/pub/category/10902.html). Once the FDA approval status for this code has been revised, the pending FDA approval symbol will be removed from the designated CPT code. This update will be posted on the AMA Web site and will be noted in subsequent CPT publications.

⊘90749 Unlisted vaccine/toxoid

▸Hydration, Therapeutic, Prophylactic, and Diagnostic Injections and Infusions (Excludes Chemotherapy)◂

▶Physician work related to hydration, injection, and infusion services predominantly involves affirmation of treatment plan and direct supervision of staff.◀

▶If a significant separately identifiable Evaluation and Management service is performed, the appropriate E/M service code should be reported using modifier 25 in addition to 90760-90779. For same day E/M service a different diagnosis is not required.◀

▶If performed to facilitate the infusion or injection, the following services are included and are not reported separately:◀

▶a. Use of local anesthesia◀

▶b. IV start◀

▶c. Access to indwelling IV, subcutaneous catheter or port◀

▶d. Flush at conclusion of infusion◀

▶e. Standard tubing, syringes, and supplies◀

▶(For declotting a catheter or port, see 36550)◀

▶When multiple drugs are administered, report the service(s) and the specific materials or drugs for each.◀

▶When administering multiple infusions, injections or combinations, only one "initial" service code should be reported, unless protocol requires that two separate IV sites must be used. The "initial" code that best describes the key or primary reason for the encounter should always be reported irrespective of the order in which the infusions or injections occur. If an injection or infusion is of a subsequent or concurrent nature, even if it is the first such service within that group of services, then a subsequent or concurrent code from the appropriate section should be reported (eg, the first IV push given subsequent to an initial one-hour infusion is reported using a subsequent IV push code).◀

▶When reporting codes for which infusion time is a factor, use the actual time over which the infusion is administered.◀

▶Hydration◀

▶Codes 90760-90761 are intended to report a hydration IV infusion to consist of a pre-packaged fluid and electrolytes (eg, normal saline, D5-$\frac{1}{2}$ normal saline +30mEq KCl/liter), but are not used to report infusion of drugs or other substances. Hydration IV infusions typically require direct physician supervision for purposes of consent, safety oversight, or intraservice supervision of staff. Typically such infusions require little special handling to prepare or dispose of, and staff that administer these do not typically require advanced practice training. After initial set-up, infusion typically entails little patient risk and thus little monitoring.◀

●**90760** Intravenous infusion, hydration; initial, up to 1 hour

▶(Do not report 90760 if performed as a concurrent infusion service)◀

+●**90761** each additional hour, up to 8 hours (List separately in addition to code for primary procedure)

▶(Use 90761 in conjunction with 90760)◀

▶(Report 90761 for hydration infusion intervals of greater than 30 minutes beyond 1 hour increments)◀

▶(Report 90761 to identify hydration if provided as a secondary or subsequent service after a different initial service [90760, 90765, 90774, 96409, 96413] is provided)◀

▶Therapeutic, Prophylactic, and Diagnostic Injections and Infusions◀

▶A therapeutic, prophylactic, or diagnostic IV infusion or injection (90765-90799) (other than hydration) is for the administration of substances/drugs. The fluid used to administer the drug(s) is incidental hydration and is not separately reportable. These services typically require direct physician supervision for any or all purposes of patient assessment, provision of consent, safety oversight, and intra-service supervision of staff. Typically, such infusions require special consideration to prepare, dose or dispose of, require practice training and competency for staff who administer the infusions, and require periodic patient assessment with vital sign monitoring during the infusion.◀

▶Intravenous or intra-arterial push is defined as: a) an injection in which the health care professional who administers the substance/drug is continuously present to administer the injection and observe the patient, or b) an infusion of 15 minutes or less.◀

▶(Do not report 90765-90779 with codes for which IV push or infusion is an inherent part of the procedure (eg, administration of contrast material for a diagnostic imaging study))◀

●90765 Intravenous infusion, for therapy, prophylaxis, or diagnosis (specify substance or drug); initial, up to 1 hour

+●90766 each additional hour, up to 8 hours (List separately in addition to code for primary procedure)

►(Report 90766 in conjunction with 90765, 90767)◄

►(Report 90766 for additional hour(s) of sequential infusion)◄

►(Report 90766 for infusion intervals of greater than 30 minutes beyond 1 hour increments)◄

+●90767 additional sequential infusion, up to 1 hour (List separately in addition to code for primary procedure)

►(Report 90767 in conjunction with 90765, 90774, 96409, 96413 if provided as a secondary or subsequent service after a different initial service. Report 90767 only once per sequential infusion of same infusate mix)◄

+●90768 concurrent infusion (List separately in addition to code for primary procedure)

►(Report 90768 only once per encounter)◄

►(Report 90768 in conjunction with 90765, 96413)◄

●90772 Therapeutic, prophylactic or diagnostic injection (specify substance or drug); subcutaneous or intramuscular

►(For administration of vaccines/toxoids, see 90465-90466, 90471-90472)◄

►(Report 90772 for non-antineoplastic hormonal therapy injections)◄

►(Report 96401 for anti-neoplastic nonhormonal injection therapy)◄

►(Report 96402 for anti-neoplastic hormonal injection therapy)◄

►(Do not report 90772 for injections given without direct physician supervision. To report, use 99211)◄

●90773 intra-arterial

●90774 intravenous push, single or initial substance/drug

►(90772-90774 do not include injections for allergen immunotherapy. For allergen immunotherapy injections, see 95115-95117)◄

+●90775 each additional sequential intravenous push of a new substance/drug (List separately in addition to code for primary procedure)

►(Use 90775 in conjunction with 90765, 90774, 96409, 96413)◄

►(Report 90775 to identify intravenous push of a new substance/drug if provided as a secondary or subsequent service after a different initial service is provided)◄

●90779 Unlisted therapeutic, prophylactic or diagnostic intravenous or intra-arterial injection or infusion

►(For allergy immunizations, see 95004 et seq)◄

►(90780 and 90781 have been deleted. To report, see 90760, 90761, 90765-90768)◄

▶(90782 has been deleted. To report, use 90772)◀

▶(90783 has been deleted. To report, use 90773)◀

▶(90784 has been deleted. To report, use 90774)◀

▶(90788 has been deleted. To report, use 90772)◀

▶(90799 has been deleted. To report, use 90779)◀

Rationale

Seven codes were deleted and 11 codes, guidelines, and related cross-references were established for reporting hydration and therapeutic, prophylactic, or diagnostic intravenous (IV) infusions or injections.

The drug administration codes are grouped into three categories: (1) hydration; (2) therapeutic, prophylactic, or diagnostic injections and intravenous (IV) infusions (other than hydration); and (3) chemotherapy administration. The new codes clarify those services that are appropriately reported by the chemotherapy administration codes expanding the definition of chemotherapy services. Previously, the chemotherapy administration services codes were considered to be appropriately reported only when the administered drug was anti-neoplastic and the diagnosis was cancer.

In order to more accurately report infusion services, several secondary service categories of new codes have been established to report additional sequential infusions, sequential intravenous pushes and intravenous chemotherapy pushes for additional drugs for hydration and therapeutic, prophylactic, or diagnostic IV infusions or injections. Previously, reporting for additional sequential infusion services was indistinguishable from additional hours of infusion.

Broad guidelines have been added that apply to both the Hydration Services and the Therapeutic, Prophylactic, and Diagnostic Injections and Infusions subsections. For each of these subsections, definitions are provided for the expected physician activity for reporting these codes; the requirements for reporting a separate evaluation and management (E/M) service; reporting sequential services and additional infusions; and reporting service time.

As indicated within the infusion guidelines, "When administering multiple infusions, injections or combinations, only one 'initial' service code should be reported, unless protocol requires that two separate IV sites must be utilized. If an injection or infusion is of a subsequent or concurrent nature, even if it is the first such service within that group of services, then a subsequent or concurrent code from the appropriate section should be reported." The initial code that should be reported is the code that best describes the primary, most significant service provided for the patient. Additional codes are secondary to the primary procedure. New definitions and codes have been added related to IV push administration in the therapeutic injections codes and in the chemotherapy services section.

Definition of the intent of the references to time (1 hour, each additional hour) in the code descriptors is also provided in the guidelines. This definition indicates that reporting the time of the service should be based only upon the administration time for the infusion. This is because the time required for the infusion was used to define the range of services included in the infusion within the hydration, therapeutic, prophylactic, and diagnostic injections and infusions codes. Services leading up to and concluding the infusion have been included in the infusion service code and are not separately reported. These services will include starting the IV and monitoring the patient post-infusion.

Hydration Services

Previously, intravenous (IV) hydration infusion services were not specifically described within the CPT codebook. Codes 90780 and 90781 were reported for all diagnostic or therapeutic infusion services involving hydration or nonchemotherapy drugs under the broad description of therapeutic or diagnostic infusions. Codes 90780 and 90781 and the related guidelines have been deleted. Hydration services should be reported with 90760-90761. New guidelines and related cross-references instruct the appropriate reporting for these codes.

As indicated in the Hydration Services guidelines, 90760-90761 are intended to report a hydration IV infusion that consists of a prepackaged fluid and/or electrolyte solutions (eg, normal saline, D5-$\frac{1}{2}$ normal saline +30mEq KC1/liter) but are not used to report infusion of drugs or other substances. Hydration IV infusion typically requires direct physician supervision for purposes of consent, safety oversight, or intraservice supervision of staff. Typically, such infusions require little special handling for preparation or disposal, and staff that administer these infusions do not typically require advanced training. After initial set up, infusion typically entails little patient risk and thus little monitoring.

However, addition of electrolytes to a bag of fluid is considered a part of the services described by 90768-90775 and would be reported with these codes based upon the route of administration and the time required to administer the solution. Fluids provided as the vehicle for the substance infused are considered to be incidental hydration and are, therefore, not separately reported.

Directions for use of modifier 25 for reporting separately identifiable E/M services indicate the separate reporting of these services, when necessary.

Code 90760 is reported for the initial hydration infusion for the service, which is greater than 15 minutes and up to 1 hour or hydration infusion greater than 30 minutes and is provided as a secondary or sequential service following a different initial infusion or chemotherapy service. Since only one initial service is reported per day, an exclusionary parenthetical note instructs that since 90760 describes an initial infusion, it would not be appropriate to report this code as a concurrent infusion service. Code 90761 is an add-on code to report hydration infusion services that extend beyond the initial hour of service. At least 30 minutes of subsequent infusion service beyond the initial hour must be provided in order to justify reporting 90761. Code 90761 is reported once for each additional hour up to eight hours. Instructional parenthetical notes also indicate that 90761 is appropriately reported as a secondary or subsequent service to the initial service codes 90765, 90774 (initial subcutaneous, intramuscular, or intravenous reference has been added to support the description of 90775 as a subsequent service to these initial services. Code 90775 is not reported for IV push injection of additional agents in the same syringe. In the instance where the service consists of administration of only one syringe containing three nonchemotherapy drugs over 15 minutes, the single injection/substance IV push code 90774 would be reported one time only. A cross-reference following 90774 directs the user to the administration codes for allergenic extracts 95115-95117.

The unlisted code for the therapeutic, prophylactic, or diagnostic injections (90799) has been deleted, and code 90779 has been established in concert with the changes to the injection services previously described.

Clinical Example (90760)
A 49-year-old female has a diagnosis of viral gastroenteritis. Intravenous hydration is prescribed. A peripheral IV line needs to be established.

Description of Procedure (90760)
The physician provides direct supervision and is immediately available in the office. The patient and the patient's response to treatment is periodically assessed by the physician. This assessment is typically done through communication with the nurse.

Clinical Example (90761)
A 49-year-old female with a diagnosis of viral gastroenteritis has 2 liters of IV hydration prescribed. At the end of the first hour, another 1500 cc remain to be infused and the infusion is continued. (This is an add-on code; code 90760 includes the IV discontinuation, flush, and discharge process.)

Description of Procedure (90761)
The physician provides direct supervision and is immediately available in the office. The physician periodically assesses the patient and the patient's response to treatment; this assessment is typically done through communication with the nurse.

Clinical Example (90765)
A 69-year-old male presents with a history of a left olecranon bursitis due to oxacillin-resistant Staphylococcus aureus. He is receiving daily infusions on an outpatient basis and has been clinically improving. A peripherally inserted central catheter (PICC) line has been previously established. (Placement of the PICC line is reported separately.)

Description of Procedure (90765)
The physician provides direct supervision and is immediately available in the office. The physician periodically assesses the patient and the patient's response to treatment; this assessment is done typically through communication with the nurse.

Clinical Example (90766)
A 32-year-old male insulin-dependent diabetic, who is status post renal transplantation, is receiving an antimycotic infusion for Cryptococcus meningitis

through an established PICC line. He is now to receive another hour of infusion. (This is an add-on code; code 90765 includes the IV discontinuation, flush, and discharge process.)

Description of Procedure (90766)
The physician provides direct supervision and is immediately available in the office. The physician periodically assesses the patient and the patient's response to treatment; this assessment is done typically through communication with the nurse.

Clinical Example (90767)
A 70-year-old female, who is status post a ruptured colonic diverticula, presents for infusion of two drugs. She has a single lumen PICC line in place. (This is an add-on code; code 90765 includes the IV discontinuation, flush, and discharge process.)

Description of Procedure (90767)
The physician provides direct supervision and is immediately available in the office. The physician periodically assesses the patient and the patient's response to treatment; this assessment is done typically through communication with the nurse.

Clinical Example (90768)
A 73-year-old patient with a diabetic ulcer and osteomyelitis presents for infusion. His wound culture was positive for several bacteria, including oxacillin-resistant Staphylococcus aureus. He is to receive an infusion of two antibiotics simultaneously through his previously established two-lumen central catheter. (This is an add-on code; code 90765 includes the IV discontinuation, flush, and discharge process.)

Description of Procedure (90768)
The physician provides direct supervision and is immediately available in the office. The physician periodically assesses the patient and the patient's response to treatment; this assessment is done typically through communication with the nurse.

Clinical Example (90772)
A 19-year-old male presents with severe dysuria. A urethral swab is performed and found to be consistent with gonorrhea.

Description of Procedure (90772)
The physician provides direct supervision and is immediately available in the office. The physician assesses the patient's response to treatment.

Clinical Example (90774)
A 58-year-old woman with no major underlying health problems presents for evaluation of nausea and vomiting. She is diagnosed with gastroenteritis with mild dehydration. An intravenous anti-emetic is prescribed, along with 1 liter of IV hydration. (The liter of hydration is separately reported.)

Description of Procedure (90774)
The physician provides direct supervision and is immediately available in the office. The physician periodically assesses the patient and the patient's response to treatment; the assessment is done typically through communication with the nurse.

Clinical Example (90775)
A 58-year-old woman with no major underlying health problems presents for evaluation of nausea and vomiting and is diagnosed as having gastroenteritis with mild dehydration. An intravenous anti-emetic is prescribed, along with 1 liter of IV hydration. The nausea persists and the physician prescribes a benzodiazepine by IV push. (The physician evaluations are reported separately. Hydration is reported separately.) (This is an add-on code; code 90774 includes the IV discontinuation, flush, and discharge process.)

Description of Procedure (90775)
The physician provides direct supervision and is immediately available in the office. The physician periodically assesses the patient and patient's response to treatment; this assessment is done typically through communication with the nurse.

Psychiatry

Hospital care by the attending physician . . .

Psychiatric Therapeutic Procedures

OTHER PSYCHIATRIC SERVICES OR PROCEDURES

►(For repetitive transcranial magnetic stimulation for treatment of clinical depression, use Category III code 0018T)◄

90862 Pharmacologic management, including prescription, use, and review of medication with no more than minimal medical psychotherapy

▲90870 Electroconvulsive therapy (includes necessary monitoring)

►(90871 has been deleted)◄

Rationale
Due to lack of peer reviewed literature supporting the efficacy of "multiple seizures" in electroconvulsive therapy, code 90871 was deleted and code 90870 was revised by removing "single seizure" from the descriptor language.

Clinical Example (90870)
A 65-year-old widower hospitalized with major depression experiences a second ECT single seizure. He is stable medically.

Dialysis

Hemodialysis

▶(90939 has been deleted. To report, use 90940)◀

▲90940 Hemodialysis access flow study to determine blood flow in grafts and arteriovenous fistulae by an indicator method

(For duplex scan of hemodialysis access, use 93990)

Rationale

Code 90939 has been deleted and 90940 has been revised in order to create one generic code and eliminate unnecessary methodological specificity for reporting a hemodialysis access flow study. Code 90940 includes the conductivity dialysance method of studying hemodialysis access flow. Code 90940 is not intended nor should it be used to describe pressure-based methods of studying hemodialysis access flow.

Clinical Example (90940)

A 63-year-old dialysis patient dialyzes three times per week with blood flow from a left arm arterio-venous loop graft. During the regularly scheduled dialysis session the blood flow rate in the arteriovenous access is determined to avoid flow-limiting stenosis to ensure adequacy of dialysis and avoidance of access clotting. The typical procedure requires attaching the sensors to the arterial and venous bloodlines of the dialyzer and recording flow. Then, the blood pump is stopped, the lines reversed, the pump restarted, and an indicator injected. Blood flow is remeasured and recorded. The pump is stopped again and the bloodlines returned to their dialysis mode and dialysis is resumed. The information is appropriately logged.

Description of Procedure (90940)

The healthcare provider supervises the aspects of the attachment of the device to the blood lines and the injection of the indicator substance or the prescription change in the machine setting ultrafiltration rates with subsequent monitoring of indicator variation. The provider evaluates the quality of the resultant data with respect to variability, consistency, and reproducibility.

Gastroenterology

91020 Gastric motility (manometric) studies

●91022 Duodenal motility (manometric) study

▶(If gastrointestinal endoscopy is performed, use 43235)◀

▶(If fluoroscopy is performed, use 76000)◀

▶(If gastric motility study is performed, use 91020)◀

Rationale

Code 91022 was established to report duodenal motility studies, a technique used to evaluate the contractile activity of the proximal small bowel. In addition to language that specifies use for *duodenal* motility, parenthetical notes have been included to assist the user in identifying other digestive motility (91020) or gastrotintestinal procedures (such as gastrointestinal endoscopy). The parenthetical notes also reference the appropriate code to use for fluoroscopic imaging (76000), if performed.

Duodenal motility studies are indicated in pediatric and adult patients with unexplained nausea and vomiting, particularly when gastric emptying is normal, or equivocal, or when severe symptoms persist despite therapeutic trials. These studies are also indicated in patients with suspected pseudo-obstruction, systemic sclerosis, recurrent small bowel bacterial overgrowth, and to exclude diffuse gut motility prior to colectomy in a patient with constipation.

By demonstration of normal motor function in the small bowel, dysmotility and direct diagnostic evaluation can definitively be excluded elsewhere. The changes in the intraluminal pressure activity of the small bowel are measured through either a water-perfused or solid-state catheter, which is placed in the small bowel. The motility changes are measured both in the fasting state and after meals. In the fasting state, the presence of muscle contractions and their site of initiation, direction of propagation, frequency, and duration are assessed. After the meal, conversion to the fed state is identified, and the duration of the fed pattern is calculated. Furthermore, the responses to prokinetic challenge are assessed. The interpretation of duodenal manometric recordings requires substantial experience and recognition of normal variability. This is performed by visual inspection of motility tracings and not by computer analysis.

Clinical Example (91022)

A 53-year-old man presents for evaluation of persistent nausea, intermittent vomiting, abdominal pain, irregular bowel habits, and weight loss. He had an extensive work-up including endoscopic studies, small bowel biopsy, and radiologic studies. The studies are negative for mucosal disease or mechanical obstruction. Duodenal manometry is requested to assess for duodenal dysmotility.

Description of Procedure (91022)

The test is performed after an overnight fast. After informed consent is obtained, and following nasal spray administration of local anesthetic, a thin motility probe, incorporating pressure transducers, is introduced through one nostril, down the back of the throat, and positioned into the duodenum as the patient swallows. The tip of the catheter contains a sensor that is positioned in the duodenum so that it is distal to the ligament of treitz. The catheter protruding from the nose is connected to a recorder that registers motility pressure. At the conclusion of the procedure, the catheter is withdrawn and the patient is discharged to home.

Ophthalmology

Contact Lens Services

The prescription of contact lens includes . . .

The fitting of contact lens includes . . .

Follow-up of successfully fitted extended wear . . .

The supply of contact lenses may be reported as part of the service of fitting. ►It may also be reported separately by using the appropriate supply codes.◄

(For therapeutic or surgical use of contact lens, see 68340, 92070)

92310 Prescription of optical and physical characteristics of and fitting of contact lens, with medical supervision of adaptation; corneal lens, both eyes, except for aphakia

►(92330, 92335 have been deleted)◄

►(For prescription, fitting, and/or medical supervision of ocular prosthetic adaptation by a physician, see Evaluation and Management services or General Ophthalmological service codes 92002-92014)◄

Rationale

Codes 92330 and 92335 for prescription, fitting, and supply of ocular prosthesis have been deleted with instructions to use the evaluation and management (E/M) services codes or general ophthalmological service codes 92002-92014 when prescription, fitting, and/or medical supervision of ocular prosthetic adaptation by a physician is provided. The E/M codes and general ophthalmological codes should be reported for the service component of these codes enabling the various levels of service (eg, detailed, expanded, intermediate, comprehensive) to encompass the variability of services and physician time involved in the prescription and fitting and supervision of the adaptation while removing the supply component formerly encapsulated in these descriptions.

In concert with the deletion of the supply codes from the ophthalmology subsection of the CPT codebook, the Contact Lens Services guidelines have been revised to reflect the deletion of these codes. Supply codes should now be reported from other services (eg, Level II Healthcare Common Procedure Coding System [HCPCS] vision services codes) for the supply of spectacles, contact lenses, and other visual aids and prosthetics.

Spectacle Services (Including Prosthesis for Aphakia)

92370 Repair and refitting spectacles; except for aphakia

92371 spectacle prosthesis for aphakia

►(Codes 92390-92396 have been deleted. For supply of spectacles or contact lenses, use the appropriate supply codes)◄

Rationale

Codes 92390-92396 have been deleted and an instructional note has been added to report the appropriate supply codes for supply of spectacles or contact lenses. The Supply of Materials section has been removed from the CPT codebook, which consists of the deletion of codes for supply of spectacles, contact lenses, low vision aids, and ocular prosthesis (92390, 92391, 92392, 92393, 92395, 92396). Additionally, all references and instructional notes pertaining to this section have been deleted with new instructions added to use supply codes that are available from other sources (eg, Level II Healthcare Common Procedure Coding System [HCPCS] vision services codes) for the supply of spectacles, contact lenses, and other visual aids and prosthetics. Prescription, fitting, and/or medical supervision of ocular prosthetic adaptation by a physician should be reported using the general ophthalmological services codes 92002-92014.

Special Otorhinolaryngologic Services

Diagnostic or treatment procedures usually included . . .

Special otorhinolaryngologic services are those diagnostic . . .

All services include medical diagnostic evaluation. . . .

►Code 92506 is used to report evaluation of speech production, receptive language, and expressive language abilities. Tests may examine speech sound production, articulatory movements of oral musculature, the patient's ability to understand the meaning and intent of written and verbal expressions, and the appropriate formulation and utterance of expressive thought. In contrast, 92626 and 92627 are reported for an evaluation of auditory rehabilitation status determining the patient's ability to use residual hearing in order to identify the acoustic characteristics of sounds associated with speech communication.◄

(For laryngoscopy with stroboscopy, use 31579)

92502 Otolaryngologic examination under general anesthesia

▲92506 Evaluation of speech, language, voice, communication, and/or auditory processing

▲92507 Treatment of speech, language, voice, communication, and/or auditory processing disorder; individual

►(92510 has been deleted)◄

►(For auditory rehabilitation, prelingual hearing loss, use 92630)◄

►(For auditory rehabilitation, postlingual hearing loss, use 92633)◄

►(For cochlear implant programming, see 92601-92604)◄

Rationale

Code 92506 was revised by adding "and/or" language and removing the phrase "aural rehabilitation status" from the descriptor. Code 92506 is intended for use by speech language pathologists for assessment of speech-reading (lip-reading) abilities.

Auditory rehabilitation, as previously described by 92507, was intended to report speech-reading (lip-reading) training. Code 92507 was revised by removing "aural rehabilitation" from the descriptor language. Revised code 92507 is now intended to be reported for services provided for the hearing impaired individual who does not use a hearing aid or cochlear implant and needs assistance to improve listening under adverse environmental conditions.

New guidelines were added to the Special Otorhinolaryngologic Services subsection to clarify the reporting of 92506, 92626, and 92627.

Code 92510 was deleted and a parenthetical note was added to delineate the deletion and to direct users to 92630 and 92633 for auditory rehabilitation for prelingual and postlingual hearing loss. Another cross-reference was added to direct users to 92601-92604 for cochlear implant programming.

Clinical Example (92506)

A 3-year-old boy with a history of frequent otitis media has poor articulation and language skills. Having previously undergone evaluation, he presents for treatment.

▲92520 Laryngeal function studies (ie, aerodynamic testing and acoustic testing)

►(For performance of a single test, use modifier 52)◄

►(To report flexible fiberoptic laryngeal evaluation of swallowing and laryngeal sensory testing, see 92611-92617)◄

►(To report other testing of laryngeal function (eg, electroglottography), use 92700)◄

Rationale

Code 92520 has been revised to clarify that this code is intended to describe aerodynamic testing and acoustic testing. Aerodynamic testing measures average airflow, peak airflow, vocal efficiency, and subglottal pressure. Acoustic testing measures pitch, loudness, jitter, shimmer, signal-to-noise ratio, and spectral analysis. In the instance when only one of these two tests is performed, modifier 52, *Reduced services*, should be appended. Code 92520 is not used to report fiber optic laryngeal evaluation of swallowing or laryngeal sensory testing. These studies are reported using the 92611-92617 series of codes. Other types of laryngeal function studies not described by codes 92520 or 92611-92617, such as electroglottography, should be reported using code 92700. Three new parenthetical notes were added instructing users on the proper use of code 92520.

Clinical Example (92520)

A 40-year-old elementary schoolteacher presents with 6 months of hoarseness unresponsive to voice rest and a short course of systemic steroids. Her symptoms began during a viral upper respiratory infection but vocal problems remained long after the other symptoms resolved, and she is unable to teach the entire day. Otherwise, her history is unremarkable. Physical examination reveals bowing of the right vocal fold and sluggish movement on phonation. Aerodynamic and acoustic analysis of the patient's voice is obtained to quantify the degree of impairment and form a basis for further testing and therapy.

Description of Procedure (92520)

The patient is taken to the voice laboratory where the health care professional asks the patient to perform tasks, such as pitch matching, easy onset of phonation, and phonation with better breath support, to determine if any of these has an effect on the voice measures. The tasks are performed by speaking into a microphone connected to a computer and an audio recording device. In addition, her voice is recorded, analyzed acoustically, and stored by the computer software. Tests include pitch and loudness of the voice as well as jitter (inconsistency or perturbation of pitch) and shimmer (inconsistency or perturbation of loudness). The computer also analyzes the amount of extraneous noise in her voice (signal-to-noise ratio) and the harmonic frequency distribution (spectral analysis). Other assessments include average airflow, peak airflow, vocal efficiency, and subglottal pressure. A report of the findings is rendered.

Audiologic Function Tests With Medical Diagnostic Evaluation

▲92568 Acoustic reflex testing; threshold

▲92569 decay

Rationale

Codes 92568 and 92569 were editorially revised in order to clarify that 92568 is intended to report the threshold portion of the acoustic reflex testing.

Clinical Example (92568)

A 49-year-old female was referred for an audiologic evaluation with the chief complaint of progressive hearing loss and tinnitus in her right ear. No episodes of vertigo or imbalance were reported. Air-conduction and bone-conduction pure-tone thresholds showed a mild–to-moderate, gradually decreasing (low frequency to high frequency) sensorineural type hearing loss for her right ear and normal pure-tone thresholds for her left ear. In addition, word recognition scores were 44% for her right ear and 100% for her left ear. Acoustic reflex thresholds were measured to determine sensory (cochlear) from neural (8th nerve) locus of origin of the hearing loss.

Description of Procedure (92568)

After the audiogram is completed, the patient is moved to a separate area of the audiology laboratory and re-seated. A headset is placed on the patient's head with an insert earphone in each ear canal. A loud sound (approximately 95 dB at 1000 Hz) is presented monaurally for approximately 1.5 seconds to the patient's right ear. The meter of the acoustic immittance measurement unit is monitored for time-locked changes in impedance at the point of the tympanic membrane. Changes in tympanic membrane impedance are consistent with stapedius muscle contraction. If time-locked changes are seen, then the intensity of the of the stimulus tone is decreased in 5 dB to 10 dB steps, presented again for approximately 1.5 seconds, and the immittance measurement unit is monitored again for impedance change. This procedure is repeated until the evidence of stapedius muscle contraction is no longer evident. At that point, the intensity is increased in 5 dB steps to validate the minimum intensity necessary to evoke stapedius muscle reflex contraction. After the threshold of the acoustic reflex is established for 1000 Hz, the procedure is repeated in like manner for 500 Hz, 2000 Hz, and 4000 Hz for ipsilateral stimulation (the stimulus tone and reflex recording occurs in the same ear) and contralateral stimulation (the stimulus tone is presented to the ear opposite the ear of recording). The test results are recorded on the appropriate form, interpreted, and a report prepared and forwarded to the referring physician.

Evaluative and Therapeutic Services

92601 Diagnostic analysis of cochlear implant, patient under 7 years of age; with programming

92602 subsequent reprogramming

(Do not report 92602 in addition to 92601)

(For aural rehabilitation services following cochlear implant, including evaluation of rehabilitation status, ►see 92626-92627, 92630-92633◄)

92625 Assessment of tinnitus (includes pitch, loudness matching, and masking)

(Do not report 92625 in conjunction with 92562)

(For unilateral assessment, use modifier 52)

●92626 Evaluation of auditory rehabilitation status; first hour

+●92627 each additional 15 minutes (List separately in addition to code for primary procedure)

►(Use 92627 in conjunction with 92626)◄

►(When reporting 92626, 92627, use the face-to-face time with the patient or family)◄

●92630 Auditory rehabilitation; pre-lingual hearing loss

●92633 post-lingual hearing loss

Rationale

Codes 92626 and 92627 were added to describe evaluation of auditory rehabilitation status for the first hour and each additional 15 minutes. These services were formerly reported with 92506. A parenthetical note was added to instruct users to report add-on code 92627 in conjunction with 92626. The objective of this assessment is to determine current abilities to instruct the use of residual hearing provided by a cochlear implant or hearing aid. The assessment addresses, in children and adults, dimensions of impairment, activity limitation, participation restriction, and applicable environmental and contextual factors.

Code 92630 was established for reporting auditory rehabilitation for patients with prelingual hearing loss, and 92633 was established for reporting auditory rehabilitation in patients with postlingual hearing loss.

The auditory training process focuses on a variety of procedures designed to teach the individual how to use auditory input (eg, how to hear) covering a range of functional activities beginning with the identification and characteristics of sound and continuing to more complex tasks of speech discrimination and identification. Codes 92630 and 92633 will be reported to describe services performed primarily for pediatric patients who have no prior experience with hearing and are learning to hear through the use of hearing aids or cochlear implants. Rehabilitation services provided for children will assist in the development of their listening and auditory discrimination abilities. The specific techniques used as part of this overall process are intended to achieve eventual speech understanding abilities. Codes 92630 and 92633 will also be reported for rehabilitation of adults who have received a cochlear implant after a long period of time during which they had no functional hearing to assist in achieving speech understanding and identification of sounds in a shorter time span.

A child is diagnosed as hearing impaired and receives either a hearing aid or a cochlear implant. It cannot be assumed that the use of only the amplification device (hearing aid) or neural stimulator (cochlear implant) will be sufficient unto itself to allow the child to hear and understand speech in a manner appropriate to develop language. The child must be taught how to hear beginning with sound identification and discrimination between two sounds, identification of distinct speech sounds, and eventually learning how to understand speech. The basis for the necessity of this instruction is that neither hearing aids nor cochlear implants restore normal auditory function. Hearing aids provide sound input at stimulation levels much louder than the ear was designed to receive and over-stimulate an impaired transducer system. As a result, the perceived input is full of distortion and is not distinct in comparison to normal hearing input. Cochlear implants stimulate the auditory nerve using pulses of electricity trying to mimic as closely as possible distribution patterns of sound input and stimulation. But the perceived quality of "sound" does not resemble that of a normal auditory system. To offer some idea of the sound quality of an implant, adults who regained hearing abilities via a cochlear implant informally describe the initial stimulation as a "metallic version of Donald Duck," meaning it does not resemble "hearing" in the same manner as they remember. Consequently training is necessary, especially for children, to teach them how to hear using these devices to overcome the effects of an impaired auditory system. As implied above, this type of training is also necessary for some adults to facilitate and accelerate their learning to use this new type of auditory input.

Aural rehabilitation code 92507 is intended to be reported for speech-reading (lip-reading) training only and not the elements of auditory habilitation previously described.

Clinical Example (92626)

A 3-year-old male with a history of profound sensorineural hearing loss received a cochlear implant. After activation and programming of the implant device for minimum and maximum stimulation across the electrodes, the child is referred for an evaluation of auditory rehabilitation status to determine current auditory perceptual abilities and to develop an individualized plan of aural rehabilitation.

Description of Procedure (92626)

The audiologist greets the child and family in the waiting room and escorts them to the auditory training area. The audiologist and child sit at a table while the other family members are seated across the room or in an observation room. After establishing rapport with the child, the audiologist begins the assessment of current listening and discrimination abilities using the following activities:

1. Determination of sound awareness (presence or absence of sound)
2. Determination of sound duration patterns (long, short, and rhythmic patterns)
3. Evaluation of supra-segmental features (loud vs soft, high pitch vs low pitch, vocal inflection)
4. Achievement of sound discrimination for a variety of environmental sounds
5. Achievement of sound discrimination for speech sounds (phonemes)
6. Achievement of word discrimination for naming words (nouns)
7. Achievement of listening abilities in noise
8. Determination of differential listening abilities between the child's cochlear implant and a personal frequency modulation (FM) system.

Clinical Example (92630)

A 4-year-old child with profound sensorineural hearing loss who also has impaired speech and language received a cochlear implant. Following the cochlear implantation and after sufficient wound healing, the patient returned to the cochlear implant center for external device fitting and programming in addition to diagnostic evaluation of the status of the auditory nerve (diagnostic analysis and programming of cochlear implant reported separately). Following an initial assessment to determine his current level of function, a therapeutic plan of auditory training was developed and the child was referred for auditory rehabilitation designed for a child with prelingual onset of his hearing loss.

Clinical Example (92633)

A 46-year-old woman with moderate sensorineural hearing loss due to autoimmune disease received a hearing aid that has been evaluated and fitted previously. She now returns to the audiology center for auditory skills training.

Cardiovascular

Cardiography

93015 Cardiovascular stress test using maximal or submaximal treadmill or bicycle exercise, continuous electrocardiographic monitoring, and/or pharmacological stress; with physician supervision, with interpretation and report

93018 interpretation and report only

▶(For inert gas rebreathing measurement, see Category III codes 0104T, 0105T)◀

Rationale

Two Category III codes, 0104T and 0105T, were established for reporting inert gas rebreathing measurement. A cross-reference was added following 93018 to direct users to these new codes.

Intracardiac Electrophysiological Procedures/Studies

+93662 Intracardiac echocardiography during therapeutic/diagnostic intervention, including imaging supervision and interpretation (List separately in addition to code for primary procedure)

(Use 93662 in conjunction with ▶92987, 93527, 93532,◀ 93580, 93581, 93621, 93622, 93651, or 93652, as appropriate)

(Do not report 92961 in addition to 93662)

Rationale

The parenthetical cross-reference following 93662 was revised to instruct that 93662 (intracardiac echocardiography) is appropriately reported in conjunction with 92987 (mitral valve valvuloplasty), 93527 (right heart and transseptal left heart catheterization through intact septum), and 93532 (right heart and transseptal left heart catheterization through intact septum for congenital cardiac anomalies) in addition to the codes already listed for percutaneous treatments for congenital defects (93580, 93581), electrophysiologic evaluation with left atrial and ventricular pacing and recording (93621, 93622), and intracardiac catheter ablation of arrhythmogenic focus (93651, 93652).

Performance of mitral valve valvuloplasties, right heart and transseptal left heart catheterizations through intact septum, and right heart and transseptal left heart catheterizations through intact septum for congenital cardiac anomalies commonly require puncturing the inter-atrial septum, and use of intracardiac echocardiography (ICE) has become common to guide the atrial puncture and avoid complications resulting from misplaced punctures. For this reason, 92987, 93527, and 93532 have also been included in the parenthetical cross-reference.

Intracardiac echocardiography (ICE) code 93662 is reported as an add-on code for cardiac electrophysiology and interventional cardiology procedures that require crossing the interatrial septum of the heart (ie, 93580, 93581, 93621, 93622, 93651, or 93652). For 93580 and 93581, intracardiac echo is used to accurately place the atrial or ventricular closure device and confirm its position. For the other codes, intracardiac echo is used to identify the area of the atrial septum where needle puncture can be safely performed. (Without intracardiac echo, fluoroscopy is used to guide the needle puncture of the atrial septum.)

Non-Invasive Vascular Diagnostic Studies

Cerebrovascular Arterial Studies

93880 Duplex scan of extracranial arteries; complete bilateral study

93882 unilateral or limited study

►(To report common carotid intima-media thickness (IMT) study for evaluation of atherosclerotic burden or coronary heart disease risk factor assessment, use Category III code 0126T)◄

Rationale

In tandem with the addition of Category III code 0126T, a cross-reference was added following extracranial artery duplex scan code 93882 to direct users to the new code.

Allergy and Clinical Immunology

Allergy Testing

95078 Provocative testing (eg, Rinkel test)

(For allergy laboratory tests, see 86000-86999)

(For intravenous therapy for severe or intractable allergic disease, see ►90765-90768, 90772, 90774, 90775◄)

Rationale

In tandem with the revisions to the infusion codes, the parenthetical cross-reference following 95078 was revised to reflect the deletion and establishment of new codes in this subsection.

Endocrinology

▲95250 Ambulatory continuous glucose monitoring of interstitial tissue fluid via a subcutaneous sensor for up to 72 hours; sensor placement, hook-up, calibration of monitor, patient training, removal of sensor, and printout of recording

(Do not report 95250 in conjunction with 99091)

●95251 physician interpretation and report

►(Do not report 95250, 95251 in conjunction with 99091)◄

Rationale

Code 95251 was established and 95250 revised to allow reporting of the physician review, interpretation, and written report associated with continuous glucose monitoring. Code 95250 was revised to clarify that this code is intended to report (1) the technical components of continuous glucose monitoring and (2) continuous ambulatory glucose monitoring. The parenthetical cross-reference that previously instructed that the physician review, interpretation, and report should be reported with the evaluation and management services codes was deleted. Code 95251 was established for reporting the physician interpretation and report component of the glucose monitoring. An exclusionary parenthetical note was added to preclude reporting 99091 for collection and interpretation of physiologic data.

Clinical Example (95251)

A 45-year-old female with type I diabetes mellitus has been unable to manage her disease and has had frequent episodes of hypoglycemia symptoms, including a recent hospitalization for ketoacidosis. Continuous ambulatory glucose monitoring is ordered to assist with management of her disease. The 72-hour recording printouts are interpreted and a report is written.

Description of Procedure (95251)

The health provider interprets more than 900 glucose values, overlayed with a patient log of several variables (caloric intake, physical activity, symptoms of hypo- or hyperglycemia, and other symptoms as they occur) and reviews the self-monitoring blood glucose measurements.

Neurology and Neuromuscular Procedures

Neurologic services are typically consultative, and any of the levels of consultation (99241-►99255◄) may be appropriate.

In addition, services and skills outlined . . .

The EEG, autonomic function, evoked potential, reflex tests, EMG, NCV, and MEG services (95812-95829 and 95860-95967) include recording, interpretation by a physician, and report. For interpretation only, use modifier 26. ►For EMG guidance, see 95873, 95874.◄

Rationale

In tandem with the addition of two codes to report EMG guidance for chemodenervation, the Neurology and Neuromuscular Procedures guidelines have been revised to direct the user to these new codes.

Muscle and Range of Motion Testing

95857 Tensilon test for myasthenia gravis

►(95858 has been deleted)◄

Rationale

Due to lack of evidence of performance of electromyographic recording at the same time as a Tensilon (edrophonium chloride) test in the diagnosis of myasthenia gravis, 95858 has been deleted.

Electromyography and Nerve Conduction Tests

►Needle electromyographic procedures include the interpretation of electrical waveforms measured by equipment that produces both visible and audible components of electrical signals recorded from the muscle(s) studied by the needle electrode.◄

95860 Needle electromyography; one extremity with or without related paraspinal areas

95864 four extremities with or without related paraspinal areas

●**95865** larynx

►(Do not report modifier 50 in conjunction with 95865)◄

►(For unilateral procedure, report modifier 52 in conjunction with 95865)◄

●**95866** hemidiaphragm

95867 cranial nerve supplied muscle(s), unilateral

Rationale

Two codes were established for reporting needle electromyography (EMG) of the larynx (95865) and of the hemidiaphragm (95866) and new introductory text was added to the Electromyography Nerve Conduction Tests guidelines to define needle EMG procedures. Needle EMG of the larynx is performed in order to diagnose laryngeal nerve and muscle disorders, for intraoperative monitoring during procedures performed on the larynx, and during botox injections in the laryngeal muscles. Needle EMG of the larynx is typically performed on both sides of the larynx; therefore, it is not appropriate to append modifier 50 to 95865. A parenthetical note has been added to instruct the bilateral intent of this code. In the instance when a unilateral or hemi-larynx study is performed, modifier 52 should be appended.

Needle EMG of the diaphragm is performed in order to diagnose respiratory muscle disorders and, less frequently, for intraoperative monitoring.

Clinical Example (95865)

A 36-year-old man complains of a raspy voice after being intubated for a number of days following a drug-induced coma. The condition does not improve 2 months after the hospitalization. His otolaryngologist is uncertain if the cord has a mechanical problem or has sustained damage to its peripheral innervation. He requests electromyography for laryngeal muscle assessment.

Description of Procedure (95865)

The needle electrode is inserted through the skin and then the cricothyroid membrane until muscle activity is located. Placement can be confirmed by phonation of high-pitched vowels. Activation of the neck strap muscles without phonation should produce no EMG activity. The muscles being studied are quite small and swallowing or coughing may displace the needle. Localization is often prolonged, particularly in circumstances of vocal fold paresis or paralysis, because phonation to assist localization may not be possible. When the correct muscles are identified, electrodiagnostic properties of the muscle are reviewed including insertion activity, spontaneous activity, and voluntary activity. Motor unit action potentials may be analyzed according to morphology, amplitude, frequency, and recruitment. After the appropriate muscles have been localized and evaluated, the needle is withdrawn and direct pressure is applied to prevent bleeding.

Clinical Example (95866)

A 59-year-old woman who has a 50-pack-per-year history of smoking develops painless weakness of intrinsic hand muscles on both sides, fasciculations of upper and lower limb muscles, and shortness of breath. Her physical examination shows diffuse weakness of upper more than lower limb muscle groups, widespread fasciculations, and hyperreflexia. The clinician suspects amyotrophic lateral sclerosis but wishes to know whether her dyspnea is due to chronic obstructive pulmonary disease or to involvement of the diaphragm in her neuromuscular disorder, which might improve with positive pressure assisted ventilation (BiPAP). She refers the patient for electromyography (EMG)/nerve coaduction study, which includes needle EMG examination of the diaphragm.

Description of Procedure (95866)

Ground and reference electrodes are attached. Localization is performed by depressing the patient's abdomen to locate the inferior border of the ninth rib. The EMG needle is inserted at the paramidclavicular line under and beneath the ninth rib. The needle is advanced through the skin and abdominal fascia and then through the abdominal wall muscles into the costal insertion of the diaphragm where muscle electrical activity is encountered. The patient may need to temporarily be taken off of the ventilator if he or she is intubated. Electrical activity of the muscle is evaluated both with breathing and during silent periods. In some instances, particularly when the patient is comatose, an assistant may employ a needle to stimulate the phrenic nerve percutaneously to activate motor unit potentials. After the data is collected and analyzed, the needle is withdrawn. In some circumstances, a postprocedure chest X ray may be desired to exclude pneumothorax or pneumoperitoneum.

+●95873 Electrical stimulation for guidance in conjunction with chemodenervation (List separately in addition to code for primary procedure)

+●95874 Needle electromyography for guidance in conjunction with chemodenervation (List separately in addition to code for primary procedure)

►(Use 95873, 95874 in conjunction with 64612-64614)◄

▶(Do not report 95874 in conjunction with 95873)◀

▶(Do not report 95873, 95874 in conjunction with 95860-95870)◀

Rationale

Two add-on codes were established in the Electromyography and Nerve Conduction Tests section for reporting needle EMG guidance with chemodenervation and electrical stimulation guidance with chemodenervation. Prior to the chemodenervation procedure, it is sometimes necessary to perform a more precise localization for needle placement before the chemical is injected. Therefore, the physician may perform electrical stimulation or needle EMG to achieve this localization. Code 95873 describes electrical stimulation and 95874 describes needle EMG. Either 95873 or 95874 should be reported, as appropriate, in conjunction with chemodenervation codes 64612-64614 when electrical stimulation or needle EMG is performed for guidance prior to injection of the chemical. Codes 95873 and 95874 should not be reported in conjunction with needle electromyography procedure codes 95860-95870. Codes 95873 and 95874 should never be reported together. Three parenthetical notes have been added following 95874 that instruct users on the proper use of these codes.

Clinical Example (95873)

A 50-year-old man presents with a 2-year history of progressive task-specific dystonia associated with writing (writer's cramp). He is now unable to sign checks or make handwritten notes, which are important functions of his job. Botulinum toxin treatment is discussed and precise localization with electrical stimulation of the small hand and forearm muscles is determined to be necessary to avoid incapacitating weakness.

Description of Procedure (95873)

The physician attaches the stimulating needle electrode and hypodermic containing botulinum toxin to the stimulating apparatus. The targeted forearm muscles are identified by anatomical surface markers and the needle is advanced through the skin. The stimulating apparatus is activated at low frequency and relatively higher intensity, and the needle is relocated until muscle contraction is seen or palpated by the physician. The stimulus is decreased and the needle position is adjusted to achieve the maximal muscle contraction at that intensity. This procedure is repeated until a maximal muscle contraction is achieved at a minimal stimulus intensity. This procedure ensures that the needle tip is in the correct small muscle and is also closest to the motor endplate so the minimum amount of toxin achieves the maximum clinical response. Toxin is injected cautiously to avoid any movement of the needle tip. The needle is withdrawn and reinserted into a different muscles and the localization procedure is repeated until all of the targeted muscle groups are injected.

Clinical Example (95874)

A 60-year-old man with rotational cervical dystonia (chin to right shoulder) is seen. Prior treatment trials include muscle relaxers and range of motion exercises without benefit. Previous treatment with botulinum toxin resulted in a very good outcome. He presents for follow-up injection 90 days following his most recent injection. He has some focal atrophy in the neck muscles in the site of the previous injection, and physical examination or identification of the involved muscles only identifies the sternocleidomastoid as being taut on the left and some nonspecific tautness over his posterior right neck area.

Description of Procedure (95874)

Prior to injecting a muscle with botulinum toxin, the muscle must be precisely localized, which can be initially done based on anatomical knowledge, but in many cases further physiologic information is required to determine the specific muscle to be injected. After attaching a recording and injection hypodermic, the needle is advanced into the body of the sternocleidomastoid and a small amount of the botulinum toxin is injected. The needle is advanced further to spread the toxin through this long muscle, and the presence of persistent electromyography motor unit activity guarantees that the needle is still in the muscle and has not perforated into nearby vessels or has moved into a nonspastic muscle. The needle is inserted lower in the muscle and the process repeated. Following this, the needle is inserted into the right splenius capitis; the first muscle entered is the trapezius, which is electrically silent, and the needle is advanced until active motor unit potentials from the splenius capitis are identified and injections are made. The needle is advanced further through the substance of the electrically quiet semispinalis capitis. As it is advanced further, distant motor units become apparent. The needle, now at 35 mm of depth, encounters an area of no insertional activity, but the distant motor unit activity is louder. With a small additional push, the needle enters the oblique capitis inferioris muscle as confirmed by the rise time and amplitude of the motor unit potentials (a muscle that, according to Gray's anatomy, ". . . owing to the length of the transverse process of the atlas exerts considerable [rotational] mechanical leverage"), and an additional injection is made. Similar injections are carried out in the right posterior scalene muscle and left semispinalis capitis. Careful notation is made of the muscles involved, their degree of motor unit activity, and the specific location of injections. Appropriate clinical comments are determined based on the patient's presenting problem.

95875 Ischemic limb exercise test with serial specimen(s) acquisition for muscle(s) metabolite(s)

►(For listing of nerves considered for separate study, see Appendix J)◄

⊘95900 Nerve conduction, amplitude and latency/velocity study, each nerve; motor, without F-wave study

⊘95903 motor, with F-wave study

⊘95904 sensory

(Report 95900, 95903, and/or 95904 only once when multiple sites on the same nerve are stimulated or recorded)

Rationale

The language explaining the proper use of existing nerve conduction codes 95900, 95903, and 95904 was revised with the addition of a reference to Appendix J. This appendix provides a listing of the nerves that published in the April 2003 *CPT Assistant*.

Central Nervous System Assessments/Tests (eg, Neuro-Cognitive, Mental Status, Speech Testing)

The following codes are used to report the services provided during testing of the cognitive function of the central nervous system. The testing of cognitive processes, visual motor responses, and abstractive abilities is accomplished by the combination of several types of testing procedures. It is expected that the administration of these tests will generate material that will be formulated into a report.

(For development of cognitive skills, see 97532, 97533)

(For mini-mental status examination performed by a physician, see **Evaluation and Management** services codes)

►(96100 has been deleted. To report, see 96101, 96102, 96103)◄

►(96100 has been deleted. To report, see 96101, 96102, 96103)◄

●**96101** Psychological testing (includes psychodiagnostic assessment of emotionality, intellectual abilities, personality and psychopathology, eg, MMPI, Rorshach, WAIS), per hour of the psychologist's or physician's time, both face-to-face time with the patient and time interpreting test results and preparing the report

●**96102** Psychological testing (includes psychodiagnostic assessment of emotionality, intellectual abilities, personality and psychopathology, eg, MMPI and WAIS), with qualified health care professional interpretation and report, administered by technician, per hour of technician time, face-to-face

●**96103** Psychological testing (includes psychodiagnostic assessment of emotionality, intellectual abilities, personality and psychopathology, eg, MMPI), administered by a computer, with qualified health care professional interpretation and report

Rationale

Code 96100 was deleted and three codes (96101, 96102, and 96103) were established to more accurately describe the services performed in psychological testing. These codes have been added to discern between the testing administration and to provide clear guidance concerning the performance and inclusion of the interpretation and report. Code 96101 is reported for the test administration by the psychologist or psychiatrist, with subsequent interpretation and report. Code 96102 is reported for the technician-administered testing, with subsequent interpretation and report by the psychologist or psychiatrist. Code 96103 is reported for the computer-administered testing, with subsequent interpretation and report by the psychologist or psychiatrist.

Since codes 96102 and 96103 were added to define the technical aspects of the testing, the physician interpretation and report of the results of these tests are separately reported with code 96101.

Clinical Example (96102)

A 35-year-old woman is referred by her primary care physician due to significant changes in behavior. A series of tests (standardized and/or projective) is administered to evaluate emotionality, intellectual abilities, personality, and psychopathology. The administration of the tests is completed by a technician for the purposes of a mental health diagnosis.

Description of Procedure (96102)

The qualified health care professional meets with the patient and conducts a diagnostic interview, including a comprehensive history. In particular, he or she focuses upon the patient's own questions for the assessment in order to shape the assessment process. The health professional attempts to establish rapport in order to ensure maximum involvement and cooperation on the part of the patient with the testing procedures. On the basis of the information gathered from the interview, the qualified health care professional may modify the selection of testing instruments (eg, if the patient raises a question that had not been part of the initial referral, addition instruments may be added to the battery to address this).

The qualified health care professional introduces the patient to the technician who conducts the remainder of the assessment.

The qualified health care professional meets again with the patient in order to answer any last questions about the procedures and to inform him or her about the timetable for the results.

Clinical Example (96103)

A 35-year-old woman is referred by her primary care physician due to significant changes in behavior. A series of tests (standardized and/or projective) is administered to evaluate emotionality, intellectual abilities, personality, and psychopathology. The administration of the tests is completed by a computer for the purpose of a mental health diagnosis.

Description of Procedure (96103)

The qualified health care professional meets with the patient and conducts an interview, including a comprehensive history. In particular, he or she focuses upon the patient's own questions for the assessment in order to shape the assessment process. The health professional attempts to establish rapport in order to ensure maximum involvement and cooperation on the part of the patient with the testing procedures. On the basis of the information gathered from the interview, the psychologist may modify the selection of testing instruments (eg, if the patient raises a question that had not been part of the initial referral, addition instruments may be added to the battery to address this).

The qualified health care professional sets up the computer program and instructs the patient on the use of the computer. The psychologist checks frequently with the patient to ensure that he or she is completing the test correctly. The psychologist sets up the next instrument and continues as before until all tests are completed.

The qualified health care professional meets again with the patient in order to answer any last questions about the procedures and to inform him or her about the timetable for the results.

96105 Assessment of aphasia (includes assessment of expressive and receptive speech and language function, language comprehension, speech production ability, reading, spelling, writing, eg, by Boston Diagnostic Aphasia Examination) with interpretation and report, per hour

96110 Developmental testing; limited (eg, Developmental Screening Test II, Early Language Milestone Screen), with interpretation and report

96111 extended (includes assessment of motor, language, social, adaptive and/or cognitive functioning by standardized developmental instruments) with interpretation and report

►(96115 has been deleted. To report, use 96116)◄

●**96116** Neurobehavioral status exam (clinical assessment of thinking, reasoning and judgment, eg, acquired knowledge, attention, language, memory, planning and problem solving, and visual spatial abilities), per hour of the psychologist's or physician's time, both face-to-face time with the patient and time interpreting test results and preparing the report

►(96117 has been deleted. To report, see 96118, 96119, 96120)◄

●**96118** Neuropsychological testing (eg, Halstead-Reitan Neuropsychological Battery, Wechsler Memory Scales and Wisconsin Card Sorting Test), per hour of the psychologist's or physician's time, both face-to-face time with the patient and time interpreting test results and preparing the report

●**96119** Neuropsychological testing (eg, Halstead-Reitan Neuropsychological Battery, Wechsler Memory Scales and Wisconsin Card Sorting Test), with qualified health care professional interpretation and report, administered by technician, per hour of technician time, face-to-face

●**96120** Neuropsychological testing (eg, Wisconsin Card Sorting Test), administered by a computer, with qualified health care professional interpretation and report

Rationale

Codes 96115 and 96117 have been deleted, and four new codes (96116, 96118, 96119, 96120) have been established to clarify the various modalities of performance of neuropsychological examinations in order to more clearly differentiate between the modalities used to provide the central nervous system assessment/tests, the varied levels of face-to-face time, current test descriptions, computerized testing, and interpretive services.

The neurobehavioral status exam, reported with 96116, is intended to describe the performance of gathering information to provide an important first analysis of brain dysfunction and the progression and changes in the symptoms over time.

Neuropsychological assessment is defined as testing that is intended to diagnose and characterize the neurocognitive effects of medical disorders that impinge directly or indirectly on the brain. Neuropsychological testing procedures differ from psychological testing in that neuropsychological testing consists primarily of individually administered ability tests that comprehensively sample ability domains that are known to be sensitive to the functional integrity of the brain (eg, abstraction, memory and learning, attention, language, problem solving, sensorimotor functions, constructional praxis). These tests are objective and quantitative and require the patient to directly demonstrate his or her level of competence in a particular cognitive domain.

With the deletion of 96115, code 96116 was established for reporting the neurobehavioral status examination by the psychologist or psychiatrist, with subsequent interpretation and report. Codes 96118-96120 were established for reporting the procedures previously reported with deleted code 96117. Code 96118 is reported for the neuropsychological test administration by the psychologist or psychiatrist, with subsequent interpretation and report. Code 96119 is reported for the technician-administered neuropsychological testing, with subsequent interpretation and report by the psychologist or psychiatrist. Code 96120 is reported for the computer-administered neuropsychological testing, with subsequent interpretation and report by the psychologist or psychiatrist. Since codes 96119 and 96120 were established to describe the technical aspects of neuropsychological testing, the physician interpretation and report of the results of these tests are separately reported with code 96118.

Clinical Example (96116)

A 68-year-old woman is referred by her neurologist due to family reports of changes in her behavior, including attention difficulties, memory problems, and difficulties with problem solving. A neurobehavioral status exam is completed for the purpose of making a medical diagnosis.

Description of Procedure (96116)

The physician meets with the patient and, if appropriate, significant others to perform a neurobehavioral status exam, which includes screening for impairments in acquired knowledge, attention, language, learning, memory, problem solving, and visual-spatial abilities. The physician observes behavior and records responses.

Clinical Example (96118)

A 23-year-old man is referred by his neurologist due to postconcussion symptoms secondary to a motor vehicle accident. A series of neuropsychological tests is administered by a provider for the purpose of making a medical diagnosis.

Description of Procedure (96118)

Standardized test procedures are administered by a qualified health professional. These include observation of test-taking behavior and recording observations and creating a record of patient responses to test questions and procedures.

Clinical Example (96119)

A 23-year-old man is referred by his neurologist due to postconcussion symptoms secondary to a motor vehicle accident. A series of neuropsychological tests is administered by a technician for the purpose of making a medical diagnosis.

Description of Procedure (96119)

The patient arrives for the appointment and meets with the qualified health care professional, who conducts a comprehensive clinical interview. The qualified health care professional gathers additional information from the patient about the nature of the complaint and the history of the presenting problems. Based on the clinical history, a final selection of tests to be administered is made. The procedures are explained to the patient, and the patient is introduced to the technician, who administers the objective tests. During testing, the qualified health care professional frequently checks with the technician to monitor the patient's performance and make any necessary modifications to the test battery or assessment plan. When all tests have been administered, the qualified health care professional meets with the patient again to answer any questions.

Clinical Example (96120)

A 23-year-old man is referred by his neurologist due to postconcussion symptoms secondary to a motor vehicle accident. A series of individualized neuropsychological tests is administered by a computer for the purpose of making a medical diagnosis.

Description of Procedure (96120)

The patient arrives for the appointment and meets with the qualified health care professional who conducts a comprehensive clinical interview and review of the presenting complaints. The qualified health care professional explains the computerized testing procedures as part of a more comprehensive test battery that also includes face-to-face testing. The computer test is explained to the patient, and a practice trial is administered to ensure adequate understanding of the test and response requirements. The computer test is administered under the supervision of the qualified health care professional who monitors performance to ensure continued engagement in the task. Upon completion, the next test is introduced and the procedures are repeated until all tests are administered.

Health and Behavior Assessment/Intervention

Health and behavior assessment procedures are . . .

The focus of the assessment is . . .

Codes 96150-96155 describe services offered to patients who present with ►primary physical◄ illnesses►, diagnoses,◄ or symptoms and may benefit from ►assessments and interventions ◄that focus on the biopsychosocial factors related to the patient's health status. These services do not represent preventive medicine counseling and risk factor reduction interventions.

96150 Health and behavior assessment (eg, health-focused clinical interview, behavioral observations, psychophysiological monitoring, health-oriented questionnaires), each 15 minutes face-to-face with the patient; initial assessment

Rationale

The guidelines related to 96150-96155 for the Health and Behavior Assessment/Intervention services were revised to clarify the appropriate use of the health and behavior codes in order to allow reporting these services for those patients with a past diagnosis of mental illness or a concurrent mental diagnosis that is not the primary diagnosis, but requiring the Health and Behavior Assessment/ Intervention services to deal with the biopsychosocial factors related to the patient's health status.

Chemotherapy Administration

▶Chemotherapy administration codes 96401-96549 apply to parenteral administration of non-radionuclide anti-neoplastic drugs; and also to anti-neoplastic agents provided for treatment of noncancer diagnoses (eg, cyclophosphamide for auto-immune conditions) or to substances such as monoclonal antibody agents, and other biologic response modifiers. These services can be provided by any physician. Chemotherapy services are typically highly complex and require direct physician supervision for any or all purposes of patient assessment, provision of consent, safety oversight and intra-service supervision of staff. Typically, such chemotherapy services require advanced practice training and competency for staff who provide these services; special considerations for preparation, dosage or disposal; and commonly, these services entail significant patient risk and frequent monitoring. Examples are frequent changes in the infusion rate, prolonged presence of nurse administering the solution for patient monitoring and infusion adjustments, and frequent conferring with the physician about these issues.◀

▶If performed to facilitate the infusion or injection, the following services are included and are not reported separately:◀

▶a. Use of local anesthesia◀

▶b. IV start◀

▶c. Access to indwelling IV, subcutaneous catheter or port◀

▶d. Flush at conclusion of infusion◀

▶e. Standard tubing, syringes and supplies◀

▶f. Preparation of chemotherapy agent(s)◀

▶(For declotting a catheter or port, use 36550)◀

▶Report separate codes for each parenteral method of administration employed when chemotherapy is administered by different techniques. The administration of medications (eg, antibiotics, steroidal agents, antiemetics, narcotics, analgesics) administered independently or sequentially as supportive management of chemotherapy administration should be separately reported using 90760, 90761, 90765, 90779 as appropriate.◀

▶Report both the specific service as well as code(s) for the specific substance(s) or drug(s) provided. The fluid used to administer the drug(s) is considered incidental hydration and is not separately reportable.◀

▶When administering multiple infusions, injections or combinations, only one "initial" service code should be reported, unless protocol requires that two separate IV sites must be used. The "initial" code that best describes the key or primary reason for the encounter should always be reported irrespective of the order in which the infusions or injections occur. If an injection or infusion is of a subsequent or concurrent nature, even if it is the first such service within that group of services, then a subsequent or concurrent code from the appropriate section should be reported (eg, the first IV push given subsequent to an initial one-hour infusion is reported using a subsequent IV push code).◀

▶When reporting codes for which infusion time is a factor, use the actual time over which the infusion is administered.◀

If a significant separately identifiable Evaluation and Management service is performed, the appropriate E/M service code should be reported ▶using modifier 25◀ in addition to ▶96401◀-96549. ▶For same day E/M service, a different diagnosis is not required.◀

Regional (isolation) chemotherapy perfusion should be reported using the codes for arterial infusion (96420-96425). Placement of the intra-arterial catheter should be reported using the appropriate code from the **Cardiovascular Surgery** section. Placement of arterial and venous cannula(s) for extracorporeal circulation via a membrane oxygenator perfusion pump should be reported using 36823. Code 36823 includes dose calculation and administration of the chemotherapy agent by injection into the perfusate. Do not report 9640▶9◀-96425 in conjunction with 36823.

▶(For home infusion services, see 99601-99602)◀

▸Injection and Intravenous Infusion Chemotherapy◂

▶Intravenous or intra-arterial push is defined as: a) an injection in which the healthcare professional who administers the substance/drug is continuously present to administer the injection and observe the patient, or b) an infusion of 15 minutes or less.◀

▶(96400 has been deleted. To report, see 96401, 96402)◀

●96401 Chemotherapy administration, subcutaneous or intramuscular; non-hormonal anti-neoplastic

●96402 hormonal anti-neoplastic

▲96405 Chemotherapy administration; intralesional, up to and including 7 lesions

▲96406 intralesional, more than 7 lesions

▶(96408 has been deleted. To report, use 96409)◀

●96409 intravenous, push technique, single or initial substance/drug

▶(96410 has been deleted. To report, use 96413)◀

+●96411 intravenous, push technique, each additional substance/drug (List separately in addition to code for primary procedure)

▶(Use 96411 in conjunction with 96409, 96413)◀

▶(96412 has been deleted. To report, use 96415)◀

●96413 Chemotherapy administration, intravenous infusion technique; up to 1 hour, single or initial substance/drug

▶(96414 has been deleted. To report, use 96416)◀

+●96415 each additional hour, 1 to 8 hours (List separately in addition to code for primary procedure)

▶(Use 96415 in conjunction with 96413)◀

▶(Report 96415 for infusion intervals of greater than 30 minutes beyond 1-hour increments)◀

▶(Report 90761 to identify hydration, or 90766, 90767, 90775 to identify therapeutic, prophylactic, or diagnostic drug infusion or injection, if provided as a secondary or subsequent service in association with 96413)◀

●96416 initiation of prolonged chemotherapy infusion (more than 8 hours), requiring use of a portable or implantable pump

▶(For refilling and maintenance of a portable pump or an implantable infusion pump or reservoir for drug delivery, see 96521-96523)◀

+●96417 each additional sequential infusion (different substance/drug), up to 1 hour (List separately in addition to code for primary procedure)

▶(Use 96417 in conjunction with 96413)◀

▶(Report only once per sequential infusion. Report 96415 for additional hour(s) of sequential infusion)◀

▸Intra-Arterial Chemotherapy◂

96420 Chemotherapy administration, intra-arterial; push technique

96422 infusion technique, up to one hour

+▲96423 infusion technique, each additional hour up to 8 hours (List separately in addition to code for primary procedure)

(Use 96423 in conjunction with 96422)

▶(Report 96423 for infusion intervals of greater than 30 minutes beyond 1-hour increments)◀

(For regional chemotherapy perfusion via membrane oxygenator perfusion pump to an extremity, use 36823)

96425 infusion technique, initiation of prolonged infusion (more than 8 hours), requiring the use of a portable or implantable pump

(For refilling and maintenance of a portable pump or an implantable infusion pump or reservoir for drug delivery, see ▶96521-96523◀)

▸Other Chemotherapy◂

▶Code 96523 does not require direct physician supervision. Codes 96521-96523 may be reported when these devices are used for therapeutic drugs other than chemotherapy.◀

▶(For collection of blood specimen from a completely implantable venous access device, use 36540)◀

96440 Chemotherapy administration into pleural cavity, requiring and including thoracentesis

96445 Chemotherapy administration into peritoneal cavity, requiring and including peritoneocentesis

96450 Chemotherapy administration, into CNS (eg, intrathecal), requiring and including spinal puncture

(For intravesical (bladder) chemotherapy administration, use 51720)

(For insertion of subarachnoid catheter and reservoir for infusion of drug, see 62350, 62351, 62360-62362; for insertion of intraventricular catheter and reservoir, see 61210, 61215)

►(96520 has been deleted. To report, use 96521)◄

●96521 Refilling and maintenance of portable pump

●96522 Refilling and maintenance of implantable pump or reservoir for drug delivery, systemic (eg, intravenous, intra-arterial)

►(For refilling and maintenance of an implantable infusion pump for spinal or brain drug infusion, use 95990-95991)◄

●96523 Irrigation of implanted venous access device for drug delivery systems

►(Do not report 96523 if an injection or infusion is provided on the same day)◄

►(96530 has been deleted. To report, use 96522)◄

96542 Chemotherapy injection, subarachnoid or intraventricular via subcutaneous reservoir, single or multiple agents

►(96545 has been deleted)◄

(For radioactive isotope therapy, use 79005)

96549 Unlisted chemotherapy procedure

Rationale

In tandem with the revisions made to the infusion codes 90780-90799, the Chemotherapy Administration subsection was revised with the deletion of eight codes, the addition of 11 codes, the revision of two codes, and addition of three new subheads and key guidelines for all of the Chemotherapy Administration subsection.

The new codes clarify those services that are appropriately reported by the chemotherapy administration codes thereby expanding the definition of chemotherapy services. Previously, the chemotherapy administration services codes were considered to be appropriately reported only when the drug being used was an anti-neoplastic and the diagnosis was cancer.

While the new *CPT 2006* chemotherapy administration codes continue to be reported for parenteral administration of non-radionuclide anti-neoplastic drugs, in a significant clarification and expansion of the chemotherapy administration services, these codes are also reported for anti-neoplastic agents provided for the treatment of non-cancer diagnoses (eg, cyclophosphamide for autoimmune conditions) or for substances such as monoclonal antibody agents and other biologic response modifiers.

In order to more accurately report infusion services, several "secondary service" categories of new codes have been established to report additional sequential and concurrent infusions, sequential intravenous pushes for additional drugs for hydration, and therapeutic, prophylactic, or diagnostic IV infusions or injections. Previously, reporting for additional sequential infusion services was indistinguishable from additional hours of infusion.

Three new subheads now distinguish the codes in this section according to route of administration, specifying intravenous, intra-arterial, and other chemotherapy administration. The Chemotherapy Administration guidelines direct the appropriate reporting for these services.

The guidelines identify the drug agents with which the new drug administration codes are appropriately reported. These agents are based upon the inherent risk of the agent administration, and are linked to the management of the possible toxic effects of the drug, rather than upon the cancer diagnosis most commonly associated with chemotherapy treatment. These procedures include parenteral administration of non-radionuclide anti-neoplastic drugs and anti-neoplastic agents provided for treatment of non-cancer diagnoses (eg, cyclophosphamide for auto-immune conditions) or for substances such as monoclonal antibody agents and other biologic response modifiers. The guidelines further define the efforts required of the provider in order to report these codes and define those procedural elements that are included and not separately reported.

The chemotherapy administration codes include confirmation or recalculation of doses based upon the condition of the patient on the day of chemotherapy administration.

As is true for all CPT codes, the Chemotherapy Administration guidelines reinforce the instruction that these codes are not limited for reporting by any specialty. The guidelines define the level of difficulty expected for provision of these services including direct physician supervision for patient assessment, provision of consent, safety oversight, and intra-service staff supervision; advanced practice training and competency for staff providing the services; the increased complexity of preparation, dosage, or disposal of these agents; and the potential patient risk and requirements for frequent monitoring due to the toxic nature of the drugs.

As indicated in the guidelines for the Hydration and Therapeutic, Prophylactic, and Diagnostic Injections and Infusions subsections, the Chemotherapy Administration guidelines define and list the services that are included, and therefore not separately reported, including local anesthesia; the IV start; establishment of access to an indwelling IV, subcutaneous catheter, or port; the flush at conclusion of infusion; administration supplies, including standard tubing and syringes; and the preparation of chemotherapy agents. Users are instructed to report 36550 for catheter or port declotting.

The guidelines also instruct separate reporting for each method and route of chemotherapy administration. These instructions support the intent of the codes to reflect the additional effort required for each route of administration. An infusion consisting of three substances in a single bag is not intended to be reported as three separate infusion services, because the parenteral administration codes are intended to report the separate work of administration and IV access and not the inclusion of multiple agents in a bag prepared prior to infusion. Further instructions direct the user to report administration of all other hydration, therapeutic, prophylactic, and/or diagnostic injections and infusions with the appropriate codes from the 90760-90779 series of codes. The user is cautioned, however, that the fluid used to administer drugs is considered to be incidental hydration and is not a separate service, and therefore not separately reported.

Guidelines are now provided to define the initial service, distinguishing the initial service code from the subsequent or concurrent injection and infusion, and to instruct reporting for initial, subsequent, concurrent, and multiple infusions, injections, or combinations of services. These instructions clarify that the definition of the service is based less upon the chronological order of the services than it is upon the primary service of the encounter. The definitions of *subsequent* and *initial* also indicate that an initial service code is reported only one time per encounter, and that subsequent, sequential, and concurrent codes are reported regardless of the subsection (ie, Hydration, Therapeutic, Prophylactic, and Diagnostic Injections, and Infusions; Chemotherapy Administration) in which the initial service code appears.

Definition of the intent of the references to time (1 hour, each additional hour) in the code descriptors is provided in the guidelines. This definition indicates that reporting the time of the service should be based only upon the administration time for the infusion. This is because the time required for the infusion was used to define the range of services included in the infusion within the Chemotherapy Administration codes. Services leading up to the infusion and to conclude the infusion have been included in the infusion service and are not separately reported. These services will include starting the IV and monitoring the patient post-infusion.

Directions for use of modifier 25 for reporting separately identifiable E/M services support the separate reporting of these services, when necessary.

Since the Chemotherapy Administration services are reported for the administration of agents with a toxic nature, the presence of a physician is required to report 96400-96549. Therefore, an exclusionary parenthetical note directs the user to 99601-99602 for home infusion services.

Injection and Intravenous Infusion is the first new subsection of the chemotherapy administration codes.

Guidelines specific to this subsection provide the definition of intravenous/intra-arterial push to distinguish these services from the infusion codes.

Two new codes, 96401 and 96402, were established for reporting subcutaneous or intramuscular hormonal and non-hormonal antineoplastic administration services, previously reported with deleted code 96400. Non-antineoplastic hormonal therapy injections are reported with 90772.

Code 96405 has been only editorially revised to accommodate the addition of 96409 and 96411 to this family of codes. This code continues to be reported for the injection of chemotherapeutic substances into one through seven lesions. This code describes the number of lesions treated, not the number of injections, and should be reported once when one to seven lesions are treated, even if a particular lesion is injected more than once.

Codes 96409 and 96411 were established for reporting IV push chemotherapy administration services, previously reported with deleted code 96408. These codes are distinguished by the administration of the single or initial substance and administration for additional substances. Since add-on code 96411 is reported for the administration of a sequential substance, a parenthetical cross-reference directs that this code is appropriately reported with initial intravenous chemotherapy service codes 96409 and 96413, as indicated in the Chemotherapy Administration guidelines.

Codes 96413 and 96417 were established for reporting IV infusion chemotherapy administration services, previously reported with deleted code 96410. These codes are distinguished by the administration of the single or initial substance and administration for additional substances. Code 96413 is reported for the IV infusion administration of a single or initial chemotherapeutic drug. Add-on code 96417 would be reported for the infusion of a sequential substance. A parenthetical note following 96417 directs that (1) this code is appropriately reported with initial intravenous infusion chemotherapy service code 96413; (2) this code should be reported one time for each additional substance; and (3) additional hours of infusion are reported with 96415.

Add-on code 96412 was deleted, renumbered to 96415, and revised to clarify that this code is intended to be reported one time for each additional hour of IV infusion chemotherapy administration services. A parenthetical note instructs that this code is appropriately reported only with the initial IV infusion chemotherapy service code 96413. A second parenthetical note was added to define the length of infusion required to be performed in order to report each additional hour of infusion. Since 96415 is not intended to be reported for non-chemotherapeutic subsequent IV services, a cross-reference directs the user to the appropriate non-chemotherapeutic secondary or subsequent service codes 90761, 90766, 90767, and 90775, which should be reported with 96413, when these services are provided. For instance, drugs that are incidental to chemotherapy are not reported with the chemotherapy services codes. Therefore, administration of an anti-emetic drug while often performed at the same session as chemotherapy administration would be reported with the secondary or therapeutic prophylactic subsequent services codes 90761, 90766, 90767, and 90775, based upon the route of administration.

Code 96414 was deleted, renumbered to code 96416, and editorially revised to clarify the use of this code for reporting initiation of prolonged IV infusion chemotherapy administration services defined as a service greater than eight hours and requiring use of a portable or implantable pump. A cross-reference refers the user to 96521-96523 for reporting services for refilling and maintenance of a portable pump or an implantable infusion pump or reservoir for drug delivery.

The family of IV chemotherapy infusion codes is not completely synchronous with the non-chemotherapy series 90765-90768. Due to evidence of current practice standards, there is no code for concurrent administration of chemotherapeutic drugs. Multiple drugs given at the same session are considered to be sequential injections, rather than concurrent, and are reported with 96411 for IV push administration of additional drugs/substances at the same session and 96417 for IV infusion administration of additional drugs/substances at the same session.

The second new subsection within the Chemotherapy Administration section is Intra-Arterial Chemotherapy. This title was added to define intra-arterial codes 96420, 96422, 96423, and 96425.

Code 96423 was editorially revised for consistency to clarify that this service is reported for each additional hour of up to eight hours of intra-arterial infusion. An exclusionary parenthetical note was added to instruct that this code would not be reported for an infusion interval of less than 30 minutes greater than the previously reported 1-hour segment.

The cross-reference following 96425 was revised to reflect the deletion of 96520 and 96530 and the establishment of three new codes 96521, 96522, and 96523 to report procedures for refilling and maintenance of a portable pump or an implantable infusion pump or reservoir for drug delivery.

The final subsection of the Chemotherapy Administration codes includes chemotherapy services other than intravenous, subcutaneous, intramuscular, and intra-arterial injections and infusions. These include the unlisted services, pleural cavity administration, and procedures for refilling and maintenance of a portable pump or an implantable infusion pump or reservoir for drug delivery. The new guidelines are specific to the portable pump and implantable infusion pump or reservoir services. These address the necessity of physician supervision and the broad use of these codes for non-chemotherapeutic substances. A new cross-reference refers the user to 36540 for collection of blood from the implanted venous access device.

Code 96520 was deleted and renumbered to 96521. Code 96530 was deleted and renumbered to 96522. A parenthetical cross-reference was added following 96522 referring the user to 95990-95991 for refilling and maintenance of implantable infusion pumps for spinal or brain drug infusion. Code 96523 was established for reporting irrigation required for implanted venous access devices for drug delivery systems when these services are provided on a separate day from the injection or infusion services, as indicated by the cross-reference following this code.

Code 96545 was deleted for consistency with Health Information Portability and Accounting Act (HIPAA) reporting guidelines. Chemotherapy supplies should be reported with the most specific supply code.

Clinical Example (96401)

A 34-year-old patient with testicular cancer presents with the appropriate indications for chemotherapy.

Description of Procedure (96401)

The physician provides direct supervision and is immediately available in the office. The physician assesses patient's response to the treatment.

Clinical Example (96402)

A 72-year-old man with prostate cancer presents with the appropriate indications for luteinizing hormone-releasing hormone (LHRH) agonist therapy.

Description of Procedure (96402)

The physician provides direct supervision and is immediately available in the office. The physician assesses patient's response to the treatment.

Clinical Example (96405)

A 60-year-old female presents with a well-defined biopsy-proven primary solid basal cell carcinoma of the nose and normal cardiac, liver, and renal status.

Clinical Example (96406)

A 65-year-old male presents with a multiple biopsy-proven primary superficial basal cell carcinoma of the torso. The patient is not a surgical candidate but otherwise has normal cardiac, renal, and liver status.

Clinical Example (96409)

A 67-year-old male with bladder cancer presents for an IV push administration. The patient does not have a venous access device and requires an IV initiation.

Description of Procedure (96409)

The physician provides direct supervision and is immediately available in the office. The physician assesses patient's response to the treatment.

Clinical Example (96411)

A 67-year-old male with bladder cancer is to receive the second drug for the day's treatment. The patient has just finished receiving an IV push of a first drug (reported separately under 96408) as part of the chemotherapy course. (This is an add-on code; code 96408 includes the IV discontinuation, flush, and discharge process.)

Description of Procedure (96411)

The physician provides direct supervision and is immediately available in the office. The physician assesses the patient's response to the treatment.

Clinical Example (96413)

This procedure is initiated for a 64-year-old woman with ovarian cancer or rheumatoid arthritis. The patient has a venous access device in place.

Description of Procedure (96413)

The physician provides direct supervision and is immediately available in the office. The physician periodically assesses the patient and the patient's response to the treatment. This assessment is typically done through communication with the nurse.

Clinical Example (96415)

A previously started infusion is continued for a 64-year-old woman with ovarian cancer or rheumatoid arthritis. The patient has a venous access device in place. (This is an add-on code; code 96410 includes the IV discontinuation, flush, and discharge process.)

Description of Procedure (96415)

The physician provides direct supervision and is immediately available in the office. The physician periodically assesses the patient and the patient's response to the treatment. This assessment is typically done through communication with the nurse.

Clinical Example (96416)

A 58-year-old female presents for one of several periodic prolonged infusions of fluorouracil therapy.

Description of Procedure (96416)

The physician provides direct supervision and is immediately available in the office. The physician periodically assesses the patient and the patient's response to treatment. This assessment is typically done through communication with the nurse.

Clinical Example (96417)

A 64-year-old female with ovarian cancer presents for infusion. She has completed infusion of one chemotherapy drug and is now infused with a second drug through her implanted venous access device. (This is an add-on code; the 96413 code includes the IV discontinuation, flush, and discharge process.)

Description of Procedure (96417)

The physician provides direct supervision and is immediately available in the office. The physician periodically assesses the patient and the patient's response to treatment. This assessment is typically done through communication with the nurse.

Clinical Example (96521)

A 58-year-old female having a prolonged infusion of fluorouracil presents to have her portable infusion pump refilled.

Description of Procedure (96521)

The physician provides direct supervision and is immediately available in the office. The physician assesses the patient's response to the treatment.

Clinical Example (96522)

A 66-year-old male patient with metastatic colorectal carcinoma with disease limited to the liver returns for treatment. A hepatic artery catheter has previously been placed, by a surgeon, with an attached implanted pump (eg, Infusaid pump). The pump is refilled.

Description of Procedure (96522)

The physician provides direct supervision and is immediately available in the office. The physician calculates and recalculates the dosage and the infusion rate.

Clinical Example (96523)

A 72-year-old male with lung carcinoma has an implanted venous access device for drug delivery and returns to the clinic for flushing and maintenance of the device on a day when chemotherapy or other treatments are not planned.

Description of Procedure (96523)

No physician intraservice work is required. Clinic staff complete the required device maintenance.

Physical Medicine and Rehabilitation

Modalities

SUPERVISED

97010 Application of a modality to one or more areas; hot or cold packs

97018 paraffin bath

►(97020 has been deleted. To report, use 97024)◄

97022 whirlpool

▲97024 diathermy (eg, microwave)

97026 infrared

Rationale

Code 97020 has been deleted due to infrequent use. Microwave therapy is a form of diathermy, a way of generating heat within an area of the body for therapeutic purposes. Therefore, code 97024, *Application of a modality to one or more areas; diathermy*, has been revised with added language in parentheses, "eg, microwave," and a cross-reference added to direct the use of 97024 for microwave therapy.

Clinical Example (97024)

A patient has a lumbosacral sprain with muscle guarding in her dorsal lumbar muscles. The patient is positioned in the prone position to comfort and the unit is turned on. The heat agent over the lumbosacral sprain is left in place for 20 minutes. The provider checks the dosage level at 5 minutes following institution of the treatment and checks patient's response at end of the 20-minute time period.

Description of Procedure (97024)

A status check is performed to evaluate the patient's sensation, muscle spasm, level of pain, and range of motion.

Therapeutic Procedures

(For osteopathic manipulative treatment (OMT), see 98925-98929)

►(97504 has been deleted. To report, use 97760)◄

Rationale

In tandem with the addition of a new subhead for Orthotic Management and Prosthetic Management, 97504 has been deleted and renumbered for location in the new subsection.

►(97520 has been deleted. To report, use 97761)◄

▲97542 Wheelchair management (eg, assessment, fitting, training), each 15 minutes

Rationale

Code 97542 was revised to more clearly identify the full range of services performed by the provider. The words *assessment* and *fitting* were included in the code descriptor to more completely describe the components of this service. The assessment service includes determination of the patient's need for a wheelchair and the determination of the type of equipment to best meet the needs of the patient. This assessment includes but is not limited to the patient's strength, endurance, living situation, work situation, ability to transfer in and out of the chair, level of independence, weight, skin integrity, muscle tone, and sitting balance. Following the verification of the patient's need, measurements are taken prior to ordering the equipment. This measurement occasionally involves testing the patient's abilities with various chair functions including propulsion, transferring from the chair to other situations (bed, toilet, car), and use of the chair's locking mechanism on various types of equipment for optimal determination of the appropriate equipment by the patient and caregiver. This code is reported one time for each 15 minutes of service.

Clinical Example (97542)

A 29-year-old C4 quadriplegic with complete right shoulder disarticulation and left above-knee amputation has been fitted with a powered wheelchair and custom seating system. After an assessment of the seating system in conjunction with his functional goals, the therapist determines that the system must provide stabilization, support, and balance as well as pressure management. To achieve these goals, the therapist trains the patient in the safe operation and management of the wheelchair in order to achieve independent mobility in the home and community environment.

Description of Procedure (97542)

The patient's abilities are observed, maneuverability skills are practiced. Instructions are provided for adjustment of seating and other wheelchair components. The patient is trained in problem solving for real-life situations in work, home, and recreation areas.

Tests and Measurements

(For muscle testing, manual or electrical, joint range of motion, electromyography or nerve velocity determination, see 95831-95904)

►(97703 has been deleted. To report, use 97762)◄

Rationale

In tandem with the addition of a new subhead for Orthotic Management and Prosthetic Management, 97703 has been deleted and renumbered for location in the new section.

97750 Physical performance test or measurement (eg, musculoskeletal, functional capacity), with written report, each 15 minutes

97755 Assistive technology assessment (eg, to restore, augment or compensate for existing function, optimize functional tasks and/or maximize environmental accessibility), direct one-on-one contact by provider, with written report, each 15 minutes

(To report augmentative and alternative communication devices, see 92605, 92607)

▸Orthotic Management and Prosthetic Management◂

●**97760** Orthotic(s) management and training (including assessment and fitting when not otherwise reported), upper extremity(s), lower extremity(s) and/or trunk, each 15 minutes

▶(Code 97760 should not be reported with 97116 for the same extremity)◀

●**97761** Prosthetic training, upper and/or lower extremity(s), each 15 minutes

●**97762** Checkout for orthotic/prosthetic use, established patient, each 15 minutes

Rationale

A new heading for Orthotic Management and Prosthetic Management has been added to the Medicine section with a revised code for reporting orthotic training of upper extremities, lower extremities, and the trunk. Codes 97504 and 97703 have been renumbered and relocated to this new section. Prior to 2006, there has been no mechanism for reporting the assessment and management of a patient using an orthotic (prefabricated or custom made). Orthotic management includes assessing the patient; determining the most appropriate orthotic (eg, static vs dynamic); and designing, selecting, and fabricating the orthotic. Code 97760 also includes further orthotic training during follow-up visits including exercises performed in the orthotic, instruction in skin care, and orthotic wearing time. Code 97762 (formerly 97703) is intended to report the assessment for determination of an established patient's response to the orthotic including redness and/or pressure areas and making any necessary adjustments.

Clinical Example (97760)

A 65-year-old woman lacerated the volar side of her left middle finger at the level of the proximal interphalangeal (PIP) (flexor tendon zone II) while cutting a bagel. She sustained a full laceration of the flexor digitorum profundus and superficialis tendons and underwent surgical repair of both tendons. The patient was referred to therapy for postoperative rehabilitation that initially included protected passive range of motion within the surgical dressings.

Description of Procedure (97760)

The therapist removed the postoperative surgical dressing and fabricated a customized dorsal forearm-based wrist-hand low temperature thermoplastic orthotic. The orthotic's purpose was to protect the tendon repair and permit limited but progressive active and passive range of motion as the tendon heals. Initially, the orthotic was positioned with the wrist in 60° of flexion, the metacarpophalangeal (MCP) in 90° of flexion, the PIP joint in 90° of flexion, and the distal interphalangeal (DIP) joint in 50° of flexion. The therapist had to assess the patient's skin condition, degree of edema, and ability to follow directions. A decision had to be made regarding the type of low-temperature thermoplastic material to use, and fabrication (including measuring, molding, padding, and applying the straps) had to be completed. The orthotic design included dynamic tension on the finger to protect the tendon repair and allow for limited exercise once enough healing occurs. The patient was trained in the wear and care of the orthotic. This education included safety information for preserving skin integrity as well as precautions to facilitate tendon healing and minimize the risk of rupture.

At subsequent visits during a 6-week period, the orthotic was remolded to permit a greater degree of excursion of the flexor tendon by permitting greater extension of the wrist, MCP, and finger IP joints.

Other Procedures

(For extracorporeal shock wave musculoskeletal therapy, ►see◄ Category III code►s◄ 0019T►, 0101T, 0102T◄)

Rationale

In tandem with the establishment of Category III codes 0101T and 0102T, the cross-reference prior to unlisted code 97799 has been revised to refer the user to these codes.

97799 Unlisted physical medicine/rehabilitation service or procedure

Acupuncture

Acupuncture is reported based on 15-minute increments of personal (face-to-face) contact with the patient, not the duration of acupuncture needle(s) placement.

If no electrical stimulation is used during a 15-minute increment, use 97810, 97811. If electrical stimulation of any needle is used during a 15-minute increment, use 97813, 97814.

►Only one code may be reported for each 15-minute increment. Use either 97810 or 97813 for the initial 15-minute increment. Only one initial code is reported per day.◄

►Evaluation and Management services may be reported separately, using modifier 25, if the patient's condition requires a significant separately identifiable E/M service, above and beyond the usual preservice and postservice work associated with the acupuncture services. The time of the E/M service is not included in the time of the acupuncture service.◄

97810 Acupuncture, 1 or more needles; without electrical stimulation, initial 15 minutes of personal one-on-one contact with the patient

►(Do not report 97810 in conjunction with 97813)◄

+▲97811 without electrical stimulation, each additional 15 minutes of personal one-on-one contact with the patient, with re-insertion of needle(s) (List separately in addition to code for primary procedure)

⊘=Modifier 51 Exempt ⊙=Conscious Sedation ✚=Add-on Code ⁄⁄=FDA approval pending

▶(Use 97811 in conjunction with 97810, 97813)◀

▲97813 with electrical stimulation, initial 15 minutes of personal one-on-one contact with the patient

▶(Do not report 97813 in conjunction with 97810)◀

+▲97814 with electrical stimulation, each additional 15 minutes of personal one-on-one contact with the patient, with re-insertion of needle(s) (List separately in addition to code for primary procedure)

▶(Use 97814 in conjunction with 97810, 97813)◀

Rationale

A guideline, parenthetical notation, and descriptor language were all revised for acupuncture codes 97811-97814 to alert users to report (1) these codes according to time spent providing the service (15-minute increments), (2) only one code per 15-minute increment according to the specific type of acupuncture treatment provided during that period, and (3) only a single initial service code (ie, either 97811 or 97813) according to the specific acupuncture service that was performed to initiate the session. Language included in the guideline specifically limits the user to report only one initial code for acupuncture because these services include both the treatment, set-up, and evaluation necessary to identify the specific acupuncture service(s) necessary for the patient; therefore, when reporting this service, only one initial code should be used per session to identify the complete initial service provided. In addition to the guidelines, specific descriptor language revisions have been made to simplify use of the codes via (1) development of the parent-child indentation of related services and (2) removal of references to the amount of needles used in favor of identifying the types of treatment provided and the ability to use more than one type of treatment per session. To accommodate this, parenthetical notes have also been changed to identify the specific codes for which the add-on procedures may be reported (ie, 97811 to be used with 97810 or 97813; 97814 to be used with 97810 or 97813). Revising this section to reflect each of the noted changes allows users the ability to report in a more granular method, identifying a single type of acupuncture according to the method used during that 15-minute increment (eg, a patient that requires an initial electrical application on his or her ventral abdomen and, via use of separate needles, nonelectrical stimulation on his or her back during a separate 15-minute increment).

Clinical Example (97813)

A 49-year-old female receiving chemotherapy for breast cancer was previously referred for acupuncture to relieve post-chemo nausea. This treatment is part of an ongoing series of treatments for this condition. The patient is weak but not faint and has not vomited since chemotherapy was received earlier in the day.

Description of Procedure (97813)

The practitioner reviews the chart, greets the patient, and obtains a brief account of the results of the previous treatment and any significant changes that have occurred since the last visit. One point is selected for the day's treatment (proximal to the palmar surface of the wrist, bilaterally). The patient is placed in the supine position. The points are located by palpation. As points may be no larger than a millimeter in diameter, the process of point location requires considerable skill. Once the points are located, they are marked by pressing the skin and then cleaned with alcohol swabs. The practitioner selects the appropriate needle lengths and gauges for this treatment. After hand-washing, the practitioner inserts and mildly stimulates the needles. The process of insertion requires care to actually obtain the dull, aching sensation of a correctly needled point, while at the same time avoiding puncture of vital structures. In this case, the point P6 is on the medial wrist, between the flexor carpi tendons and blood vessels and directly over the median nerve. Electrodes are attached to the shafts of the needles and an appropriate frequency (Hz) and waveform are selected. The practitioner slowly increases the amplitude of the signal until the patient's tolerance is reached. The patient is instructed to rest for 20 minutes while the needles are retained.

After charting the procedure, the practitioner leaves the patient to rest while the needles are retained. The practitioner returns periodically to monitor the patient, readjust the electrical stimulation, and inquire about patient's comfort and treatment response. When the desired effect is achieved, the practitioner removes the electrodes and needles, and presses on the points with a cotton ball to prevent bruising or bleeding. The needles are disposed in accordance with Occupational Safety and Health Administration guidelines. The practitioner then assists the patient to an upright position, making sure that the patient does not feel faint. Any final charting that may be required is performed. The patient is instructed to maintain hydration and to beware of the possibility of fainting.

►Education and Training for Patient Self-Management◄

►The following codes are used to report educational and training services prescribed by a physician and provided by a qualified, nonphysician healthcare professional using a standardized curriculum to an individual or a group of patients for the treatment of established illness(s)/disease(s) or to delay comorbidity(s). Education and training for patient self-management may be reported with these codes only when using a standardized curriculum as described below. This curriculum may be modified as necessary for the clinical needs, cultural norms and health literacy of the individual patient(s).◄

►The purpose of the educational and training services is to teach the patient (may include caregiver(s)) how to effectively self-manage the patient's illness(s)/disease(s) or delay disease comorbidity(s) in conjunction with the patient's professional healthcare team. Education and training related to subsequent reinforcement or due to changes in the patient's condition or treatment plan are reported in the same manner as the original education and training. The type of education and training provided for the patient's clinical condition will be identified by the appropriate diagnosis code(s) reported.◄

►The qualifications of the nonphysician healthcare professionals and the content of the educational and training program must be consistent with guidelines or standards established or recognized by a physician society, nonphysician healthcare professional society/association, or other appropriate source.◄

►(For counseling and education provided by a physician to an individual, see the appropriate Evaluation and Management codes)◄

►(For counseling and education provided by a physician to a group, use 99078)◄

►(For counseling and/or risk factor reduction intervention provided by a physician to patient(s) without symptoms or established disease, see 99401-99412)◄

►(For medical nutrition therapy, see 97802-97804)◄

►(For health and behavior assessment/intervention that is not part of a standardized curriculum, see 96150-96155)◄

●**98960** Education and training for patient self-management by a qualified, nonphysician health care professional using a standardized curriculum, face-to-face with the patient (could include caregiver/family) each 30 minutes; individual patient

●**98961** 2-4 patients

●**98962** 5-8 patients

Rationale

In order to report educational and training services designed to teach patients how to effectively self-manage illness(es) or disease(es), a new subsection was established in Medicine and titled Education and Training for Patient Self-Management. This new subsection includes three codes and guidelines for reporting education and training for patient self-management by a qualified nonphysician health care professional using a standardized curriculum. These codes allow a comprehensive reporting mechanism for education and training services for patients with diseases, which include asthma and diabetes.

There are two critical elements necessary to understanding the intent and appropriate applications of the education and training for patient self-management code family. The first fundamental element lies in the fact that these services are prescribed by a physician and provided by a qualified nonphysician health care professional. It is important to note that when (1) counseling and education services are provided by a physician to an individual, the appropriate evaluation and management codes should be reported; (2) counseling and education are provided by a physician to a group, code 99078 should be reported; (3) counseling and/or risk factor reduction intervention are provided by a physician, codes 99401-99412 should be reported; (4) medical nutrition therapy services are performed, codes 97802-97804 should be reported; and (5) health and behavior assessment or intervention that is not part of a structured curriculum are performed, codes 96150-96155 should be reported. To address these special circumstances, appropriate instructional cross-references have been included following the guidelines.

The second critical component is that the qualifications of the nonphysician health care professionals and the content of the educational and training program must be consistent with guidelines or standards established or recognized by a physician society or nonphysician health care professional society or association or other appropriate source.

Code 98960 is intended to describe education and training for patient self-management by a qualified, nonphysician health care professional using a standardized curriculum for each 30 minutes spent face-to-face with an individual patient.

Codes 98961 is intended to describe education and training for patient self-management by a qualified, nonphysician health care professional using a standardized curriculum, face-to-face with the patient (could include caregiver/family); 2-4 patients.

Code 98962 is intended to describe education and training for patient self-management by a qualified, nonphysician health care professional using a standardized curriculum, face-to-face with the patient (could include caregiver/family); 5-8 patients.

Clinical Example 1 (98960)

A 35-year-old woman with disease (eg, diabetes or asthma) is a working mother with a history of multiple emergency room visits because of signs and symptoms of the disease. After evaluation by a physician, the patient is referred to a disease educator/counselor/coordinator.

Description of Procedure (98960)

The patient and her accompanying family members are taught from a standardized curriculum the fundamental concepts about disease and the effect of environmental factors, including effects on her individual home and work environment and beneficial changes in her lifestyle habits. The patient also is instructed in the importance of self-monitoring and the proper use of medications and/or devices that have been prescribed in order to maintain or improve health, avoid loss of work, and eliminate frequent emergency room visits. The educator assesses the patient, provides the intervention (curriculum), and establishes a plan for follow-up evaluation and ongoing assessment of outcomes to identify necessary modifications in treatment in order to improve quality of life. The disease educator documents the training and service provided at the session and describes the plan for follow-up education and training.

Disease education is a comprehensive service that requires knowledge and skills beyond classroom teaching about basic facts of disease. Educational expertise is required to reach both the individual with the disease and his or her family and/or caregiver(s). Educational emphasis is on imparting the knowledge and skills necessary to minimize the effect of disease on one's quality of life. The successful disease educator possesses comprehensive, current knowledge of the pathophysiology and management of disease including developmental theories, cultural dimensions, the effect of chronic illness, and principles of teaching-learning. The disease educator is able to assess health literacy and learning style and tailors the curriculum to compliment the patient's abilities in this regard. The disease educator also is knowledgeable about objective and subjective evaluations used to diagnose disease and assess its control. He or she capably instructs individuals with disease on the optimal use of medications and/or delivery devices, explaining complex technical concepts to individuals in a manner each can understand.

The disease educator conducts thorough assessments of individuals and families to identify strengths and resources as well as negative psychological factors, the social and economic effect of disease, educational needs, and barriers to optimal health and self-management including lifestyle habits and referrals for beneficial lifestyle habit changes. He or she works with an individual with disease, his or her family, and other health care professionals to develop, implement, monitor, and revise a disease action plan customized to the individual's needs, environment, disease severity, and lifestyle to optimize the individual's self-management skills. The disease educator monitors disease education program outcomes and recommends modifications to improve quality and effectiveness. The disease educator serves as a resource to the community by providing information about disease as well as health care and community resources.

Clinical Example 2 (98960)

A 35-year-old woman with asthma is a working mother with a history of multiple emergency room visits because of acute shortness of breath. After evaluation by a physician, the patient is referred to an asthma educator/counselor/coordinator.

Description of Procedure (98960)

The patient and her accompanying family members are taught from a standardized curricula the fundamental concepts about asthma and the effect of environmental factors, focusing on her individual home and work environment including tobacco control. The patient also is instructed in the importance of self-monitoring and the proper use of medications and devices that have been prescribed in order to avoid loss of work and frequent emergency room visits. The asthma educator assesses the patient, provides the intervention (curriculum), and establishes a plan for follow-up evaluation and ongoing assessment of outcomes to identify necessary modifications in treatment in order to improve quality of life. The educator documents the training and service provided at the session and describes the plan for follow-up education and training.

Clinical Example 3 (98960)

A 56-year-old female patient with type I diabetes on two insulin injections per day is referred to an endocrinologist because of frequent severe hypoglycemic reactions with emergency room visits approximately every 2 months.

She is referred to the endocrinologist's diabetes educator for intensive insulin therapy training under an approved curriculum. After her insulin regimen is changed to four injections per day (glargine insulin at bedtime with lispro insulin at meals), she continues to have uncontrolled blood glucose levels with frequent hypoglycemia. A decision is made to convert the patient to subcutaneous insulin pump therapy.

Description of Procedure (98960)

The diabetes educator discusses the patient's history with the endocrinologist and reviews the patient's medical record.

The diabetes educator, under the endocrinologist's supervision, provides intensive insulin therapy training under an approved curriculum. This intensive insulin training includes the provision of needs assessment and blood glucose testing and adjusting insulin dosages as needed. This service also includes performance of protocols for prevention, detection, and treatment of potential complications; management of hypo- and hyperglycemia; the determination of the role of exercise and physical activity in adjusting insulin dosage; and management of other illnesses within the context of insulin requirements. Carbohydrates are counted to match or adjust the insulin dose to food consumption at the proper insulin-to-carbohydrate ratio and a calculation and titration of basal rates is performed.

If the patient's diabetes remains uncontrolled, the physician may prescribe insulin pump therapy with an additional nationally approved education curriculum that includes calculation, adjustment, and correction of meal boluses; calculation of basal rates to meet diurnal variation of blood sugar and establish pattern control; and use of the catheter, including infusion set preparation and insertion techniques for the insulin pump.

The content, type (individual or group), duration, and patient response to the intensive insulin training is documented in the patient's medical record.

Clinical Example (98961)

A 56-year-old female patient and a 62-year-old male patient, both with type I diabetes, have been followed by their endocrinologist for several years. They are referred to the endocrinologist's diabetes educator for group intensive insulin therapy training under an approved curriculum. Despite changes to their insulin regimens, they continue to have uncontrolled blood glucose levels with frequent hypoglycemia. Decisions are made to convert them to subcutaneous insulin pump therapy.

Description of Procedure (98961)

The diabetes educator discusses the patients' histories with the endocrinologist and reviews the patients' medical records.

Under the endocrinologist's supervision, the educator provides intensive insulin therapy training under an approved curriculum. This intensive insulin training includes blood glucose testing and adjusting insulin dosages as needed; protocols for prevention, detection, and treatment of potential complications; and management of hypo- and hyperglycemia. It is also necessary to assess the role of exercise and physical activity in adjusting insulin dosage and the management of other illnesses within the context of insulin requirements. Carbohydrates are counted to match or adjust the insulin dose to food consumption at the proper insulin-to-carbohydrate ratio and calculation and titration of basal rates.

If any of the patients' diabetes remains uncontrolled, the physician may prescribe insulin pump therapy with additional, nationally approved education curriculum including calculating, adjusting, and correcting meal boluses; calculating the basal rates to meet diurnal variation of blood sugar and establish pattern control; and using the catheter, including infusion set preparation and insertion techniques for the insulin pump.

The content, type (individual or group), duration, and patient response to the intensive insulin training is documented in the patients' medical records.

Special Services, Procedures and Reports

The procedures with code numbers 99000 . . .

Code 99091 should be reported no . . .

If the services described by 99091 . . .

Do not report 99091 if it . . .

▶Codes 99050-99060 are reported in addition to an associated basic service. Typically only a single adjunct code from among 99050-99060 would be reported per patient encounter. However, there may be circumstances in which reporting multiple adjunct codes per patient encounter may be appropriate.◀

MISCELLANEOUS SERVICES

▲99050 Services provided in the office at times other than regularly scheduled office hours, or days when the office is normally closed (eg, holidays, Saturday or Sunday), in addition to basic service

●99051 Service(s) provided in the office during regularly scheduled evening, weekend, or holiday office hours, in addition to basic service

▶(99052 has been deleted)◀

●99053 Service(s) provided between 10:00 PM and 8:00 AM at 24-hour facility, in addition to basic service

▶(99054 has been deleted)◀

▲99056 Service(s) typically provided in the office, provided out of the office at request of patient, in addition to basic service

▲99058 Service(s) provided on an emergency basis in the office, which disrupts other scheduled office services, in addition to basic service

●99060 Service(s) provided on an emergency basis, out of the office, which disrupts other scheduled office services, in addition to basic service

99070 Supplies and materials (except spectacles), provided by the physician over and above those usually included with the office visit or other services rendered (list drugs, trays, supplies, or materials provided)

▶(For supply of spectacles, use the appropriate supply codes)◀

Rationale

Codes 99050, 99056, and 99058 were revised to reflect the current practice environment in clarifying historically the recognized intent of these codes; three codes—99051, 99053, 99060—were established to allow greater granularity in reporting, and codes 99052 and 99054 were deleted in the revision of this section of codes to clarify reporting of the special services codes. Each of these codes is intended to be reported in addition to the service provided, as indicated in their descriptors. The revisions to the existing codes and additions of the new codes are intended to describe as many as possible of the combinations in which a service is

▲=Revised Code ●=New Code ▶◀=New or Revised Text

provided outside of the usual timeframe and location in order to allow a wider use of these codes. Guidelines have been added to the Special Services, Procedures, and Reports subsection to indicate that while these codes are typically reported with only one code per encounter, there may be occasions in which more than one code is appropriately reported due to the dual nature of these codes in reporting unusual times and sites in providing services.

Qualifying Circumstances for Anesthesia

(For explanation of these services, see **Anesthesia Guidelines**)

+99100 Anesthesia for patient of extreme age, under 1 year and over 70 (List separately in addition to code for primary anesthesia procedure)

Moderate (Conscious) Sedation

►Moderate (conscious) sedation is a drug induced depression of consciousness during which patients respond purposefully to verbal commands, either alone or accompanied by light tactile stimulation. No interventions are required to maintain a patent airway, and spontaneous ventilation is adequate. Cardiovascular function is usually maintained.◄

►Moderate sedation does not include minimal sedation (anxiolysis), deep sedation or monitored anesthesia care (00100-01999).◄

►When providing moderate sedation, the following services are included and NOT reported separately:◄

►• Assessment of the patient (not included in intraservice time);◄

►• Establishment of IV access and fluids to maintain patency, when performed;◄

►• Administration of agent(s);◄

►• Maintenance of sedation;◄

►• Monitoring of oxygen saturation, heart rate and blood pressure; and◄

►• Recovery (not included in intraservice time).◄

►Intraservice time starts with the administration of the sedation agent(s), requires continuous face-to-face attendance, and ends at the conclusion of personal contact by the physician providing the sedation.◄

►Do not report 99143-99150 in conjunction with 94760-94762.◄

►Do not report 99143-99145 in conjunction with codes listed in Appendix G. Do not report 99148-99150 in conjunction with codes listed in Appendix G when performed in the nonfacility setting.◄

►When a second physician other than the healthcare professional performing the diagnostic or therapeutic services provides moderate sedation in the facility setting (eg, hospital, outpatient hospital/ambulatory surgery center, skilled nursing facility) for the procedures listed in Appendix G, the second physician reports 99148-99150. However, for the circumstance in which these services are performed by the second physician in the nonfacility setting (eg, physician office, freestanding imaging center), codes 99148-99150 are not reported.◀

▶(99141, 99142 have been deleted. To report, see 99143-99145)◀

⊘●99143 Moderate sedation services (other than those services described by codes 00100-01999) provided by the same physician performing the diagnostic or therapeutic service that the sedation supports, requiring the presence of an independent trained observer to assist in the monitoring of the patient's level of consciousness and physiological status; under 5 years of age, first 30 minutes intra-service time

⊘●99144 age 5 years or older, first 30 minutes intra-service time

+●99145 each additional 15 minutes intra-service time (List separately in addition to code for primary service)

▶(Use 99145 in conjunction with 99143, 99144)◀

⊘●99148 Moderate sedation services (other than those services described by codes 00100-01999), provided by a physician other than the health care professional performing the diagnostic or therapeutic service that the sedation supports; under 5 years of age, first 30 minutes intra-service time

⊘●99149 age 5 years or older, first 30 minutes intra-service time

+●99150 each additional 15 minutes intra-service time (List separately in addition to code for primary service)

▶(Use 99150 in conjunction with 99148, 99149)◀

Rationale

New guidelines, six codes, and associated cross-references were established to report moderate sedation services. Moderate sedation is the same service that was previously described in the CPT codebook as conscious sedation. With the evolution of medical practice of these services, moderate sedation is the most clinically relevant term used to describe the services provided. For this reason, the subhead and guidelines have been revised to reference conscious sedation as the secondary less preferred term to describe moderate sedation services. The range of anesthesiology codes has been included as an exclusionary list within the moderate sedation code descriptors and in the guidelines in order to clarify that the new codes describe services that are distinct from the anesthesiology codes.

Instructions have been included in the guidelines for the moderate sedation codes to define the upper and lower levels of moderate sedation, to distinguish these services from minimal sedation (anxiolysis) in the lower range of services and from deep sedation and monitored anesthesia care in the upper range of services, and to assist in directing documentation regarding the services provided. Services that are included in moderate sedation and, therefore, not separately reported include patient assessment; establishment of IV access; administration of agents; sedation maintenance; oxygen saturation, heart rate, and blood pressure monitoring; and recovery. The service time included in the descriptor is defined in the guidelines and starts at the time of the administration of the sedation agent. Exclusionary parenthetical notes in the guidelines indicate the inappropriate use of these codes with those codes listed in Appendix G. Codes 99148-99150, requiring a second physician, are appropriately reported with the codes in Appendix G only in the facility setting. An exclusionary note in the guidelines indicates the inappropriate use of these codes with the oxygen saturation measurement codes 94760-94762, supporting the directions provided in the guidelines.

Codes 99141 and 99142 that were previously used to describe moderate (conscious) sedation services have been deleted. While these codes were distinguished only by route of administration, they have been replaced with two separate families of codes, distinguished by provision of sedation services by a single physician and a trained observer (99143-99148) or two physicians (other than an anesthesiologist) and a trained observer (99148-99150). These families consist of two separate time-based base codes in each family, distinguished by patient age (younger or older than 5 years of age), with a single add-on code in each family to report additional time beyond the first 30 minutes of intraservice time. As indicated in the guidelines for these codes, the service time included in the descriptor starts at the time of the administration of the sedation agent. The new codes continue to include all of the six possible routes of administration (intramuscular, intravenous, oral, rectal, intranasal, inhalation).

Clinical Example (99143)

A 2-year-old patient undergoes a procedure that requires moderate sedation to complete safely and with minimal emotional trauma. The physician will supervise and direct an independent trained observer who will assist in monitoring the patient's level of consciousness and physiologic status throughout the procedure.

Description of Procedure (99143)

The physician supervises the administration and induction of the sedating agent, with or without an analgesic, initiated by the independent trained observer. The patient is assessed continuously until an effective and safe level of moderate sedation and/or analgesia is achieved. Additional doses of sedating and/or analgesic agent(s) are ordered by the physician as needed. The physician's intraservice time ends when the procedure is complete, the patient is physiologically stable, and face-to-face physician time is no longer required.

Clinical Example (99144)

A patient 5 years of age or older presents with a complaint necessitating performance of some procedure or service (ie, the "supported procedure"), in support for which moderate sedation is deemed clinically appropriate. The treating physician will perform both the supported procedure and the moderate sedation service.

Description of Procedure (99144)

The physician supervises the administration and induction of the sedating agent, with or without an analgesic, initiated by the independent trained observer. The patient is observed until a safe and effective level of moderate sedation is achieved. The physician, assisted by the independent trained observer, continually assesses the patient's level of consciousness and physiological status throughout the performance of the supported procedure. Additional doses of sedating agent are ordered by the physician, as needed, to maintain the achieved level of sedation for the supported procedure.

Clinical Example (99145)

A patient 5 years of age or older presents with a complaint necessitating performance of some procedure or service (ie, the "supported procedure"), in support for which moderate sedation is deemed clinically appropriate. The treating physician will perform both the supported procedure and the moderate sedation service.

Description of Procedure (99145)

The physician, assisted by the independent trained observer, continually assesses the patient's level of consciousness and physiological status throughout the performance of the supported procedure. Additional doses of sedating agent are ordered by the physician, as needed, to maintain the achieved level of sedation for the supported procedure.

Clinical Example (99148)

A 3-year-old patient undergoes a procedure that requires moderate sedation for safety reasons and to minimize emotional trauma. The physician performing the procedure requests that the sedation be delivered and monitored by a second physician.

Description of Procedure (99148)

The sedating agent(s) with or without an analgesic agent is administered and the patient is assessed continuously until an effective and safe level of moderate sedation and/or analgesia is achieved. The patient is closely monitored by the sedating physician and additional doses of sedating and/or analgesic agent(s) are delivered as needed. The sedating physician's intraservice time ends when the procedure is complete, the patient is physiologically stable, and face-to-face time with the sedating physician is no longer required.

Clinical Example (99149)

A patient 5 years of age or older presents with a complaint necessitating performance of some procedure or service (ie, the "supported procedure"), in support for which moderate sedation is deemed clinically appropriate. One health care professional will perform the supported procedure while a different physician will provide the moderate sedation service.

Description of Procedure (99149)

Administration of the sedating agent, with or without an analgesic, is initiated. The patient is observed until a safe and effective level of moderate sedation is achieved. During this face-to-face time, the physician continuously assesses the patient's level of consciousness and physiological status throughout performance of the supported procedure. Additional doses of sedating agent are ordered by the physician, as needed, to maintain the achieved level of sedation for the supported procedure.

Clinical Example (99150)

A patient 5 years of age or older continues to require the presence of a physician to provide moderate conscious sedation.

Description of Procedure (99150)

The patient is closely monitored by the sedating physician and additional doses of sedating and/or analgesic agent(s) are delivered as needed. The sedating physician's intraservice time ends when the procedure is complete, the patient is physiologically stable, and face-to-face time with the sedating physician is no longer required.

Other Services and Procedures

99170 Anogenital examination with colposcopic magnification in childhood for suspected trauma

(For conscious sedation, use 99143-99150)

Category II

The revisions of the Category II section consist of the addition of the first code measures to the Composite Measures and Diagnostic/Screening Process or Results subsections. Most notable is the addition of two Category II specific modifiers to report for performance measures considered but not provided.

Category II Codes

These codes describe clinical components that may be typically included in evaluation and management services or clinical services and, therefore, do not have a relative value associated with them. Category II codes may also describe results from ►clinical◄ laboratory ►or radiology◄ tests and ►other◄ procedures, ►identified◄ processes intended to address patient safety practices, or services reflecting compliance with state or federal law.

Category II codes described in this section make use of alphabetical character►s◄ as the 5th character in the string (ie, 4 digits followed by the letter **F**). These digits are not intended to reflect the placement of the code in the regular (Category I) part of the CPT codebook. To promote understanding of these codes and their associated measures, users are referred to Appendix H, which contains information about ►performance measurement exclusion modifiers,◄ measures, and ►source◄.

Cross-references to the measures associated with each Category II code and its ►source◄ are included for reference in Appendix H. Users should review the complete measure(s) associated with each code prior to ►implementation.◄

Category II codes are reviewed by the Performance Measures Advisory Group (PMAG), an advisory body to the CPT Editorial Panel and the CPT/HCPAC Advisory Committee. The PMAG is comprised of performance measurement experts representing the Agency for Healthcare Research and Quality (AHRQ), the American Medical Association (AMA), the Centers for Medicare and Medicaid Services (CMS), the Joint Commission on Accreditation of Healthcare Organizations (JCAHO), the National Committee for Quality Assurance (NCQA), and the Physician Consortium for Performance Improvement. The PMAG may seek additional expertise and/or input from other national health care organizations, as necessary, for the development of ►tracking◄ codes. These may include national medical specialty societies, other national health care professional associations, accrediting bodies, and federal regulatory agencies.

►(For blood pressure measured, use 2000F)◄

►(For tobacco use cessation intervention, pharmacologic therapy, use 4001F)◄

Modifiers

►The following performance measurement modifiers may be used for Category II codes to indicate that a service specified in the associate measure(s) was considered but, due to either medical or patient circumstance(s) documented in the medical record, the service was not provided. These modifiers serve as denominator exclusions from the performance measure.◄

►Category II modifiers should only be reported with Category II codes—they should not be reported with Category I or Category III codes. In addition, unless otherwise noted in special guidelines, parenthetic notes, or code descriptor language, the modifiers included in the Category II section may be used with any code listed in the Category II section.◄

►**1P** Performance Measure Exclusion Modifier due to Medical Reasons:◄

▶Includes, for example:◀

▶• Patient allergic history,◀

▶• Potential adverse drug interaction,◀

▶• Acquired or congenital absence of organ/limb,◀

▶• Other documented clinical contraindication.◀

▶**2P** Performance Measure Exclusion Modifier due to Patient Choice:◀

▶Includes, for example:◀

▶• Patient refusal,◀

▶• Economic,◀

▶• Social,◀

▶• Religious.◀

Rationale

Two modifiers have been established to report exclusionary circumstances. These modifiers are used to note services identified by a performance measure that were considered but not provided due to (1) medical reasons or (2) patient choice. They are intended to be appended only to Category II codes. They should not be used in addition to Category I codes. Each is reported according to whether the cause for exclusion is due to medical reasons (1P) or patient reasons (2P). Medical reasons include (1) exclusions due to patient allergic history, (2) potential adverse drug interactions, (3) acquired or congenital absence of an organ or limb, and/or (4) other documented clinical contraindications. Patient reasons include (1) patient refusal of treatment, (2) economic issues (eg, lack of follow-up by patient due to inability to pay), (3) social issues, and (4) religious reasons. As is true with other CPT modifiers, these modifiers should be appended to the specific Category II code(s) for which they apply.

Composite Measures

●**0001F** Heart failure assessed (includes assessment of all the following components):

▶Blood pressure measured (2000F)[1]◀

▶Level of activity assessed (1003F)[1]◀

▶Clinical symptoms of volume overload (excess) assessed (1004F)[1]◀

▶Weight, recorded (2001F)[1]◀

▶Auscultation of the heart performed (2003F)[1]◀

▶Clinical signs of volume overload (excess) assessed (2002F)[1]◀

▶(To report blood pressure measured, use 2000F)◀

●**0005F** Osteoarthritis assessed

Includes assessment of all the following components:

Osteoarthritis symptoms and functional status assessed (1006F)[1]

Use of anti-inflammatory or over-the-counter (OTC) analgesic medications assessed (1007F)[1]

Initial examination of the involved joint(s) (includes visual inspection, palpation, range of motion) (2004F)[1]

(To report tobacco use cessation intervention, use 4001F)

Rationale

Two codes have been included in the Composite Measures section of Category II codes. Code 0001F has been established to identify heart failure assessment, and code 0005F has been added to identify assessment of osteoarthritis. As indicated in the guidelines included for Composite Measure codes, these codes combine several measures and their identifying Category II codes grouped within a single code descriptor to facilitate reporting for a clinical condition when all components are met. Code 0001F for assessment of heart failure includes (1) the performance of blood pressure measurement (2000F), (2) assessment of the level of activity (1003F), (3) assessment of the clinical symptoms of volume overload (1004F), (4) recording of weight (2001F), and (5) an auscultation of the heart (2003F). Code 0005F for assessment of osteoarthritis includes (1) assessment of osteoarthritis symptoms and functional status (1006F), (2) assessment of use of anti-inflammatory or analgesic over-the-counter (OTC) medications for symptom relief (1007F), and (3) an initial examination of the involved joint (2004F). Also indicated in the guidelines is the fact that these codes should be used only if all of the individual component measures for that specific composite measure are met. If only some of the components are met, then individual Category II codes should be used to identify the services measured. Similarly, if services are provided in addition to those included in the composite measure code, then those additional services may be reported individually using the corresponding CPT Category II codes for those services.

Patient History

Patient history codes describe measures for select aspects of patient history or review of systems.

●**1003F** Level of activity assessed[1]

●**1004F** Clinical symptoms of volume overload (excess) assessed[1]

●**1005F** Asthma symptoms evaluated (includes physician documentation of numeric frequency of symptoms or patient completion of an asthma assessment tool/survey/questionnaire)[1]

●**1006F** Osteoarthritis symptoms and functional status assessed (may include the use of a standardized scale or the completion of an assessment questionnaire, such as the SF-36, AAOS Hip & Knee Questionnaire)[1]

▶[Instructions: Report when osteoarthritis is addressed during the patient encounter]◀

●1007F Use of anti-inflammatory or analgesic over-the-counter (OTC) medications for symptom relief assessed[1]

●1008F Gastrointestinal and renal risk factors assessed for patients on prescribed or OTC non-steroidal anti-inflammatory drug (NSAID)[1]

Rationale

Six new codes have been included in the Patient History section for Category II codes. These include codes for assessment of level of activity (1003F), assessment of clinical symptoms of volume overload (1004F), evaluation of asthma symptoms (1005F), assessment of osteoarthritis symptoms and functional status (1006F), assessment of the use of anti-inflammatory or analgesic over-the-counter medications for symptom relief (1007F), and assessment of gastrointestinal and renal risk factors (1008F). Each code should be reported according to the specific type of assessment provided.

Physical Examination

Physical examination codes describe aspects of physical examination or clinical assessment.

2000F Blood pressure, measured[1]

●2001F Weight recorded[1]

●2002F Clinical signs of volume overload (excess) assessed[1]

●2003F Auscultation of the heart performed[1]

●2004F Initial examination of the involved joint(s) (includes visual inspection, palpation, range of motion)[1]

▶[Instructions: Report only for initial osteoarthritis visit or for visits for new joint involvement]◀

Rationale

Four codes have been established for measurement of physical examination. These include codes to identify recording of weight (2001F), assessment of the clinical signs of volume overload (excess) (2002F), performance of heart auscultation (2003F), and initial examination of joint(s) (2004F). Each of these codes should be reported according to the specific type of examination provided.

Diagnostic/Screening Processes or Results

Diagnostic/screening processes or results codes describe results of tests ordered (clinical laboratory tests, radiological or other procedural examinations).

●3000F Blood pressure $\leq$ 140/90 mm Hg[2]

●3002F Blood pressure > 140/90 mm Hg[2]

⊘=Modifier 51 Exempt ⊙=Conscious Sedation ✚=Add-on Code ⁄⁄=FDA approval pending

Rationale

Codes 3000F and 3002F were established to report blood pressure measurement and are included in the Diagnostic/Screening Processes or Results section of Category II codes. They vary according to the specific pressure measurement indicated in each descriptor. Each of these codes should be reported according to the result of the value of the measurement necessary/provided.

Therapeutic, Preventive or Other Interventions

Therapeutic, preventive or other interventions codes describe pharmacologic, procedural, or behavioral therapies, including preventive services such as patient education and counseling.

4000F Tobacco use cessation intervention, counseling[1]

4001F Tobacco use cessation intervention, pharmacologic therapy[1]

4002F Statin therapy, prescribed[1]

●**4003F** Patient education, written/oral, appropriate for patients with heart failure performed[1]

4006F Beta-blocker therapy, prescribed[1]

4009F Angiotensin converting enzyme (ACE) inhibitor therapy, prescribed[1]

4011F Oral antiplatelet therapy prescribed (eg, aspirin, clopidogrel/Plavix, or combination of aspirin and dipyridamole/Aggrenox)[1]

●**4012F** Warfarin therapy prescribed[1]

●**4014F** Written discharge instructions provided to heart failure patients discharged home. (Instructions include all of the following components: activity level, diet, discharge medications, follow-up appointment, weight monitoring, what to do if symptoms worsen)[3]

▶[Excludes patients < 18 years of age]◀

●**4015F** Persistent asthma, long term control medication [inhaled corticosteroids or an acceptable alternative treatment, (cromolyn sodium, leukotriene modifier, nedocromil, OR sustained release theophylline)], prescribed[1]

▶[Note: There are no medical exclusion criteria]◀

▶(Do not report modifier 1P with 4015F)◀

▶(To report patient reasons for not prescribing, use modifier 2P)◀

●**4016F** Anti-inflammatory/analgesic agent prescribed[1]

▶[Use for prescribed or continued medication(s), including over-the-counter medication(s)]◀

●**4017F** Gastrointestinal prophylaxis for NSAID use prescribed[1]

●**4018F** Therapeutic exercise for the involved joint(s) instructed or physical or occupational therapy prescribed[1]

✍ Rationale

Seven new codes were established in the Therapeutic, Preventive, or Other Interventions of the Category II codes to report measures associated with interventions (including preventative or other interventions). Each of these codes should be reported according to the intervention performed.

Category III

Several series of codes have been added to the Category III codes, including those to report total disc arthroplasty, quantitative sensory testing, inert gas re-breathing, and extracorporeal shock wave therapy procedures. One new series, Medication Therapy Management, also includes guidelines to instruct appropriate reporting for these procedures. In addition, 14 other codes have been added, 11 deleted, and two revised for *CPT 2006*.

Category III Codes

▶(0010T has been deleted. To report, use 86480)◀

Rationale

In tandem with the conversion of 0010T to Category I code 86480, a cross-reference has been included to note the deletion of code 0010T and direct the user to report 86480.

▲0019T Extracorporeal shock wave involving musculoskeletal system, not otherwise specified, low energy

▶(For application of high energy extracorporeal shock wave involving musculoskeletal system not otherwise specified, use 0101T)◀

▶(For application of high energy extracorporeal shock wave involving lateral humeral epicondyle, use 0102T)◀

▶(0020T has been deleted. To report, use 28890)◀

Rationale

CPT Category III code 0019T has been revised to clarify its usage for low-energy modalities. In tandem with the establishment of 0101T and 0102T, and the deletion and conversion of 0020T to 28890, cross-references have been added to direct users to the appropriate codes for high-energy extracorporeal shock wave treatments of the plantar fascia.

Clinical Example **(0019T)**

Tennis elbow is a condition in which there is inflammation or degeneration of the tendons attached to the outside (lateral side) of the elbow. This disease process is generally characterized as an abrupt or subtle tearing of the tendonous area around the lateral aspect of the elbow and normally affects people between the ages of 30 and 50. Although many tennis players suffer with tennis elbow, the majority of people affected are not involved in sports. Because pain occurs from injured or damaged tendons near the elbow, people in occupational settings that require repetitive wrist and forearm movements such as painters, mechanics, and clerical workers are also likely to suffer from lateral epicondylitis.

The diagnosis of lateral epicondylitis is normally made through a physical examination, and radiographic studies if necessary. Patients with tennis elbow experience pain at the lateral aspect of the elbow that can radiate or travel into the forearm and occasionally the hand. The pain occurs with grasping activities and may be accompanied by a sense of weakness.

The patient normally presents with such symptoms as pain along the lateral aspect of the elbow, difficulty lifting, and a weakened grip.

High-energy ESW surgery is indicated for use in patients with chronic lateral epicondylitis who have failed to respond to conservative treatment such as physical therapy and stretching exercises, orthotics, bracing, NSAIDs, cortisone injections, or previous surgery.

Description of Procedure **(0019T)**

Prior to the administration of anesthesia, the area of tenderness on the affected area is palpated, and clearly designated with a marking pen. High-energy ESW surgery with appropriate delivery devices is painful; therefore, the procedure should be performed with anesthesia. The choice of anesthesia (local, regional, MAC, bier block, or general), after discussion with the patient, is the responsibility of the physician or anesthesiologist. The patient is placed supine on the stretcher with the affected arm placed in the lateral position. The head of the device is pointed downward towards the floor, and the table is raised to bring the elbow into the F2 area (F2 is the focal zone/treatment area of the shock wave).

Coupling gel is applied to the area of maximum tenderness or the treatment head. The shock head is coupled to the patient's elbow and positioned by the physician. It is important that there is good contact between the patient's elbow and the shock head to ensure that the treatment area remains within F2 throughout the procedure. The physician instructs the technician to set the device shock wave delivery rate to 4 Hz.

The procedure starts at 14 kV and the power is increased in increments until reaching a maximum power of 18 kV level to evaluate the effect of anesthesia. (The power level is not to exceed 18 kV.) The treatment protocol for soft tissue application of high-energy ESW surgery is as follows:

25 shocks @ 14 kV

25 shocks @ 15 kV

50 shocks @ 16 kV

1400 shocks @ 18 kV (Total 1500 shocks)

Ensuring that the elbow remains in constant contact with the shock head, the physician moves the affected area within the shock wave path (F2), and pronates and supinates the patient's hand during the procedure to ensure the entire tendon is treated to the proper depth based on the individual patient's anatomy and pathophysiology.

▶(0023T has been deleted. To report, use 87900)◀

Rationale

In tandem with the conversion of 0023T to Category I code 87900, a cross-reference has been added to note the deletion of code 0023T.

▶(0033T has been deleted. For endovascular repair of descending thoracic aorta, involving coverage of left subclavian artery origin, use 33880)◀

▶(0034T has been deleted. For endovascular repair of descending thoracic aorta, not involving coverage of left subclavian artery origin, use 33881)◀

▶(0035T has been deleted. For proximal extension during endovascular repair of descending thoracic aorta, use 33883. Distal extensions are included in 33880, 33881. Distal extensions performed after endovascular repair of descending thoracic aorta are reported with 33886)◀

▶(0036T has been deleted. For additional proximal extensions use 33884. Additional distal extensions during endovascular repair of descending thoracic aorta are included in 33880, 33881. Additional distal extensions placed after endovascular repair of thoracic aorta are included in 33886)◀

▶(0037T has been deleted. For open subclavian to carotid artery transposition performed in conjunction with endovascular thoracic aortic repair by neck incision, use 33889)◀

▶(0038T has been deleted. For endovascular repair of descending thoracic aorta, involving coverage of left subclavian artery origin, radiological supervision and interpretation, use 75956)◀

▶(0039T has been deleted. For endovascular repair of descending thoracic aorta, not involving coverage of left subclavian artery origin, radiological supervision and interpretation, use 75957)◀

▶(0040T has been deleted. For placement of proximal extension prosthesis for endovascular repair of descending thoracic aorta, radiological supervision and interpretation, use 75958. For placement of distal extension prosthesis after thoracic endovascular repair of descending thoracic aorta, radiological supervision and interpretation, use 75959)◀

Rationale

Category III codes 0033T-0037T have been deleted in tandem with the establishment of Category I codes 33880-33889 to report the performance of procedures related to endovascular repair of descending thoracic aorta. Similarly, Category III codes 0038T-0040T have been deleted in tandem with the establishment of Category I codes 75956-75959 to report the radiological supervision and interpretation procedures related to descending thoracic aorta endovascular repair procedures. Cross-references have been added to denote these deletions and to refer the user to the appropriate Category I code.

▲0078T Endovascular repair using prosthesis of abdominal aortic aneurysm, pseudoaneurysm or dissection, abdominal aorta involving visceral branches (superior mesenteric, celiac and/or renal artery(s))

(Report 0078T in conjunction with 35454, 37205-37208 when these procedures are performed outside the target zone of the endoprosthesis)

Rationale

Category III code 0078T has been editorially revised to reflect the recent revisions of the endograft device to a two-piece body with one iliac docking limb. References to the "fenestration" of the graft have been removed with the understanding that the references to the visceral arteries are sufficient to address the use of the endograft for communication between the aorta and the listed arteries in the repair of abdominal aortic aneurysm.

Clinical Example (0078T)

A 67-year-old male with coronary artery disease status post myocardial infarction and chronic obstructive pulmonary disease was found to have a 6.8-cm diameter abdominal aortic aneurysm (AAA). Imaging studies (CT scan, MRI, and/or angiography) indicate that the aneurysm has a configuration unsuitable for infrarenal repair but amenable to a fenestrated aortic endograft with covered extension stents to both renals and the superior mesenteric artery. Distally the aneurysm extends to the very end of the aorta, indicating that a bifurcated prosthesis will be required.

Note: Code 0078T does not include open femoral or iliac artery exposure, arterial catheterization, placement of the fenestrated graft limbs to visceral vessels, or radiological supervision and interpretation. These services are reported separately. See CPT Instructions for Endovascular Repair of Abdominal Aortic Aneurysm.

Description of Procedure (0078T)

Work begins after the decision to operate is made, from the day before the operation until the skin incision. This activity includes obtaining and reviewing the previous work-up, with special attention to potential cardiovascular risks. In addition, an extensive and detailed review of the preoperative imaging studies (CT, CT angiogram, CT with 3D reconstructions, MRI, and/or contrast angiogram) is required to determine the exact measurements of the aneurysm. This is necessary because an accurate preoperative choice of component diameters and lengths is one of the primary determinants of whether the endovascular procedure will be successful.

Initial work for aneurysm repair involving the visceral arteries also includes determining the exact location of the visceral artery orifices so appropriate fenestrations can be placed in the main component of the endograft. There can be no error in loading the graft into the delivery system, because the graft fenestrations must align exactly with the visceral artery orifices when deployed.

Informed consent is obtained from the patient following a discussion of surgical risks and benefits with the patient and the family. Other preservice work includes scrubbing, donning lead apparel, patient positioning, waiting for the anesthetic to become effective, prepping, and draping the patient.

Note: Reporting the deployment of 0078T will follow the coding guidelines in the CPT introductory notes for Endovascular Repair of Abdominal Aortic Aneurysm. In addition, deployment of the visceral extension prostheses will be reported using 0079T. The intraservice work of 0078T includes performing road-mapping arteriogram with specific attention to renal artery origins, final examination of endovascular components for correct models, sizing, exchange of soft J-wires for superstiff wires, and reconfirming that the appropriate device has been chosen. The main-body component is then unpackaged and the device is prepared for insertion. The patient is anticoagulated with IV heparin. The main-body component is then loaded onto the ipsilateral superstiff wire and advanced to the femoral artery. The tip of main device is introduced into arteriotomy site, the proximal vascular clamp is opened, and the front of the device is advanced into the artery. Rubber constrictors are used to limit blood loss. Under fluoroscopic guidance, the main-body device is directed through the external iliac and advanced into the common iliac artery and, subsequently, into the aorta. The device is pushed through the aneurysm carefully such that the tip lies above visceral artery origins and the circular orientation aligns fenestrations with visceral artery origins. Arteriography is repeated as needed to absolutely confirm orientation, and deployment is begun. Final precise adjustments are made to align top of device at desired visceral level with fenestrations lying exactly over visceral artery origins. The main-body device is deployed with constant attention to exact positioning, making final position adjustments as needed, keeping the proximal anastomosis and fenestrations as required, and checking distally to determine that the position above the aortic bifurcation is correct. Next, the main-body device is deployed to the point of opening the contralateral docking port. The contralateral docking port is cannulated using a selective catheter/guidewire combination, and the catheter advanced into the main body of the graft to the level of the proximal anastomosis. Inject contrast and image graft is provided to confirm placement of the catheter within the graft. A final angiogram is performed to confirm positioning of the proximal anastomosis, and any final adjustments to position of the proximal anastomosis are made at this time. The suprarenal fixation portion of the main body component is deployed. At this point in the procedure, one to four visceral artery extensions are deployed through the previously placed aortic graft fenestrations. This work is reported separately as 0079T for each vessel.

Sterile dressings are applied, and the physician ensures that the patient is stable and able to leave the suite. Help is provided to transfer the patient to a post-procedure recovery unit.

Depending on the preexisting comorbidities and operative course, it is determined if the patient requires admission to the intensive care unit. The physician writes orders, dictates the operative note, and communicates with the patient's family and referring and consulting physicians. Assistance is provided for the anesthesiologist to ensure smooth emergence from anesthesia. After this, the physician discusses the procedure results with the patient once he is fully awake and determines when the patient is adequately recovered for transfer to floor. Daily visits are provided during postoperative care, and orders and notes are written, etc.

Discharge day management includes communicating with all support services such as visiting nurse, meals on wheels, etc, communication with the referring physician, provision of activity advice, warnings to the patient and family, and arranging office follow-ups for wound checks, suture/staple removal, etc. All related office visits for 90 days are included in the postservice work of 0078T.

●0089T Actigraphy testing, recording, analysis and interpretation (minimum of three-day recording)

Rationale

Code 0089T was established to report the performance of actigraphy testing. Actigraphy is a method for assessing sleep and activity patterns in a variety of sleep-related disorders to assist in their diagnosis and treatment.

Actigraphy monitors movements only. This procedure does not define stages of sleep. No EEG monitoring or cardiopulmonary monitoring is performed. Therefore, separate codes should be reported if these procedures are performed.

Clinical Example (0089T)

A 26-year-old business manager presents for evaluation of difficulty falling asleep. He goes to bed at approximately 11 PM but says that he can lie there "for hours" unable to sleep. He often leaves his bed to play or work on the computer. The patient reports that his sleep schedule is erratic. He has extreme difficulty awakening in the morning and has missed or been late for work on a number of occasions. His supervisor has indicated that this is beginning to compromise his work responsibilities. On occasion, he will stay up virtually all night, go to work, and then sleep from 5 PM until 6 AM the next morning. On weekends he stays up "very late" and usually sleeps until 1-2 PM the following day. This pattern has been worsening for 18-24 months. He frequently falls asleep at morning meetings. He admits to "occasional" naps in the late afternoon following work because he is "just so exhausted," although minimizes the frequency and duration of the naps.

He denies other medical or psychiatric problems. He takes no medications. Physical and mental status examinations suggest no underlying medical or psychiatric illness.

The attending sleep specialist orders actigraphic recording in order to obtain an objective measure of the patient's sleep-wake schedule, sleep duration, and napping behavior. A 7-day actigraphy recording demonstrates an average time of sleep onset at approximately 2:50 AM. On 4 of 5 weekdays, his arising time was between 7 AM and 7:20 AM. On one weekday and both weekend mornings, his arising times ranged from 12:30 PM to1:45 PM. From estimated sleep-onset to estimated time of final awakening, there are no sustained awakenings. The recording also shows evidence of napping on 3 afternoons, with a mean nap duration of approximately 1.75 hours.

Based on the history and actigraphic recording, a diagnosis of delayed sleep phase is made. Specific behavioral recommendations are made regarding napping and sleep scheduling, and a program of morning high-intensity light treatment and evening melatonin is prescribed.

Following initiation of the treatment, the actigraphy recording is repeated for the purpose of tracking the treatment response and compliance with schedule recommendations. The recording demonstrates continued daytime napping on 2 afternoons. Sleep logs show an average bedtime of 11:30 PM with a shift of estimated sleep onset time (from actigraphic recording) to a mean of approximately 1:15 AM. The patient rises at 7 AM-7:20 AM except on weekends, when his rising times were 10:30 AM and 11:15 AM. Based on these results, the patient was advised to eliminate napping and to rise no later than 8:30 AM on weekends.

Description of Procedure (0089T)

This procedure consists of placement of a wristwatch-like device on an upper extremity (or, in the case of monitoring primarily for periodic limb movement disorder, a lower extremity) for a period of three or more days. The device monitors movement continuously during the period of use. Following removal of the actigraph, recorded data are downloaded into a computer and analyzed by visual inspection and/or by software algorithms that provide quantitative estimates of sleep-wake schedule, total sleep time, and napping behavior. These data are analyzed and interpreted in the clinical context by the evaluating professional. Some actigraphs are now equipped with light-monitoring instrumentation that allows determination of light exposure patterns as well. Actigraphy can provide diagnostic information that is not readily obtainable by means of polysomnography, subjective reports, or other means.

●0090T Total disc arthroplasty (artificial disc), anterior approach, including diskectomy to prepare interspace (other than for decompression); single interspace, cervical

●0091T single interspace, lumbar

+●0092T each additional interspace (List separately in addition to code for primary procedure)

►(Use 0092T in conjunction with 0090T, 0091T)◄

●0093T Removal of total disc arthroplasty, anterior approach; single interspace, cervical

●0094T single interspace, lumbar

+●0095T each additional interspace (List separately in addition to code for primary procedure)

►(Use 0095T in conjunction with 0093T, 0094T)◄

●0096T Revision of total disc arthroplasty, anterior approach; single interspace, cervical

►(Do not report 0096T in conjunction with 0093T)◄

●0097T single interspace, lumbar

►(Do not report 0097T in conjunction with 0094T)◄

+●0098T each additional interspace (List separately in addition to code for primary procedure)

►(Use 0098T in conjunction with 0096T, 0097T)◄

►(Do not report 0098T in conjunction with 0095T)◄

►(0090T-0097T include fluoroscopy when performed)◄

►(Do not report 0090T-0097T in conjunction with 22851, 49010, when performed at the same level)◄

►(For decompression, see 63001-63048)◄

Rationale

Three codes (0090T-0092T) have been added to report total disc arthroplasty, three codes (0093T-0095T) added to report the removal of a total disc arthroplasty, and three codes (0096T-0098T) added to report the revision of a total disc arthroplasty.

Total disc arthroplasty is performed on patients with degenerative disc disease. In a total disc arthroplasty, the degenerated disc is replaced with an artificial disc. This technique is an alternative to spinal fusion.

When the total disc is removed and replaced, this is considered to be a revision of the total disc arthroplasty. When reporting a revision, the revision codes 0096T-0098T should not be reported in conjunction with the removal codes 0093T-0095T. Removal of a total disc arthroplasty may be performed without replacement. In this instance, the removal codes are appropriate. Parenthetical notes have been added below codes 0096T-0098T to exclude the use of the arthroplasty revision codes with the arthroplasty removal codes.

When fluoroscopy is performed, it is included in codes 0096T-0098T and not separately reported as indicated in the parenthetical instructions. Decompression, when performed in addition to the total disc arthroplasty procedures, is reported separately using codes 63001-63048. Parenthetical notes have been added following code 0098T instructing users on the appropriate reporting of these circumstances.

Clinical Example (0090T)

A 45-year-old woman presents with progressive neck pain for several years unresponsive to multiple modalities of conservative treatment. Plain X rays and MRI scan show degenerative disc disease at the C5/6 level. At surgery a total disc arthroplasty is performed using an anterior approach. Postoperative hospital care and office visits are conducted as necessary through the 90-day global period.

Description of Procedure (0090T)

The medical record is reviewed to ensure that the patient is stable for the planned surgical procedure. The radiographic studies are reviewed. Radiographic findings are correlated with the clinical exam and the surgical plan is confirmed. The surgeon confers with the patient and family; explaining the current condition and the need for surgical intervention. Questions are answered, consent obtained, and a note written in the record. He confers with the anesthesiologist and the operating room to review positioning, the intraoperative plan, and equipment needs. After the patient is anesthetized, monitoring lines are placed, the patient is positioned, and the surgical site is prepped and draped into a sterile field.

An anterior approach to the spine is performed. The esophagus and trachea are mobilized and retracted exposing the spine. Intraoperative imaging is used to correctly identify levels. The disc is removed and the disc space is distracted. Decompression if required is performed (coded separately). The vertebral body endplates are shaped to accommodate the disc arthroplasty. The height, depth, and width are measured and an appropriate size prosthesis selected. The components are inserted and final intraoperative imaging obtained to confirm alignment. Hemostasis is obtained and a multi-layer closure performed.

Dressings are applied and the patient is rolled onto a recovery bed and examination shows her to be moving her extremities equivalent to preop. The surgeon calls the family and describes the findings during the operation and answers their questions. Orders are written and a note is dictated. During the postoperative hospitalization, the patient is examined for neurologic function. The dressing is inspected and changed as needed. Postoperative X rays are reviewed showing the alignment of the spine. Daily visits are made while on the hospital floor and notes are written documenting the in-hospital progress. Activity parameters are modified to advance the patient's ambulation and mobility. The patient's diet is advanced as tolerated. Questions from the physiotherapy staff are answered. Discharge instructions are reviewed and follow-up care coordinated.

After discharge, the patient returns to the office for suture removal and wound check. Questions regarding physiotherapy and activity levels are answered. Phone calls are answered concerning pain levels and activity restrictions. Subsequent follow-up office visits are scheduled to review activity levels and physiotherapy. X rays of the spine are ordered and reviewed showing the alignment of the spine. Prescription medication refills are reviewed and written. An exercise program is recommended and printed material regarding therapy is provided to the patient.

Clinical Example (0091T)

A 41-year-old man with progressive lower back pain for several years is unresponsive to multiple modalities of conservative treatment. Plain X rays and MRI scan show degenerative disc disease at the L5/S1 level. Discograms reproduce concordant pain at the affected level. At surgery a total disc arthroplasty is performed using an anterior approach. Postoperative hospital care and office visits are conducted as necessary through the 90-day global period.

Description of Procedure (0091T)

The medical record is reviewed to ensure that the patient is stable for the planned surgical procedure. The radiographic studies are reviewed. Radiographic findings are correlated with the clinical exam and the surgical plan is confirmed. The surgeon confers with the patient and family; explaining the current condition and the need for surgical intervention. Questions are answered, consent obtained, and a note written in the record. He confers with the anesthesiologist and the operating room to review positioning, the intraoperative plan, and equipment needs. After the patient is anesthetized, monitoring lines are placed, the patient is positioned, and the surgical site is prepped and draped into a sterile field.

An anterior retroperitoneal approach to the spine is performed. The abdominal contents are mobilized exposing the spine. Intraoperative imaging is used to correctly identify levels. The disc is removed and the disc space is distracted. The vertebral body endplates are shaped to accommodate the disc arthroplasty. The height, depth, and width are measured and appropriate size prosthesis selected. The components are inserted and final intraoperative imaging obtained to confirm alignment. Hemostasis is obtained and a multi-layer closure performed.

Dressings are applied and the patient is rolled onto a recovery bed and examination shows him to be moving his legs equivalent to preop. The surgeon calls the family and describes the findings during the operation and answers their questions. Orders are written and a note is dictated. During the postoperative hospitalization, the patient is examined for neurologic function and to determine the presence of bowel sounds. The dressing is inspected and changed as needed. Drain output, fluid balance, and postoperative laboratory values are reviewed and blood transfusion is ordered if needed. Postoperative X rays are reviewed showing the alignment of the spine. Daily visits are made while on the hospital floor and notes are written documenting the in-hospital progress. Activity parameters are modified to advance the patient's ambulation and mobility. The patient's diet is advanced as tolerated. Questions from the physiotherapy staff are answered. Calls are made to arrange for physiotherapy visits after discharge. Discharge instructions are reviewed and follow-up care coordinated.

After discharge, the patient returns to the office for suture removal and wound check. Questions regarding physiotherapy and activity levels are answered. Phone calls are answered concerning pain levels and activity restrictions. Subsequent follow-up office visits are scheduled to review activity levels and physiotherapy. Neurologic examinations confirm improvement in leg strength and sensation. Postoperative X rays of the spine are ordered and reviewed showing the alignment of the spine. Prescription medication refills are reviewed and written. An exercise program is recommended and printed material regarding therapy is provided to the patient.

Clinical Example (0092T)

A 45-year-old man with progressive low back pain for several years is unresponsive to multiple modalities of conservative treatment. Plain X rays and MRI scan show degenerative disc disease at the L4/L5 and L5/S1 levels. Discograms reproduce concordant pain at the affected levels. At surgery a total disc arthroplasty is performed using an anterior approach.

Description of Procedure (0092T)

Using the existing incision, additional mobilization of the tissues anterior to the spine is performed exposing the adjacent intervertebral disc. The disc is removed and the disc space is distracted. The vertebral body endplates are shaped to accommodate the disc arthroplasty. The height, depth, and width are measured and appropriate size prosthesis selected. The components are inserted and final intraoperative imaging obtained to confirm alignment. Hemostasis is obtained and a multi-layer closure performed.

Clinical Example (0093T)

A 45-year-old woman with progressive neck pain for several years unresponsive to multiple modalities of conservative treatment underwent a total disc arthroplasty 3 weeks previously at the C5/C6 level. Postoperatively the patient develops sepsis and wound infection unresponsive to intravenous antibiotics. At surgery the wound is irrigated and debrided and the total disc arthroplasty is removed using an anterior approach. Postoperative hospital care and office visits are conducted as necessary through the 90-day global period.

Description of Procedure (0093T)

The medical record is reviewed to ensure that the patient is stable for the planned surgical procedure. The radiographic studies are reviewed. Radiographic findings are correlated with the clinical exam and the surgical plan is confirmed. The surgeon confers with the patient and family; explaining the current condition and the need for surgical intervention. Questions are answered, consent obtained, and a note written in the record. He confers with the anesthesiologist and the operating room to review positioning, the intraoperative plan, and equipment needs. After the patient is anesthetized, monitoring lines are placed, the patient is positioned, and the surgical site is prepped and draped into a sterile field.

An anterior approach to the spine is performed. The esophagus and trachea are mobilized and retracted exposing the spine. The disc arthroplasty is removed. The wound and spine are thoroughly debrided. Hemostasis is obtained, drains are placed, and a multi-layer closure performed.

Dressings are applied and the patient is rolled onto a recovery bed and examination shows her to be moving her extremities equivalent to preop. The surgeon calls the family and describes the findings during the operation and answers their questions. Orders are written and a note is dictated. During the postoperative hospitalization, the patient is examined for neurologic function. The dressing is inspected and changed as needed. Postoperative X rays are reviewed showing the alignment of the spine. Daily visits are made while on the hospital floor and notes are written documenting the in-hospital progress. Activity parameters are modified to advance the patient's ambulation and mobility. The patient's diet is advanced as tolerated. Questions from the physiotherapy staff are answered. Discharge instructions are reviewed and follow-up care coordinated.

After discharge, the patient returns to the office for suture removal and wound check. Questions regarding physiotherapy and activity levels are answered. Phone calls are answered concerning pain levels and activity restrictions. Subsequent follow-up office visits are scheduled to review activity levels and physiotherapy. Postoperative X rays of the spine are ordered and reviewed showing the alignment of the spine. Prescription medication refills are reviewed and written. An exercise program is recommended and printed material regarding therapy is provided to the patient.

Clinical Example (0094T)

A 41-year-old man with progressive low back pain for several years unresponsive to multiple modalities of conservative treatment underwent a total disc arthroplasty 3 weeks previously at the L5/S1 level. Postoperatively, the patient develops sepsis and wound infection unresponsive to intravenous antibiotics. At surgery the wound is irrigated, debrided, and the total disc arthroplasty is removed using an anterior approach. Postoperative hospital care and office visits are conducted as necessary through the 90-day global period.

Description of Procedure (0094T)

The medical record is reviewed to ensure that the patient is stable for the planned surgical procedure. The radiographic studies are reviewed. Radiographic findings are correlated with the clinical exam and the surgical plan is confirmed. The surgeon confers with the patient and family; explaining the current condition and the need for surgical intervention. Questions are answered, consent obtained, and a note written in the record. He confers with the anesthesiologist and the operating room to review positioning, the intraoperative plan, and equipment needs. After the patient is anesthetized, monitoring lines are placed, the patient is positioned, and the surgical site is prepped and draped into a sterile field.

An anterior retroperitoneal approach to the spine is performed. The abdominal contents are mobilized exposing the spine. The disc arthroplasty is removed. The wound and spine are thoroughly debrided. Hemostasis is obtained, drains are placed, and a multi-layer closure performed.

Dressings are applied and the patient is rolled onto a recovery bed and examination shows him to be moving his legs equivalent to preop. The surgeon calls the family and describes the findings at operation and answers their questions. Orders are written and a note is dictated. During the postoperative hospitalization, the patient is examined for neurologic function and to determine the presence of bowel sounds. The dressing is inspected and changed as needed.

Drain output, fluid balance, and postoperative laboratory values are reviewed and blood transfusion is ordered if needed. Postoperative X rays are reviewed showing the alignment of the spine. Daily visits are made while on the hospital floor and notes are written documenting the in-hospital progress. Activity parameters are modified to advance the patient's ambulation and mobility. The patient's diet is advanced as tolerated. Questions from the physiotherapy staff are answered. Calls are made to arrange for physiotherapy visits after discharge. Discharge instructions are reviewed and follow-up care coordinated.

After discharge, the patient returns to the office for suture removal and wound check. Questions regarding physiotherapy and activity levels are answered. Phone calls are answered concerning pain levels and activity restrictions. Subsequent follow-up office visits are scheduled to review activity levels and physiotherapy. Neurologic examinations confirm improvement in leg strength and sensation. Postoperative X rays of the spine are ordered and reviewed showing the alignment of the spine. Prescription medication refills are reviewed and written. An exercise program is recommended and printed material regarding therapy is provided to the patient.

Clinical Example (0095T)

A 41-year-old man with progressive low back pain for several years unresponsive to multiple modalities of conservative treatment underwent a total disc arthroplasty 3 weeks previously at the L4/L5 and L5/S1 levels. Postoperatively the patient develops sepsis and wound infection unresponsive to intravenous antibiotics. At surgery the wound is irrigated and debrided and both total disc arthroplasties are removed using an anterior approach.

Description of Procedure (0095T)

Using the existing incision, additional mobilization of the tissues anterior to the spine is performed exposing the adjacent intervertebral disc. The disc arthroplasty is removed. The wound and spine are thoroughly debrided. Hemostasis is obtained, drains are placed, and a multi-layer closure is performed.

Clinical Example (0096T)

A 45-year-old woman with progressive neck pain for several years unresponsive to multiple modalities of conservative treatment underwent a total disc arthroplasty at the C5/C6 level. Two weeks postoperatively the patient develops increasing pain. X rays identify loss of fixation of the arthoplasty components and progressive migration. At surgery the total disc arthroplasty is removed and replaced using an anterior approach. Postoperative hospital care and office visits are conducted as necessary through the 90-day global period.

Description of Procedure (0096T)

The medical record is reviewed to ensure that the patient is stable for the planned surgical procedure. The radiographic studies are reviewed. Radiographic findings are correlated with the clinical exam and the surgical plan is confirmed. The surgeon confers with the patient and family; explaining the current condition, and the need for surgical intervention. Questions are answered, consent obtained, and a note written in the record. He confers with the anesthesiologist and the operating room to review positioning, the intraoperative plan, equipment needs. After the patient is anesthetized, monitoring lines are placed and the patient is positioned, and the surgical site is prepped and draped into a sterile field.

An anterior approach to the spine is performed. The esophagus and trachea are mobilized and retracted exposing the spine. The disc arthroplasty is removed. The vertebral body endplates are reshaped and prepared for reinsertion of the arthroplasty components. The disc space is distracted, and the height, depth, and width are measured and an appropriate size prosthesis selected. The components are inserted and final intraoperative imaging obtained to confirm alignment. Hemostasis is obtained and a multi-layer closure performed.

Dressings are applied and the patient is rolled onto a recovery bed and examination shows her to be moving her extremities equivalent to preop. The surgeon calls the family and describes the findings at operation and answers their questions. Orders are written and a note is dictated. During the postoperative hospitalization, the patient is examined for neurologic function. The dressing is inspected and changed as needed. Postoperative X rays are reviewed showing the alignment of the spine. Daily visits are made while on the hospital floor and notes are written documenting the in-hospital progress. Activity parameters are modified to advance the patient's ambulation and mobility. The patient's diet is advanced as tolerated. Questions from the physiotherapy staff are answered. Discharge instructions are reviewed and follow-up care coordinated.

After discharge, the patient returns to the office for suture removal and wound check. Questions regarding physiotherapy and activity levels are answered. Phone calls are answered concerning pain levels and activity restrictions. Subsequent follow-up office visits are scheduled to review activity levels and physiotherapy. Postoperative X rays of the spine are ordered and reviewed showing the alignment of the spine. Prescription medication refills are reviewed and written. An exercise program is recommended and printed material regarding therapy is provided to the patient.

Clinical Example (0097T)

A 41-year-old man with progressive lower back pain for several years unresponsive to multiple modalities of conservative treatment underwent a total disc arthroplasty at the L5/S1 level. Three weeks postoperatively the patient develops increasing pain. X rays identify loss of fixation of the arthoplasty components and progressive migration. At surgery the total disc arthroplasty is removed and replaced using an anterior approach. Postoperative hospital care and office visits are conducted as necessary through the 90-day global period.

Description of Procedure (0097T)

The medical record is reviewed to ensure that the patient is stable for the planned surgical procedure. The radiographic studies are reviewed. Radiographic findings are correlated with the clinical exam and the surgical plan is confirmed. The surgeon confers with the patient and family; explaining the current condition and the need for surgical intervention. Questions are answered, consent obtained, and a note written in the record. He confers with the anesthesiologist and the operating room to review positioning, the intraoperative plan, and equipment needs. After the patient is anesthetized, monitoring lines are placed, the patient is positioned, and the surgical site is prepped and draped into a sterile field.

An anterior retroperitoneal approach to the spine is performed. The abdominal contents are mobilized exposing the spine. The disc arthroplasty is removed. The vertebral body endplates are reshaped and prepared for reinsertion of the arthroplasty components. The disc space is distracted, and the height, depth, and width are measured and an appropriate size prosthesis selected. The components are inserted and final intraoperative imaging obtained to confirm alignment. Hemostasis is obtained and a multi-layer closure performed.

Dressings are applied and the patient is rolled onto a recovery bed and examination shows him to be moving his legs equivalent to preop. The surgeon calls the family and describes the findings at operation and answers their questions. Orders are written and a note is dictated. During the postoperative hospitalization, the patient is examined for neurologic function and to determine the presence of bowel sounds. The dressing is inspected and changed as needed. Drain output, fluid balance, and postoperative laboratory values are reviewed and blood transfusion is ordered if needed. Postoperative X rays are reviewed showing the alignment of the spine. Daily visits are made while on the hospital floor and notes are written documenting the in-hospital progress. Activity parameters are modified to advance the patient's ambulation and mobility. The patient's diet is advanced as tolerated. Questions from the physiotherapy staff are answered. Calls are made to arrange for physiotherapy visits after discharge. Discharge instructions are reviewed and follow-up care coordinated.

After discharge, the patient returns to the office for suture removal and wound check. Questions regarding physiotherapy and activity levels are answered. Phone calls are answered concerning pain levels and activity restrictions. Subsequent follow-up office visits are scheduled to review activity levels and physiotherapy. Neurologic examinations confirm improvement in leg strength and sensation. Postoperative X rays of the spine are ordered and reviewed showing the alignment of the spine. Prescription medication refills are reviewed and written. An exercise program is recommended and printed material regarding therapy is provided to the patient.

Clinical Example (0098T)

A 41-year-old man with progressive lower back pain for several years unresponsive to multiple modalities of conservative treatment underwent a total disc arthroplasty at the L4/L5 and L5/S1 level. Three weeks postoperatively the patient develops increasing pain. X rays identify loss of fixation of the arthoplasty components at both levels and progressive migration. At surgery, both total disc arthroplasties are removed and replaced using an anterior approach.

Description of Procedure (0098T)

Using the existing incision, additional mobilization of the tissues anterior to the spine is performed exposing the adjacent intervertebral disc. The disc arthroplasty is removed. The vertebral body endplates are reshaped and prepared for reinsertion of the arthroplasty components. The disc space is distracted, and the height, depth, and width are measured and an appropriate size prosthesis selected. The components are inserted and final intraoperative imaging obtained to confirm alignment. Hemostasis is obtained and a multi-layer closure performed.

●0099T Implantation of intrastromal corneal ring segments

Rationale

Code 0099T was established to report implantation of intrastromal corneal ring segments (two thin crescent-shaped implants made of durable material) into the cornea to protect the sight, improve visual functional quality, and delay the need for complex surgical intervention (eg, corneal transplant) for patients with keratoconus.

Keratoconus is characterized by a progressive thinning and steepening of the central and inferior areas of the cornea. As the cornea steepens and thins, the patient experiences a decrease in functional vision, which can be mild or severe depending on the degree to which the corneal tissue is affected. Typically, spectacles or soft contact lenses are prescribed early on to provide a uniform refracting surface and therefore improve vision. However, as the disease progresses further, and the degree of irregular astigmatism increases, the rigid contact lenses are less effective. Some of these patients will need a corneal transplant. Implantation of the corneal ring segments can be offered as an alternative to transplant surgery.

This procedure preserves corneal tissue and requires remodeling of the cornea by creation of small incisional channels into which the implants are inserted. The implants are then threaded into the channels and positioned to achieve maximum effect and incisions are sutured. The placement and dimensions of the implants help to reshape the cornea to its original, natural shape, thereby normalizing the cornea's architecture and adjusting for the myopia and irregular astigmatism caused by keratoconus.

Clinical Example (0099T)

A 25-year-old female with fluctuating vision caused by a combination of myopia and irregular astigmatism has for several years needed and worn custom-made rigid gas-permeable contact lenses to achieve and maintain functional vision. During a periodic eye examination with an optometrist, the patient explains her difficulty in performing everyday tasks with current lenses; she also complains of ongoing eye irritation that makes daily wear of her contact lenses difficult. The optometrist has identified that patient's keratoconus has progressed and now requires further intervention. He refers the patient to a corneal surgeon with diagnosis of keratoconus.

Description of Procedure (0099T)

At an evaluation of the patient, the corneal surgeon reviews the patient's history with her optometrist, performs a separate evaluation of the patient's visual acuity with existing correction using a Snellen visual acuity chart, takes a corneal topography image of the eye, checks the patient's intra-ocular pressure, and takes several pachymetry readings over the surface of the cornea. Upon confirming the diagnosis of keratoconus and discussing the patient's options, INTACS insertion procedure is scheduled.

●0100T Placement of a subconjunctival retinal prosthesis receiver and pulse generator, and implantation of intra-ocular retinal electrode array, with vitrectomy

Rationale

Code 0100T was added to describe surgical implantation of a retinal prosthetic device consisting of a stimulator and electrode array for vision restoration in patients blinded by retinal degenerative diseases. This device directly stimulates the inner retinal layer with indwelling electrodes to produce visual perception for patients with diseases in which photoreceptors have been damaged (eg, retinitis pigmentosa, age-related macular degeneration). Procedural steps in this treatment include isolation of the rectus muscle and positioning of the external transmitter (receiver/pulse generator stimulator), followed by a pars plana vitrectomy and intraocular insertion of the internal receiver (electrode array) to the retinal surface.

Clinical Example (0100T)

The patient is a 70-year-old female who has been diagnosed with retinitis pigmentosa since the age of 19. The degenerative disease has progressed to a state where the patient has no light perception. The patient has a severely limited quality of life due to blindness.

Description of Procedure (0100T)

Under either monitored local or general anesthesia, the procedure begins with a 360° conjunctival peritomy and isolation of the rectus muscles. Next, the extra-ocular portion of the retinal prosthesis, which includes the receiver/pulse generator, is positioned and attached to the episclera in one quadrant in a manner similar to a scleral buckling procedure. Three pars plana incisions are made and an infusion is started through one of the sclerotomies. A vitrectomy is performed, beginning by stripping the posterior hyaloid from the retina. The internal limiting membrane may be peeled at this point. One of the pars plana incisions is then enlarged and the intra-ocular portion of the stimulator, an electrode array, is inserted. With the assistance of perfluorocarbon liquid, the array is placed over the macular region of the retina centered over the fovea centralis and affixed using a custom retinal tack. Each of the scleral wounds are closed with sutures and the conjunctiva is sutured at the limbus. Subconjunctival and topical antibiotics and steroids are administered and the eye is patched and shielded.

The patient is evaluated in a clinic or office at 1 day, 1 week (3-7 days), 2 weeks (10-14 days), 1 month, and 3 months postoperatively. These visits include a surgical evaluation, medical interview, operative site exam, and complete ophthalmic exam, including extended ophthalmoscopy.

►(For application of low energy musculoskeletal system extracorporeal shock wave, use 0019T)◄

►(For application of low energy musculoskeletal system extracorporeal shock wave, use 0019T)◄

●**0101T** Extracorporeal shock wave involving musculoskeletal system, not otherwise specified, high energy

●**0102T** Extracorporeal shock wave, high energy, performed by a physician, requiring anesthesia other than local, involving lateral humeral epicondyle

▶(For application of low energy musculoskeletal system extracorporeal shock wave, use 0019T)◀

Rationale

To more accurately reflect current practice of extracorporeal shock wave treatments, the codes in the Category III section for this treatment have been changed. Code 0019T was revised to identify low-energy extracorporeal shock wave treatments. Code 0101T was established to report high-energy procedures (other than procedures for the lateral humeral epicondyle or plantar fascia). Code 0102T was established to report high-energy extracorporeal shock wave of the lateral humeral epicondyle. Code 0020T was deleted in tandem with its conversion to Category I code 28890 to identify physician-performed, high-energy shock wave treatment of plantar fascia requiring anesthesia other than local anesthesia. The descriptor language for code 28890 specifically includes (1) the requirement of providing anesthesia other than local when performing this service, (2) the specific anatomy involved (ie, the plantar fascia), and (3) the requirement of physician performance. This language differentiates provision of high-energy procedures for plantar fasciitis from the high-energy procedures reported with codes 0101T and 0102T or that do not require the same effort for high-energy procedures (code 0019T). The procedure identified by code 28890 requires provision by a physician due to pain issues and other considerations. When performing the high-energy extracorporeal shock wave therapy described by code 28890, a certain population of patients may require only regional anesthesia. However, this treatment is commonly provided with general anesthesia. Treatment of the lateral humeral epicondyle or of other anatomic areas using high energy should be identified by use of code 0102T and 0019T because these codes are intended to identify nonplantar faciitis treatments.

Clinical Example (0102T)

Tennis elbow is a condition in which there is inflammation or degeneration of the tendons attached to the outside, lateral side of the elbow. This disease process is generally characterized as an abrupt or subtle tearing of the tendonous area around the lateral aspect of the elbow and normally affects people between the ages of 30 and 50. Although many tennis players suffer with tennis elbow, the majority of people affected are not involved in sports. Because pain occurs from injured or damaged tendons near the elbow, people in occupational settings that require repetitive wrist and forearm movements such as painters, mechanics, and clerical workers are also likely to suffer from lateral epicondylitis.

The diagnosis of lateral epicondylitis is normally made through a physical examination and radiographic studies if necessary. Patients with tennis elbow experience pain at the lateral aspect of the elbow that can radiate or travel into the forearm and occasionally the hand. The pain occurs with grasping activities and may be accompanied by a sense of weakness.

The patient normally presents with such symptoms as pain along the lateral aspect of the elbow, difficulty lifting, and a weakened grip.

High-energy extracorporeal shock wave (ESW) is indicated for use in patients with chronic lateral epicondylitis who have failed to respond to conservative treatment such as physical therapy and stretching exercises, orthotics, bracing, NSAIDs, cortisone injections, or previous surgery.

Description of Procedure (0102T)
Prior to the administration of anesthesia, the area of tenderness on the affected area is palpated, and clearly designated with a marking pen.

High-energy ESW surgery with devices such as the OssaTron is painful; therefore, the procedure should be performed with anesthesia. The choice of anesthesia (local, regional, MAC, bier block, or general), after discussion with the patient, is the responsibility of the physician or anesthesiologist. The patient is placed supine on the stretcher with the affected arm placed in the lateral position. The head of the OssaTron is pointed downward towards the floor, and the table is raised to bring the elbow into the F2 area (F2 is the focal zone/treatment area of the shock wave).

Coupling gel is applied to the area of maximum tenderness or the treatment head. The shock head is coupled to the patient's elbow and positioned by the physician. It is important that there is good contact between the patient's elbow and the shock head to ensure that the treatment area remains within F2 throughout the procedure. The physician instructs the technician to set the OssaTron shock wave delivery rate to 4 Hz.

The procedure starts at 14 kV and the power is increased in increments until reaching a maximum power of 18 kV to evaluate the effect of anesthesia. (Power level is not to exceed 18 kV.) Treatment protocol increments for soft tissue application of high-energy ESW surgery with the OssaTron is as follows:

25 shocks @ 14 kV

25 shocks @ 15 kV

50 shocks @ 16 kV

1400 shocks @ 18 kV (Total 1500 shocks)

Ensuring that the elbow remains in constant contact with the shock head, the physician moves the affected area within the shock wave path (F2), and pronates and supinates the patient's hand during the procedure to ensure the entire tendon is treated to the proper depth based on the individual patient's anatomy and pathophysiology.

●**0103T** Holotranscobalamin, quantitative

Rationale
Code 0103T has been added to report performance of quantitative measurement of holotranscobalamin (vitamin B12 bound to transcobalamin) in human serum or plasma.

The test used to identify holotranscobalamin (Holo TC) quantitatively is an in-vitro diagnostic assay for quantitative measurement of holotranscobalamin (vitamin B12 bound to transcobalamin) in human serum or plasma. Measurements obtained by this procedure are utilized in the diagnosis and treatment of vitamin B12 deficiency.

Clinical Example 1 (0103T)

A 76-year-old woman complains of tingling in the feet and toes; she also has noted increasing irritability and forgetfulness. Physical examination reveals impaired position sense and absent vibration sense in both lower extremities. A blood specimen is drawn to measure complete blood count, chemistry panel, vitamin B12 and holo TC, serum methylmalonic acid (MMA), and intrinsic factor antibody assay.

Results:

Blood count = Normal

Hemoglobin = 14.1 g/dl

MCV = 94 fl

Chemistry panel = Normal (ref 200-900 pg/μl)

Serum B12 = 135 pg/mL (ref 200-900 pg/ml)

holo TC = 15 pmol/L (ref 40-150 pmol/L)

Serum MMA = 760 nM (ref < 270 nM)

Serum antibodies to intrinsic factor present

Interpretation:

The patient has vitamin B12 deficiency (low serum vitamin B12, low holo TC, high MMA) caused by autoimmune pernicious anemia (positive IF antibodies). Myeloneuropathy is present in the absence of anemia and macrocytosis.

Clinical Example 2 (0103T)

An 81-year-old man complains of lethargy and easy forgetfulness. Physical examination is unremarkable except for mild pallor. A blood specimen is drawn to measure blood count, chemistry panel, serum B12, holo TC, methylmalonic acid (MMA), and homocysteine (Hcy).

Results:

Blood count = Hemoglobin 10.5 g/dl

MCV = 84 fl

Chemistry panel showed creatinine increased 2.2 mg/dl, otherwise normal.

Serum MMA = 802 nM

Serum Hcy = 21 M

Serum B12 = 205 pg/ml

holo TC = 50 pmol/L

Interpretation:

The patient does not have objective evidence of vitamin B12 with borderline low-normal serum B12, and normal holo TC. The elevated MMA and Hcy are caused by chronic renal disease (elevated creatinine). Anemia is caused by refractory anemia (a myelodysplastic syndrome).

Clinical Example 3 (0103T)

A 58-year-old man complains of abdominal distension with tiredness and lethargy. Four years previously he had a subtotal gastrectomy for gastric carcinoma. Blood is drawn for a blood count, serum B12, and holo TC; a bone marrow biopsy was carried out.

Results:

Blood count shows anemia

Hemoglobin = 10.1 g/dl

MCV = 101 fl

Leukocytosis = (WCC 24.6 × 103) with neutrophilia, left shift including 4% myelocytes and 7% metamyelocytes

Serum B12 = 380 pg/ml (ref 200-900)

Holo TC = 22 pmol/L

Bone marrow showed granulocytic hyperplasia and megaloblastic change.

Cytogenetic analysis showed the presence of a 9-22 reciprocal translocation (Philadelphia chromosome).

Interpretation:

Patient has chronic myelogenous leukemia with coexistent vitamin B12 deficiency caused by previous gastrectomy. Total serum B12 is spuriously normal because of increased levels of haptocorrin produced by high leukocyte count. TC levels are not affected by this and reflect the true state of B12 deficiency.

●**0104T** Inert gas rebreathing for cardiac output measurement; during rest

●**0105T** during exercise

Rationale

Two codes, 0104T and 0105T, have been established to report inert gas rebreathing measurement.

Code 0104T is intended to report an inert gas rebreathing test for cardiac output measurement during rest. Code 0105T is intended to describe this same test during exercise.

The inert gas rebreathing method accumulates non-invasive cardiac output and related parameters of hemodynamic data.

Inert gas rebreathing is used to test adults and children. It can be used during testing at rest and in maximal or submaximal exercise stress testing. A stress test, including inert gas rebreathing maneuvers, evaluates the heart's function as a pump during physical or pharmacological stress.

The test interrogates the cardiac reaction to increased demand for oxygen and therefore provides important information that cannot be obtained at rest alone. The preferred method of stress involves either bicycle or treadmill symptom-limited exercise testing. If the patient is unable to perform adequate exercise, pharmacological stress or heart rate pacing in those patients with pacemakers becomes the preferred method. Unless complications that are not perceived by the patient develop, the test continues until the patient reaches the target heart rate or experiences chest pain or fatigue.

Clinical Example (0104T)

A male patient in his early 50s has had a heart transplant half a year ago. The patient is being followed at regular intervals in the cardiology department to confirm that the new heart's mechanical pumping function remains adequate. Limitations are most likely to appear at increased cardiac output values compared to the resting values. Increased cardiac output would normally be obtained by means of exercise testing (physical stress); however, due to the recent transplantation and the resulting inability to control the heart rate and contractility, the ability to increase cardiac output was instead examined by means of pharmacological stress testing.

Description of Procedure (0104T)

The patient underwent a dobutamine stress test while lying on a bed. Dobutamine is a medication that increases heart rate and blood pressure similar to the effect of exercise. The rise in heart rate increases the oxygen demand of the heart and helps to determine if the heart muscle is getting enough blood and oxygen.

Electrodes were placed on the chest to record an electrocardiogram for monitoring the heart's rate and rhythm. At the same time, a cuff was placed on the patient's upper arm to take blood pressure measurements. First, two baseline measurements of cardiac output were performed using inert gas rebreathing. An IV line was started in the patient's arm and a nurse administered dobutamine through the vein. The cardiologist observed for any symptoms, irregular heart rhythms, an inappropriate heart rate, or blood pressure responses. The patient was instructed to report any symptoms such as chest discomfort, headache, palpitations, nausea, and shortness of breath. The dose was increased every 20 down to 5 minutes from 5 to 10, 20 and 30 mg/min to gradually increase the heart rate. The heart rate increased from approximately 90 to above the target of 150 bpm. Cardiac output as measured by inert gas rebreathing increased from 7 L/min at rest to a plateau of 10-11 L/min at the highest infusion rates. Stroke volume changed little. After the pharmacological stress test, the dobutamine was stopped and both heart rate and cardiac output quickly returned to normal (prestress level) after a few minutes.

This test helped the physician evaluate the patient's post heart transplant condition related to the functioning of the heart muscle and valves under stress.

Clinical Example (0105T)

A 36-year-old man presented with slowly progressive breathlessness over the preceding 6 months. Three months previously, he had to stop playing tennis and was now unable to work. He was now limited to walking slowly and could only manage a flight of stairs before needing to rest and recover his breath. His symptoms had initially been associated with ankle edema, but this had cleared with the prescription of bumetanide by the primary care physician.

He was a nonsmoker. He had suffered from exercise-induced asthma as a child but had not required treatment for this for the last 10 years. He had been hospitalized for 48 hours with an episode of chest pain 3 years prior to this presentation; the previous diagnosis had been due to musculoskeletal pain.

His only medication was bumetanide. There was no family history of cardiac disease. Both his parents were alive and well.

Description of Procedure (0105T)

On examination, he appeared to have lost muscle bulk. Pulse was 90 in sinus rhythm, blood pressure 128/76. There was a trace of pitting edema at the ankles and some abdominal distension. The liver edge was palpable. The jugular venous pressure was elevated 4 cm above the sternal angle. Palpation of the precordial impulse was normal, and there were no abnormal features on auscultation.

The 12-lead electrocardiogram was normal, as were a full blood count and urea and electrolytes. Bilirubin was slightly raised, and an abdominal ultrasound revealed small amounts of ascites. A chest X ray showed a normal heart size with filling in of the costophrenic angles bilaterally and evidence of pulmonary venous distension.

The initial diagnosis was felt to be heart failure, presumed due to dilated cardiomyopathy. An echocardiogram, however, showed a morphologically normal heart, with normal left ventricular systolic function. The right heart was not dilated, and the transmitral diastolic blood flow was normal.

He underwent cycle ergometer testing with ECG monitoring and measurement of cardiac output using inert gas rebreathing. The resting cardiac output was 4.6 $L.min^{-1}$, and after exercise at 25 watts for 3 minutes was 4.8 $L.min^{-1}$. After a further 3 minutes exercise at 50 watts, cardiac output was 4.2 $L.min^{-1}$. He was unable to continue exercising thereafter due to extreme breathlessness.

The failure of his cardiac output to rise in response to exercise lead to the suggestion that he might have constrictive pericarditis and that the physical signs had been masked by the use of diuretics. He underwent cardiac catheterization, and the diagnosis was confirmed; there was the characteristic "dip-and-plateau" appearance in the diastolic traces in both the left and right ventricles with equalization of the diastolic pressures in all of the cardiac chambers.

The patient underwent pericardial stripping. The pericardium was densely adherent to the myocardium with no calcification. Histological findings were nonspecific. His breathlessness resolved immediately postoperatively, and, at 3-months follow up, he has returned to his normal activities. He is playing tennis again and has returned to work.

His notes from the previous admission with chest pain were reviewed; there were no striking findings at the time, but it was felt that he may have had an acute episode of pericarditis at that time and that the constriction had followed.

●0106T Quantitative sensory testing (QST), testing and interpretation per extremity; using touch pressure stimuli to assess large diameter sensation

●0107T using vibration stimuli to assess large diameter fiber sensation

●0108T using cooling stimuli to assess small nerve fiber sensation and hyperalgesia

●0109T using heat-pain stimuli to assess small nerve fiber sensation and hyperalgesia

●0110T using other stimuli to assess sensation

Rationale

Five codes were established to report quantitative sensory testing (QST). QST measures sensory impairment in the evaluation of endocrine and neurological disorders, by providing a quantitative value of the sensations of touch-pressure, vibration, cooling, warming, and pain. Each code describes the use of one of these stimuli to assess large-diameter fiber sensation or small nerve fiber sensation.

Clinical Example 1 (0106T)

A 22-year-old woman with a 10-year history of type I diabetes complains of burning pain, periodic lancinating pains, and some degree of "asleep-numbness" of the feet for 6 months. She also reports dryness of the eyes. Careful evaluation reveals only mild background retinopathy, 24-hour microalbumin is 7 mg, and except for mild diminuation of the ankle reflexes, no other neurologic abnormalities were found. The neuromuscular physician evaluating her diagnoses small fiber sensory polyneuropathy and considers the following diagnoses: diabetic sensorimotor polyneuropathy, immune sensory neuropathy with sicca, amyloidosis (primary or transthyretin), hereditary sensory and autonomic neuropathies (especially type I), Tangiers disease, hypothyroidism, and various toxic and deficiency conditions. Further characterization of the type and severity of the modality of sensory loss and whether hyperalgesia is present (from the QST evaluation) will aid in differential diagnosis. The characteristics of electrophysiologic tests (testing of attributes of nerve conduction and needle electromyography) are also needed. Tests of autonomic dysfunction will also help. The three types of tests—NC and EMG, QST, and QAT—should reliably indicate the class of fibers, proximal to distal level of involvement, and severity and pathophysiologic abnormality of the disease. Additional specific clinical and laboratory tests may be needed. In this case, the Rose Bengal test of the eyes, the serologic tests of ANA, RhF, ENA, and ANCA, a panel of paraneoplastic antibodies, TSH, the CSF, and maybe even nerve biopsy may be needed to make a firm and correct diagnosis.

Clinical Example 2 (0106T)

A 64-year-old woman with type II diabetes for 8 years visits a physician because of pigmentation and edema of the legs and bothersome calluses of the feet. On clinical examination, she has bilateral bunions, a high instep of each foot, and blackened plantar calluses over the head of the first metatarsal bone. No obvious retinopathy was observed and the serum creatinine is 1 mg/dl. On physical examination, no weakness, absent ankle reflexes, and using QST only slight diminution of vibration sensation of the toe is found. The HbA1c is 10%. Because the symptoms and pattern of clinical involvement is in keeping with very poor glycemic control, the physician diagnoses diabetic sensory polyneuropathy and institutes a remedial program of (1) improved glycemic control, (2) improved foot care, and (3) surveillance of the effect of these measures. For the third objective, using QST he assesses sensation of the foot to test for the sensation and the degree of sensation loss. Depending on the degree of protective sensation loss, the physician makes a decision about the degree of weight bearing that should be allowed, the frequency of further evaluation, the degree and kind of treatment of the calluses, and what foot wear should be used.

Clinical Example 3 (0106T)

A 16-year-old boy is admitted to the hospital for intractable vomiting and diarrhea the day after a meal that included chicken. The physician's first thought is that it is food poisoning, from an endotoxin or from an infective agent. The boy recovers from the gastrointestinal upset in 36 hours but complains of some leg weakness and increasing discomfort of the feet in walking. On examination, only mild weakness of legs, absent knee and ankle reflexes, and no sensory loss is found. The physician observes that the patient's feet appear to be unusually sensitive. The consulting neurologist considers acute intermittent pophyria, acute inflammatory demyelinating polyradiculoneuropathy, vasculitic polyneuropathy, and acute poisoning (arsenic, mercury, or thallium). To evaluate the patient further, the neurologist elects to test NC, EMG, and QST (to see whether sensation loss is present, which class of fibers is dysfunctional, and whether there is sensory loss and hyperalgesia). The CSF will need to be examined and tests will be needed to rule out various intoxications and metabolic disorders. Nerve tissue may also be needed. The case illustrates how the QST is used to characterize type and severity of sensory loss by modality of sensation and whether hyperalgesia is present. This characterization influences the degree of further evaluation and the kind of treatment that might be used.

Description of Procedure (0106T)

QST is accomplished by a number of devices or systems that vary considerably in design, complexity, degree of quantitation, and standardization. Typically, the stimulus probe(s) is/are placed on the patient's extremity or anatomical part to be tested. The level of stimulus is given in ramps or in steps from small to large, the latter in increments of just noticeable steps, with use of null stimuli or forced choice algorithms. The algorithm of testing varies by device but should be validated and expressed as a threshold as a just noticeable difference (JND) value, actual physical units, and percentile and/or normal deviate values considering site, age, sex, and anthropomorphic characteristics.

●0111T Long-chain (C20-22) omega-3 fatty acids in red blood cell (RBC) membranes

▶(For very long chain fatty acids, use 82726)◀

Rationale

Code 0111T was established to report long-chain omega-3 fatty acid testing. This is a test for long-chain (C20-22) omega-3 fatty acids (eicosapentaenoic [EPA] and docosahexaenoic acids [DHA]) in red blood cell (RBC) membranes. Results are reported as the EPA + DHA content of RBCs expressed as a percent of total fatty acids. This test seeks to detect deficient tissue levels of EPA + DHA (based on RBC as a surrogate). This condition has been shown to be associated with increased risk for death from coronary heart disease in ecological, case-control, and prospective cohort studies. This test measures a new analyte (long-chain [C20-22] fatty acids) by a current method (gas chromatography) but in a new specimen source (RBC membrane).

Existing code 82726 is intended to report an assessment of very long chain fatty acids (greater than C22). Similarly, code 82725 is intended to report the measurement concentration of unesterified fatty acids in serum, not their composition, nor all fatty acids in plasma (ie, fatty acids that are sterified in triglycerides, phospholipids, and cholesteryl esters are excluded from this measurement).

Clinical Example (0111T)

A 57-year-old white female with a history of a previous myocardial infarction visits her cardiologist. She naturally wants to avoid a future event. She asks for the most complete risk factor evaluation available. Her physician orders a cardiac risk panel, which includes an assessment of the RBC EPA + DHA, in addition to cholesterol, LDL, HDL, triglycerides, homocysteine, and C-reactive protein. The former is an independent risk factor for death from CHD, especially sudden cardiac death. If her value is less than 8%, then she would be encouraged to eat fatty fish or take fish oil supplements.

Description of Procedure (0111T)

The test is done on the RBC pellet from any anticoagulated specimen. There are no special or unusual collection, storage, analytical, or reporting requirements.

▶MEDICATION THERAPY MANAGEMENT◀

▶Medication Therapy Management Service(s) (MTMS) describe face-to-face patient assessment and intervention as appropriate, by a pharmacist. MTMS is provided to optimize the response to medications or to manage treatment-related medication interactions or complications.◀

▶MTMS includes the following documented elements: review of the pertinent patient history, medication profile (prescription and non-prescription), and recommendations for improving health outcomes and treatment compliance. These codes are not to be used to describe the provision of product-specific information at the point of dispensing or any other routine dispensing-related activities.◀

●**0115T** Medication therapy management service(s) provided by a pharmacist, individual, face-to-face with patient, initial 15 minutes, with assessment, and intervention if provided; initial encounter

●**0116T** subsequent encounter

+●0117T each additional 15 minutes (List separately in addition to code for primary service)

►(Use 0117T in conjunction with 0115T, 0116T)◄

Rationale

Three codes—0115T, 0116T, and add-on code 0117T—and guidelines have been established to report the provision of medication therapy management services (MTMS). These services are provided by a pharmacist to optimize the response to medications or for the management of treatment-related medication interactions or complications. MTMS services are initiated at the request of the patient. These services are not intended to describe a pharmacist providing counter discussion concerning dispensed medications, but rather to describe services that are out of the ordinary.

In provision of MTMS, the review of the pertinent patient history and medication profile will include evaluation of prescription medications, over-the-counter (OTC) medications, and herbal medications, and physician samples. The pharmacist will inventory the medications list to determine duplications, under- or overdosing, and drug interactions. The pharmacist may discover medications that need to be added or stopped. This service will include communication of management recommendations to the prescriber.

Each medication is assessed to determine the effectiveness and the side effects. A follow-up monitoring call is included in MTMS to determine if the symptoms are resolving, if the patient is experiencing side effects, and to assess the patient's compliance.

Assessment will be performed to determine the patient's adherence to medication recommendations. The pharmacist will educate the patient and monitor reaction to new and changed prescriptions and OTC medications.

Similar to other codes series in the CPT codebook, these codes have been structured to report the initial and more intensive encounter service with code 0115T. The subsequent encounter, reported with code 0116T, is intended to be reported for services provided that are similar to the initial encounter, with an emphasis on updating information provided at the initial encounter, assessment of the patient compliance and reactions, and further evaluation of medications that have been added to the patient's therapy with those previously assessed. Add-on code 0117T is reported in addition to codes 0115T, 0116T for each additional 15 minutes of service beyond the initial service.

Clinical Example (0115T)

A 66-year-old female with pre-existing osteoporosis has been diagnosed with type II diabetes and hyperlipidemia. Initial medication therapy assessment and intervention is performed.

Description of Procedure (0115T)

Patient intake information is obtained; materials that will be used during the patient encounter are gathered and prepared; and the physician coordinates other support staff.

Assessment of the patient may include obtaining a patient medical and medication (eg, prescription and nonprescription) history; determining the appropriateness of medication therapy (supra- or suboptimal); performing a review of relevant systems; evaluating pertinent laboratory data; assessing potential or existing drug-drug, drug-disease, and drug-nutrient interactions; establishing and/or obtaining such additional information (eg, obtaining information from other medical records) as may be necessary; and developing a care plan that includes recommendations for optimizing medication therapy.

Pharmacist interventions may include providing education, training, and resources; administering medication; formulating a treatment and/or follow-up plan; providing recommendations for disease prevention; and evaluating the patient's knowledge of medication and willingness to implement recommendations.

Additionally, the visit includes documentation of the patient encounter; non-face-to-face interventions and recommendations; referrals; communication with other health care professionals; administrative functions (including patient and family communications) relative to the patient's care; and, as appropriate, scheduling of follow-up appointment(s).

Clinical Example (0116T)

A 66-year-old female with osteoporosis, type II diabetes, and hyperlipidemia is receiving follow-up reassessment after receiving a prior medication therapy management service.

Description of Procedure (0116T)

Patient intake information is obtained; materials that will be used during the patient encounter are gathered and prepared; and the physician coordinates other support staff.

Assessment of the patient may include obtaining or updating a patient medical and medication (prescription and nonprescription) history; performing reviews of relevant systems; reviewing pertinent laboratory data; assessing potential or existing drug-drug, drug-disease, and drug-nutrient interactions; evaluating medication-related adverse events and toxicities; assessing medication effectiveness, organizing and interpreting the data; establishing and/or obtaining such additional information (eg, obtaining information from other medical records) as may be necessary; assessing any recent change in medication therapy or a new medication therapy-related problem; and developing a care plan that includes recommendations for optimizing medication therapy.

Pharmacist interventions may include providing reinforcement of education, training, and resources; modifying therapy; administering medication; formulating a treatment and/or follow-up plan; providing recommendations for disease prevention; re-evaluating the patient's knowledge of medication; and evaluating the patient's knowledge and willingness to follow new recommendations.

Additionally, the visit includes documentation of the patient encounter interventions and recommendations; referrals; communication with other health care professionals; administrative functions (including patient and family communications) relative to the patient's care; and, as appropriate, scheduling of follow-up appointment(s).

Clinical Example (0017T)

The service(s) is(are) continued for an additional 15 minutes with the same patient.

●**0120T** Ablation, cryosurgical, of fibroadenoma, including ultrasound guidance, each fibroadenoma

►(Do not report 0120T in conjunction with 90772)◄

Rationale

Code 0120T was established to report cryosurgical ablation of fibroadenomas. This procedure describes treatment of fibroadenomas in the breast with cryosurgical ablation. A parenthetical note has been added following code 0120T instructing users that code 0120T is not reported in conjunction with 90782. Code 0120T should be reported for each fibroadenoma treated.

Clinical Example (0120T)

A woman in her twenties presents with a palpable mass in her breast. She undergoes clinical and ultrasound examination that suggests a fibroadenoma, which is confirmed by a core or fine needle aspiration breast biopsy. The physician offers conservative management (watchful waiting), surgical excision, or cryoablation. The patient decides through consultation with her physician that conservative management is not an appropriate option due to the psychological and/or quality of life impact of leaving a palpable mass in the breast. The patient also does not wish to have a surgical incision, which is cosmetically disadvantageous, especially for a young woman concerned about the physical appearance of her breasts. Given a choice between (1) a surgical excision as an ambulatory surgical procedure under sedation or general anesthesia or (2) cryoablation in the physician's office under local anesthetic, the patient chooses to undergo the cryoablation procedure.

Description of Procedure (0120T)

The patient is positioned and prepped in a manner identical to that were she about to undergo an ultrasound-guided breast biopsy, with the breast cleansed and the area to be ablated numbed using local anesthesia. Ultrasound guidance from a handheld breast ultrasound transducer confirms the location of the benign tumor. A small nick in the skin is made to allow for cryoprobe introduction. The sharp cryoprobe tip is centered in 3 dimensions with the use of ultrasound guidance in the fibroadenoma. When cryoprobe placement is confirmed, the treatment cycle is initiated according to a programmed algorithm in the cryoablation system based on lesion size. If separation between the tumor and skin surface is required to protect the skin, sterile saline can be injected between them to increase separation and prevent skin injury from the cold. The ice ball formation is monitored with ultrasound throughout the treatment cycle. Two complete freeze-thaw cycles are required to complete the tissue ablation process. When the second freeze has been completed, the cryoprobe is warmed by flowing helium gas through it. It is removed from the breast once its temperature rises above the freezing point (ie, it is no longer frozen to the tissue).

Following cryoablation, the puncture entry is compressed to achieve hemostasis and a Steri-Strip or bandage is applied. Typically, postprocedure discomfort, if present, is controlled with nonsteroidal anti-inflammatory medications (NSAIDs) or acetaminophen.

●0123T Fistulization of sclera for glaucoma, through ciliary body

Rationale

Code 0123T was established to report the performance of a glaucoma filtering surgery using a pair of ablation tips utilizing a device to treat primary open angle glaucoma in phakic patients, to create a filter tract through the sclera and tissue behind the iris into the posterior chamber of the eye. Creation of this tract filters aqueous fluid from behind the iris (posterior chamber) through the ciliary body and attempts to reduce iatrogenically induced cataracts, anterior angle pathology in the form of peripheral anterior synechia, and cornea endothelial damage. Draining aqueous fluid to the posterior chamber of the eye changes the aqueous dynamics in the anterior part of the eye, thereby maintaining positive pressure in the eye and eliminating the need for an iridectomy (placement of a hole in the iris).

Clinical Example (0123T)

This procedure replaces trabeculectomy in any phakic chronic open angle glaucoma (COAG) patient but has many advantages that accommodate systemic medical diseases that afflict the age group normally involved with open angle glaucoma (ie, 50 years and older).

A 61-year-old black male with severe cardiovascular disease presents. The patient underwent prior right carotid endarterectomy and quadruple bypass surgery. The patient is a labile diabetic poorly controlled by insulin. One year ago, the patient had uncontrolled advanced glaucoma and underwent a surgical trabeculectomy of the right eye. Postoperatively, the patient developed a large choroidal detachment with positive pressure in the eye resulting in a flat anterior chamber of the eye. The flat anterior chamber persisted and caused an iatrogenic cataract formation, severe peripheral anterior synechia, and cornea endothelial cell damage requiring a corneal transplant. Trabeculectomies filter aqueous fluid from the anterior chamber of the eye (ie, in front of the iris) and, therefore, have a high incidence of postoperative flat anterior chambers. During the postoperative period, this patient had a stress-related hospitalization for acute myocardial infarction. Coronary stents were placed. Presently, the patient has uncontrolled COAG of the left eye and requires a surgical filtering procedure. The patient's labile medical status and history of post-trabeculectomy flat anterior chamber presents a difficult case that can be managed much more safely with transciliary filtration (TCF) since the FDA protocol incidence of flat anterior chambers was 0%. The FDA protocol also showed that the ocular tissue that is surgically traumatized is significantly less for TCF than for trabeculectomy, thereby making surgical revisions of a filtering procedure much safer with TCF.

Description of Procedure (0123T)

The patient undergoes a conjunctival flap, a plasma ablation through sclera above the ciliary body, a plasma ablation starting at the base of the scleral pit created above, and a plasma ablation creating a 100-micron pore through the ciliary body and into the posterior chamber of the eye. Aqueous fluid thereby drains from the posterior chamber of the eye and out under the conjunctiva, which has been sutured back into its natural position. No iridectomy is usually required.

A surgical prep of the patient for surgery under OR microscope is performed. A 5-mm conjunctival flap (fornix or limbal based) is raised. An electromagnetic plasma generator is used to produce a plasma wave coating over a 0.6-mm wide blunt, metal tip in order to create a plasma ablated pit through the sclera above the ciliary body of the eye (ie, behind the iris). This device is used to produce a plasma wave coating over a 100-micron diameter blunt, metal tip in order to create a plasma ablated pore from the base of the above-created scleral pit through the ciliary body into the posterior chamber of the eye. Posterior chamber aqueous fluid is drained to prevent a collapse of the anterior chamber postoperatively, which avoids iatrogenically induced cataracts, peripheral anterior synechia, and cornea endothelial cell damage with a subsequent cloudy cornea. Plasma ablation prevents burning of tissue while it also prevents bleeding through a process called "autostasis." The conjunctival flap is reattached with sutures. **Note:** Attempts to drain from the posterior chamber with other methods besides plasma ablation results in extensive bleeding from the highly vascular ciliary body.

●**0124T** Conjunctival incision with posterior juxtascleral placement of pharmacological agent (does not include supply of medication)

Rationale

Code 0124T was established to report the performance of a conjunctival incision, passage of a catheter to the posterior aspect of the globe in Tenon's space, and placement of a depot medication for treatment of macular degeneration.

Clinical Example (0124T)

A 67-year-old white male presents with decreased visual acuity and metaphorphopsia secondary to subfoveal choroidal neovascularization. Aposterior juxtascleral injection of an anti-angiogenic pharmacologicagent is performed.

Description of Procedure (0124T)

After reclining the patient in an examination chair, topical anesthetic is administered and a lid and conjunctival preparation with 5% povidone iodine solution is administered. A lid speculum is positioned and topical 4% lidocaine applied to the incision site. A 2- to 3-mm conjunctival and Tenon's capsule incision is made in the superior temporal quadrant, 8 mm from the limbus, and Tenon's space is entered. The injection cannula is passed into Tenon's space and follows the globe posteriorly to the macula where 0.5 cc is injected. An assistant provides pressure over the injection site to prevent reflux. The speculum is removed and a semi-pressure patch is applied.

●0126T Common carotid intima-media thickness (IMT) study for evaluation of atherosclerotic burden or coronary heart disease risk factor assessment

Rationale

Code 0126T was established to report performance of a study to determine IMT common carotid measurement of obstruction and scanning for arterial wall thickness as a precursor to narrowing. An IMT study is performed to measure the dimensions of the inner two layers of the arterial wall (the intima and the media) of the carotid artery for evidence of thickening or development and anatomical manifestation of atherosclerotic vascular disease in its early stages in the asymptomatic patient.

Clinical Example (0126T)

A 45-year-old male patient is seen for an annual, routine medical visit. The physician determines that, due to the patient's age, high-fat diet, sedentary lifestyle, and hypertension, the patient should undergo an IMT study.

Description of Procedure (0126T)

After consent, the patient's right common carotid is scanned using high-resolution B-mode ultrasound, the image analyzed, and the patient provided with his IMT measurement and interpretation. In consult with the physician, the patient may receive one or all of the following recommendations: dietary change, exercise plan, lipid-lowering therapy, antihypertensive therapy, and/or further cardiovascular testing. A follow-up IMT study is recommended every 1-2 years to measure treatment efficacy.

●0130T Validated, statistically reliable, randomized, controlled, single-patient clinical investigation of FDA approved chronic care drugs, provided by a pharmacist, interpretation and report to the prescribing health care professional

Rationale

Code 0130T was established to report the pharmacist performance of a validated, statistically reliable, randomized, single-patient clinical investigations of FDA-approved chronic care drugs, for valid prescriptions. This service includes the provision of a report to the prescribing professional. This service is intended to promote rational, cost-effective drug use and adherence.

In providing the service, the pharmacist statistically analyzes and reviews the patient's drug therapy diary. A report is provided for the prescribing physician to detail the relative effectiveness and adverse event profile of the drug treatment, to assist the physician in determining the optimal drug therapy for the patient.

Clinical Example (0130T)

A 70-year-old female osteoarthritis patient complains of "morning finger stiffness." The patient requests Celebrex because she saw a television advertisement "where all the old people were playing tennis because of Celebrex." Her sister, who is a homemaker, also recommended Celebrex because her neighbor uses it. The physician wants to prescribe naproxen but also wishes to maintain the patient's trust and goodwill. He or she, therefore, prescribes a single-patient trial test kit comparing naproxen to Celebrex for osteoarthritis.

Description of Procedure (0130T)

The prescription is received by fax at a pharmacy authorized to assemble blinded medications in compliance blister cards with easy-to-fill-out diaries for data collection on effectiveness and adverse events. The test kit is prepared and dispensed according to the prescriber's valid prescription and the pharmacy's SOPs. The pharmacy call center follows up with the patient to ensure that the test was received and to answer any questions and to record the start of test date. The patient also receives a unique patient identification card with the kit number of the test included on the card. This is provided in the rare case where the patient experiences a severe adverse event and the pharmacy must be contacted at any time in order to break the blind and identify which of the two medicines was being taken at the time of the event. During the test period, the patient contacts the pharmacy and explains that she forgot to take her medicine for a few days. She wants to know if she should continue the test. The pharmacy instructs her to continue the test and asks if she would like a periodic phone call to remind her to take the medicines. She declines and is able to complete the remainder of the test successfully. At the end of the test period, the patient returns the diaries to the pharmacy operation where the blind is broken and the data is statistically analyzed and reviewed by a pharmacist in collaboration with a biostatistician. Despite two missed days of reporting, a detailed report that contains a valid statistical analysis of effectiveness and side-effect data is prepared and e-mailed to the prescribing physician. In this case, naproxen was superior to Celebrex on certain pain relief parameters, while both drugs had similar adverse event profiles. Therefore, based on objective evidence, naproxen was shown to be the preferred treatment for this patient. Because of this objective information created by direct participation of the patient, naproxen is re-prescribed by the physician. The outcomes report is then electronically filed in the patient's file.

●0133T Upper gastrointestinal endoscopy, including esophagus, stomach, and either the duodenum and/or jejunum as appropriate, with injection of implant material into and along the muscle of the lower esophageal sphincter (eg, for treatment of gastroesophageal reflux disease)

Rationale

Code 0133T was established to report delivery of submucosal injections of multiple doses of a polymer into the intramuscular portion of the lower esophageal sphincter for the purpose of treating gastroesophageal reflux disease. As is true with other endoscopy codes, code 0133T includes the upper GI endoscopy procedure and, therefore, is not separately reported from diagnostic GI endoscopy. Code 0133T is intended to be reported one time, regardless of the number of injections required for insertion of the implant material.

Clinical Example (0133T)

A 54-year-old woman reports chronic heartburn symptoms three times or more per week. Upper gastrointestinal endoscopy (EGD), 24-hour pH testing, and esophageal manometry testing are performed. The patient demonstrates a normal manometric examination and an abnormally elevated DeMeester score of > 14.7. She has Los Angeles Grade A esophagitis and no hiatal hernia. The patient is provided a trial of daily full-dose proton pump inhibitor therapy. Her symptoms improve but are not completely relieved. Double-dose treatment is instituted with control of the symptoms but she is desirous of pursuing other means to allow her to control the disease. The patient is counseled regarding the treatment options, including pharmacologic, endoscopic, and surgical. Given the risk and benefit of each option, the patient states she is adverse to a surgical procedure. The patient and physician choose endoscopic deep intramural injection of a biopolymer into the lower esophageal sphincter for treatment of her gastroesophageal reflux disease.

Description of Procedure (0133T)

The procedure is performed on an outpatient basis in an endoscopy unit equipped for fluoroscopy. After informed consent is obtained, the patient is placed on an endoscopy gurney. Intravenous access is obtained, conscious sedation is administered, and vital signs are monitored. An EGD is performed to confirm the absence of pathology that would represent a contraindication to the performance of the proposed procedure. The upper endoscope is then positioned in the lower esophagus and the injection catheter introduced through the endoscope. The squamocolumnar junction (Z-line) is visualized, the injection needle is advanced, and the mucosa punctured 1-2 mm below the Z-line. The biopolymer solution is then injected along the muscle layer under fluoroscopic guidance. Multiple discrete injections of 1-2 cc each are performed in a circumferential manner until a total of 6-8 cc are implanted. The injection rate is no faster than 1 cc/min to allow for polymerization and heat dissipation. The needle remains in place for 1 minute after complete implantation. During the procedure, fluoroscopy is used to monitor the injection procedure and confirm intramural implant location. Following the last injection, the endoscope is removed and the procedure terminated. Postprocedure vital signs are checked and the patient is transferred to the recovery suite. The patient is monitored for signs of complications. Prescriptions for pain medication and anti-emetics are provided and the patient is discharged with instructions regarding potential delayed complications.

●**0135T** Ablation, renal tumor(s), unilateral, percutaneous, cryotherapy

Rationale

Code 0135T was established to report percutaneous cryotherapy ablation of renal tumor(s).

Percutaneous cryotherapy ablation of renal tumors is clinically indicated for a select group of patients that includes those who have tumors 4 cm or smaller and may be poor surgical candidates; or who refuse radical nephrectomy or partial nephrectomy; or have multiple comorbid illnesses, a solitary kidney, renal insufficiency; or for those patients for whom renal preservation is desired, such as those with von Hippel-Lindau disease (a rare, genetic multi-system disorder characterized by the abnormal growth of tumors in certain parts of the body; including the kidneys).

The modality of imaging used to guide percutaneous cryotherapy ablation of renal tumors is dependent on patient-specific clinical considerations and physician preference. The existing guidance codes (76362, computer tomography; 76394, magnetic resonance imaging; 76940, ultrasound guidance) are appropriately reported for the visceral tissue ablation imaging services for percutaneous cryotherapy ablation of renal tumors.

Clinical Example (0135T)

A 76-year-old man was presented to his primary care physician complaining of abdominal pain. A computed tomography (CT) scan was ordered and a 3.0-cm enhancing solid renal mass in the posterior aspect of the midpole of the left kidney was incidentally found. The patient has had previous open-heart surgery and has marginal renal function making open total or partial nephrectomy extremely risky. The patient's urologist refers the patient for cryoablation of this renal mass based on his comorbidities.

Description of Procedure (0135T)

On the day of the procedure, after an overnight fast as directed, the patient is admitted to the pre-procedural preparation area. The patient is evaluated by anesthesia and the appropriate lines placed. After premedication, the patient is transferred to the interventional suite. The patient is placed under successful general anesthesia, and all imaging compatible monitors were placed. The patient is placed in the prone position on the table and is properly protected. Imaging is performed to target the lesion (separately reportable using appropriate modality specific imaging code: 76940, ultrasound; 76362, CT; or 76394, magnetic resonance imaging). A set of images are obtained for localization purposes (included in the separately reportable modality-specific imaging code: 76940, 76362, or 76394) and for selection of the site for initial cryoprobe placement. The physician reviews these initial images and plans a skin entry site and treatment plan. The appropriate size cryoprobe(s) (2 mm or 3 mm) are placed in the lesion. The cryoprobe tip locations are confirmed and found to be safely positioned. Freezing of the lesion is then begun and monitored continuously to ensure complete coverage of the lesion with an appropriate margin, as well as avoidance of injury to other organs. After complete freezing of the lesion, the entire tumor is actively thawed. The cryoprobes are maintained in place without repositioning and the tumor is frozen a second time. A second active thaw sufficient to allow removal of the cryoprobe(s) without tearing of the tissue is performed, then the remainder of the tumor thaws passively. If the iceball coverage is judged to be inadequate, the lesion is thawed to allow repositioning of the existing cryoprobes or implantation of additional probes. Freezing is continued or probes are added until the entire tumor plus any margin receives two complete freeze/thaw cycles. The incision sites are cleaned and covered with sterile adhesive dressings.
The patient is transported to the recovery room and admitted overnight to an observation bed for pain control and monitoring of any significant hemorrhage. If stable, he is discharged home the following morning with antibiotics and narcotics. Documentation of the procedure is done for the permanent record. Cryoablation outcome and the patient's status are communicated to the patient's

family and copies of reports are sent to the patient's referring physician. Upon discharge, the patient is advised to contact the treating physician for treatment-related issues such as return of symptoms to the area, fever, or pain with breathing and scheduled for a follow-up appointment within 7-10 days.

●**0137T** Biopsy, prostate, needle, saturation sampling for prostate mapping

▶(Do not report 0137T in conjunction with 76942)◀

Rationale

Code 0137T was established to report prostate saturation biopsy. An instructional parenthetical note was added following code 0137T to preclude the use of code 0137T in conjunction with 76942.

Prostate mapping through saturation biopsies is a technique performed under general anesthesia. A transrectal ultrasound probe is used to image the prostate while a template or grid identifies the exact location of each biopsy core. Typically, a total of 20 to 40 cores are taken. Each core is individually marked so that the exact position and extent of the tumor can be mapped.

Prostrate mapping is typically performed after an initial diagnosis of prostate cancer when (1) initial biopsies obtained through the traditional method (55700) are equivocal or nondiagnostic and more extensive biopsying is needed to rule out prostate cancer (eg, a patient with a rising PSA with traditional biopsy revealing tissue suspicious but not diagnostic for prostate cancer); and (2) traditional biopsies reveal localized prostate cancer and the patient has elected focal tissue cryoablation.

Clinical Example (0137T)

A 50-year-old gentleman has a rising prostate specific antigen (PSA). He recently underwent traditional transrectal ultrasound with biopsies that revealed two suspicious biopsies suggestive, but not diagnostic, for carcinoma. In an effort to more accurately determine if he has prostate cancer and the volume of the disease, he is to undergo template-guided saturation biopsies for prostate mapping.

Description of Procedure (0137T)

The patient is taken to the operating suite and given general anesthesia. He is placed in the dorsal lithotomy position and prepped and draped. A foley catheter is inserted into the bladder. A transrectal ultrasound transducer is placed into the rectum and the prostate is visualized. A midway reference place is determined using the stepping function of the biopsy stepper. At the midway reference plane, everything toward the base is labeled "proximal" and everything toward the apex is labeled "distal." Next a coronal reference plane that divides the prostate into anterior and posterior zones is chosen, preferably at the junction of the transition and the peripheral zones. A brachytherapy grid is then placed against the perineum and rectum. Using transrectal ultrasound for needle guidance, a total of 20 to 40 biopsies are taken using the template or grid as a guide. Starting at the highest point within the prostate, biopsies are taken moving from the right to left until the row is completed. Then, moving down a row, the same sequence is performed until all rows are complete. With several deeper sections, a proximal and distal biopsy is taken from the same tract. With each biopsy, the urologist states the correct location and coordinates of that specimen. The assistant keeps track of the numbers and location of the biopsies to prevent confusion and mislabeling. After completion, the patient is taken to the recovery room and is scheduled for follow-up in 2 weeks.

●**0140T** Exhaled breath condensate pH

Rationale

Code 0140T was established to report exhaled breath condensate pH measurement. Exhaled breath condensate pH test measures exhaled breath condensate (EBC), a respiratory fluid. This measurement yields an assessment of airway chemistry and inflammation in patients with asthma.

Clinical Example (0140T)

An 18-year-old female athlete with a history of mild intermittent asthma presents by ambulance to the emergency department with acute respiratory distress beginning during a track and field competition. She has inspiratory and expiratory wheezes, a slightly elevated heart rate with normal heart sounds, and no evidence of heart disease. She has an oxygen saturation of 99% on room air. A chest X ray and spirometry are ordered and, after providing informed consent, the patient is enrolled in a research study and exhaled breath condensate collection is obtained. Therapy is instituted with beta agonists. The chest X ray is normal without evidence of hyperinflation or infiltrate. Spirometry reveals truncated inspiratory and expiratory loops without evidence of small airway disease. Exhaled breath condensate pH is 7.8 (normal 7.5-8.3). Further history is obtained and reveals that she is an A student and has frequent anxiety episodes. The patient improves rapidly in the emergency department and is discharged with the diagnosis of suspected vocal cord syndrome.

Description of Procedure (0140T)

The physician, respiratory therapist, or nurse removes a disposable breath condensate collector from its package, obtains a chilled metal condenser from a nearby freezer, and places an insulation cover over it. Alternatively, an electric exhaled breath cooling (EBC) device for the disposable collector can be used. The health care professional has the patient hold the portable device and place the mouthpiece of the EBC collector into her mouth (the mouthpiece is identical to a nebulizer mouthpiece). The patient is instructed to breathe in and out normally through the mouthpiece for 2 to 10 minutes. Ambient air (optionally supplemented with oxygen) is inhaled through a one-way valve while exhaled air is directed through the condensation chamber. The health care professional uses a specially designed syringe-style plunger to remove the EBC from the condenser. Approximately 400 microliters of EBC are obtained and placed in a micro centrifuge tube, deaerated with Argon gas (bubbling inexpensive Argon through the sample by means of a pipette), and the pH measured with a glass pH microelectrode after appropriate calibration. The sample is stored for subsequent research involving other biomarkers in EBC, such as cytokines and cysteinyl-leukotrienes.

Other applications include incorporating the collector into the exhalation limb of a ventilator circuit for either one collection and assay or for continuous minute-by-minute EBC pH monitoring for hours or days.

Collection systems other than the one described can also be employed, although the technique described is the most common method employed in the last 2 years in the United States and the technique employed in the NIH-sponsored multi-centered asthma studies.

Appendices

For *CPT 2006*, the appendix section has again been revised. Three new appendices have been added to the CPT code set. The new appendices include a listing of the codes pending FDA approval at the time of publication and two anatomic listings of nerve and vascular families as coding resources.

Appendix A

✍ Rationale

The explanatory language for modifier 25 was revised with the addition of language to expand on the phrase "significant, separately identifiable E/M services" in order to clarify those circumstances for which modifier 25 is appropriately reported.

Modifiers

▲25 **Significant, Separately Identifiable Evaluation and Management Service by the Same Physician on the Same Day of a Procedure or Other Service**

The physician may need to indicate that on the day a procedure or service identified by a CPT code was performed, the patient's condition required a significant, separately identifiable E/M service above and beyond the other service provided or beyond the usual preoperative and postoperative care associated with the procedure that was performed. ►A significant, separately identifiable E/M service is defined or substantiated by documentation that satisfies the relevant criteria for the respective E/M service to be reported (see Evaluation and Management Services Guidelines for instructions on determining level of E/M service).◄ The E/M service may be prompted by the symptom or condition for which the procedure and/or service was provided. As such, different diagnoses are not required for reporting of the E/M service. **Note:** This modifier is not used to report an E/M service that resulted in a decision to perform surgery (see modifier 57).

Appendix G

✍ Rationale

In tandem with the revision of the subsection heading and addition of guidelines, codes, and cross-references to report moderate sedation services, the guidelines that direct the use of Appendix G have been revised to include directions for appropriately reporting the listed procedures in addition to codes 99148-99150 for moderate sedation provided by a second physician.

Summary of CPT Codes That Include Moderate (Conscious) Sedation

►The following list of procedures includes conscious sedation as an inherent part of providing the procedure. These codes are identified in the CPT codebook with a ⊙ symbol.◄

►Since these services include moderate sedation, it is not appropriate for the same physician to report both the service and the sedation codes 99143-99145. It is expected that if conscious sedation is provided to the patient as part of one of these services, it is provided by the same physician who is providing the service.◄

►In the unusual event when a second physician other than the health care professional performing the diagnostic or therapeutic services provides moderate sedation in the facility setting (eg, hospital, outpatient hospital/ambulatory surgery center, skilled nursing facility) for the procedures listed in Appendix G, the second physician can report 99148–99150. However, for the circumstance in which these services are performed by the second physician in the nonfacility setting (eg, physician office, freestanding imaging center), codes 99148-99150 would not be reported. Moderate sedation does not include minimal sedation (anxiolysis), deep sedation, or monitored anesthesia care (00100-01999).◄

►The inclusion of a procedure on this list does not prevent separate reporting of an associated anesthesia procedure/service (CPT codes 00100-01999) when performed by a physician other than the health care professional performing the diagnostic or therapeutic procedure. In such cases the person providing anesthesia services shall be present for the purpose of continuously monitoring the patient and shall not act as a surgical assistant. When clinical conditions of the patient require such anesthesia services, or in the circumstances when the patient does not require sedation, the operating physician is not required to report the procedure as a reduced service using modifier 52.◄

Appendix H

Rationale

New codes and conditions have been included in Appendix H. Rationale for the new codes can be found in the Category II section. The new clinical conditions that have been added to Appendix H include asthma, congestive heart failure (CHF), hypertension (HTN), osteoarthritis (adult), and prenatal-postpartum care.

All Category II information, including Appendix H, is included on the American Medical Association Web site at www.ama-assn.org/go/cpt. In addition, information regarding the source of the original measure as well as the Web site location of the measure organization is also included in a footnote subsequent to both the listing of the Category II codes and the Appendix H section.

Alphabetic Index of Performance Measures by Clinical Condition or Topic

Note: Prior to coding, the user must review the complete description of the code in the Category II section of the CPT codebook and the complete description of its associated measure by accessing the measure developer's Web site provided in the footnoted reference.

Performance Measure Exclusion Modifiers	**-1P Performance Measure Exclusion Modifier due to Medical Reasons** Includes, for example: - patient allergic history, - potential adverse drug interaction, - acquired or congenital absence of organ/limb, - other documented clinical contraindication	Performance measurement exclusion modifiers may be used to indicate that a service specified by a performance measure was considered but, due to either medical or patient circumstance(s) documented in the medical record, the service was not provided. These modifiers serve as denominator exclusions from the performance measure.
	-2P Performance Measure Exclusion Modifier due to Patient Choice Includes, for example: - patient refusal, - economic, - social, - religious	

Brief Description of Performance Measure & Source	CPT Code(s)	Brief Code Descriptor
Asthma		
Asthma Assessment[1]—Percentage of patients aged 5-40 years with asthma who were evaluated during at least one office visit during the reporting year for the frequency (numeric) of daytime and nocturnal asthma symptoms (To be counted in calculations of this measure, symptom frequency must be numerically quantified. Measure may also be met by physician documentation or patient completion of an asthma assessment tool/survey/questionnaire. Assessment tool may include the QualityMetric Asthma Control Test™, National Asthma Education & Prevention Program (NAEPP) Asthma Symptoms and Peak Flow Diary) **Numerator:** Patients in the denominator who were evaluated during at least one office visit during the reporting year for the frequency (numeric) of daytime and nocturnal asthma symptoms **Denominator:** All patients aged 5-40 years with asthma **Inclusion(s):** None **Exclusion(s):** None	**1005F**	Asthma symptoms evaluated
Asthma Pharmacologic Therapy[1]—Percentage of patients aged 5-40 years with mild, moderate, or severe *persistent* asthma who were prescribed either the preferred long-term control medication (inhaled corticosteroids)* or an acceptable alternative treatment **Numerator:** Patients in the denominator who were prescribed either the preferred[a] long-term control medication (inhaled corticosteroids)* or an acceptable alternative treatment[b] (cromolyn sodium, leukotriene modifier, nedocromil, OR sustained release theophylline) **Denominator:** All patients aged 5-40 years with mild, moderate, or severe persistent asthma **Inclusion(s):** None **Exclusion(s):** Documentation of patient reasons (eg, economic, social, religious) for not prescribing either the preferred long-term control medication or an acceptable alternative treatment (There are no medical exclusion criteria) [a, b] Refer to complete description of measure on the Consortium's Internet site for list of medications, treatment recommendations, dosages * In patients with moderate or severe persistent asthma, strong evidence indicates that use of inhaled long-term acting $beta_2$-agonists (LABA) in combination with ICS leads to improvements in lung function and symptoms and reduced supplemental bronchodilator use. LABA is not recommended for use as monotherapy	**4015F**	Persistent asthma, long-term control medication prescribed

[1]Physician Consortium for Performance Improvement, www.ama-assn.org/go/quality
[2]National Committee on Quality Assurance (NCQA), Health Employer Data Information Set (HEDIS®), www.ncqa.org
[3]Joint Commission on Accreditation of Healthcare Organizations (JCAHO), ORYX Initiative Performance Measures, www.jcaho.org/pms

Brief Description of Performance Measure & Source	CPT Code(s)	Brief Code Descriptor
Congestive Heart Failure (CHF)		
Composite Measure: Heart Failure Assessment[1]— See individual measures listed below for: level of activity assessed (1003F), clinical symptoms of volume overload (excess) assessed (1004F), blood pressure measured (2000F), weight recorded (2001F), clinical signs of volume overload (excess) assessed (2002F), and auscultation of the heart performed (2003F)	**0001F**	Heart failure assessed (includes assessments 1003F, 1004F, 2000F, 2001F, 2002F, and 2003F)
Assessment of Activity Level[1]—Percentage of heart failure patient visits with assessment of activity level **Numerator:** Patient visits in the denominator with assessment of current level of activity OR documentation of standardized scale or completion of assessment tool (includes use of New York Heart Association Functional Classification of Congestive Heart Failure; Kansas City Cardiomyopathy Questionnaire; Minnesota™ Living with Heart Failure Questionnaire; or Guyatt's Chronic Heart Failure Questionnaire) **Denominator:** All patient visits for patients aged ≥ 18 years with heart failure **Inclusion(s):** None **Exclusion(s):** None	**1003F**	Level of activity assessed
Assessment of Clinical Symptoms of Volume Overload (Excess)[1]—Percentage of heart failure patient visits with assessment of clinical symptoms of volume overload (excess) **Numerator:** Patient visits in the denominator with assessment of clinical symptoms of volume overload (excess) OR documentation of standardized scale or completion of assessment tool (includes New York Heart Association Functional Classification of Congestive Heart Failure; Kansas City Cardiomyopathy Questionnaire; Minnesota™ Living with Heart Failure Questionnaire; or Guyatt's Chronic Heart Failure Questionnaire) **Denominator:** All patient visits for patients aged ≥ 18 years with heart failure **Inclusion(s):** None **Exclusion(s):** None	**1004F**	Clinical symptoms of volume overload (excess) assessed
Blood Pressure Measurement[1]—Percentage of patients in the denominator who had a blood pressure measurement during the last office visit **Numerator:** Patients who had a blood pressure measurement during the last office visit **Denominator:** All patients with CHF **Inclusion(s):** None **Exclusion(s):** None	**2000F**	Blood pressure measured

[1]Physician Consortium for Performance Improvement, www.ama-assn.org/go/quality
[2]National Committee on Quality Assurance (NCQA), Health Employer Data Information Set (HEDIS®), www.ncqa.org
[3]Joint Commission on Accreditation of Healthcare Organizations (JCAHO), ORYX Initiative Performance Measures, www.jcaho.org/pms

Brief Description of Performance Measure & Source	CPT Code(s)	Brief Code Descriptor
Congestive Heart Failure (CHF), *continued*		
Weight Measurement[1]—Percentage of heart failure patient visits with weight measurement **Numerator:** Patient visits in the denominator with weight measurement recorded **Denominator:** All patient visits for patients aged ≥ 18 years with heart failure **Inclusion(s):** None **Exclusion(s):** None	**2001F**	Weight recorded
Assessment of Clinical Signs of Volume Overload (Excess)[1]—Percentage of patient visits with assessment of clinical signs of volume overload (excess) **Numerator:** Patient visits in the denominator with assessment of clinical signs of volume overload (excess) **Denominator:** All patient visits for patients aged ≥ 18 years with heart failure **Inclusions(s):** None **Exclusion(s):** None	**2002F**	Clinical signs of volume overload (excess) assessed
Examination of the Heart[1]—Percentage of patient visits with examination of the heart **Numerator:** Patient visits in the denominator with examination of the heart **Denominator:** All patient visits for patients aged ≥ 18 years with heart failure **Inclusion(s):** None **Exclusion(s):** None	**2003F**	Auscultation of the heart performed
Patient Education[1]—Percentage of heart failure patients who were provided with patient education on disease management and health behavior changes during one or more visit(s) within a six-month period **Numerator:** Patients in the denominator who were provided with written and/or verbal education at one or more visit(s) during a six-month care period under evaluation Patient education (includes one or more of the following: weight monitoring; diet (sodium restriction); symptom management; physical activity; smoking cessation; medication instruction; minimizing or avoiding use of NSAIDs; follow-up plans for next appointment or visiting nurse; referral for specific educational or management programs; or prognosis/end-of-life issues) **Denominator:** All patients aged ≥ 18 years with heart failure and with one or more visit(s) during a six-month period **Inclusion(s)(Denominator):** Patients with one or more visit(s) during a six-month period **Exclusion(s):** None	**4003F**	Patient education, written/oral, appropriate for patients with heart failure performed

[1]Physician Consortium for Performance Improvement, www.ama-assn.org/go/quality
[2]National Committee on Quality Assurance (NCQA), Health Employer Data Information Set (HEDIS®), www.ncqa.org
[3]Joint Commission on Accreditation of Healthcare Organizations (JCAHO), ORYX Initiative Performance Measures, www.jcaho.org/pms

Brief Description of Performance Measure & Source	CPT Code(s)	Brief Code Descriptor
Beta-Blocker Therapy[1]—Percentage of heart failure patients who also have LVSD who were prescribed beta-blocker therapy **Numerator:** Patients in the denominator who were prescribed beta-blocker therapy **Denominator:** All heart failure patients aged ≥ 18 years with left ventricular ejection fraction (LVEF) ≤ 40% or with moderately or severely depressed left ventricular systolic function **Inclusion(s):** None **Exclusion(s):** Documentation that a beta-blocker was not indicated; documentation of medical or patient reason(s) for not prescribing beta-blocker (eg, bradycardia < 50 bpm without beta-blocker therapy, history of Class IV heart failure, history of second- or third-degree AV block without permanent pacemaker)	**4006F**	Beta-blocker therapy prescribed
Heart Failure Angiotensin Converting Enzyme (ACE) Inhibitor for left ventricular systolic dysfunction (LVSD)[1]—Percentage of heart failure patients who also have LVSD and who were prescribed ACE inhibitor therapy **Numerator:** Heart failure patients in the denominator aged ≥ 18 years who are prescribed an ACE inhibitor at hospital discharge **Denominator:** All heart failure patients with aged ≥ 18 years with left ventricular ejection fraction (LVEF) < 40% or with moderately or severely depressed left ventricular systolic function **Inclusion(s):** None **Exclusion(s) (Denominator):** Documentation that ACE inhibitor was not indicated (eg, patients on angiotensin receptor blockers (ARB)); documentation of medical reason(s) for not prescribing ACE inhibitor therapy (eg, allergy, angioedema due to ACE inhibitor, anuric renal failure due to ACE inhibitor, pregnancy, moderate or severe aortic stenosis); documentation of patient reasons for not prescribing ACE inhibitor therapy (economic, social, or religious)	**4009F**	Angiotensin Converting Enzyme (ACE) inhibitor therapy prescribed
Warfarin Therapy for Patients with Atrial Fibrillation[1]—Percentage of heart failure patients who also have paroxysmal or chronic atrial fibrillation who were prescribed warfarin therapy **Numerator:** Patients in the denominator who were prescribed warfarin therapy **Denominator:** All heart failure patients aged ≥ 18 years with paroxysmal or chronic atrial fibrillation **Inclusion(s):** None **Exclusion(s):** Documentation that warfarin was not indicated; documentation of medical reasons(s) for not prescribing warfarin (eg, allergy to warfarin, risk of bleeding or bleeding disorder, compliance, etc); documentation of patient reason(s) (eg, economic, social, and/or religious) for not prescribing warfarin	**4012F**	Warfarin therapy prescribed

[1]Physician Consortium for Performance Improvement, www.ama-assn.org/go/quality
[2]National Committee on Quality Assurance (NCQA), Health Employer Data Information Set (HEDIS®), www.ncqa.org
[3]Joint Commission on Accreditation of Healthcare Organizations (JCAHO), ORYX Initiative Performance Measures, www.jcaho.org/pms

Brief Description of Performance Measure & Source	CPT Code(s)	Brief Code Descriptor
Congestive Heart Failure (CHF), *continued*		
Heart Failure Discharge Instructions[3]—Percentage of hospitalized heart failure patients in the denominator who received written discharge instructions **Numerator:** Heart failure patients in the denominator with documentation that they or their caregivers were given written discharge instructions or other educational material addressing all of the following: activity level, diet, discharge medications, follow-up appointment, weight monitoring, what to do if symptoms worsen **Denominator:** Heart failure patients discharged home **Inclusion(s):** none **Exclusion(s):** Patients aged < 18 years	**4014F**	Written discharge instructions provided to heart failure patients discharged home
Coronary Artery Disease (CAD)		
Smoking Cessation Evaluation[1]—Percentage of patients evaluated for smoking or other tobacco use **Numerator:** Patients evaluated for smoking or other tobacco use **Denominator:** All patients **Inclusion(s):** None **Exclusion(s):** None	**1000F** **1001F**	Tobacco use, smoking, assessed Tobacco use, non-smoking, assessed
Symptom & Activity Assessment[1]—Percentage of CAD patients who were evaluated for both level of activity and anginal symptoms during one or more office visits **Numerator:** Patients who were evaluated for both level of activity and anginal symptoms during one or more office visits **Denominator:** All patients with CAD **Inclusion(s):** None **Exclusion(s):** None	**1002F**	Anginal symptoms and level of activity assessed
Blood Pressure Measurement[1]—Percentage of patients who had a blood pressure measurement during the last office visit **Numerator:** Patients who had a blood pressure measurement during the last office visit **Denominator:** All patients with CAD **Inclusion(s):** None **Exclusion(s):** None	**2000F**	Blood pressure measured
Smoking Cessation Intervention[1]—Percentage of patients identified as cigarette smokers who received smoking cessation intervention **Numerator:** Patients identified as smokers or other tobacco users who were offered an intervention for tobacco use cessation, either counseling or pharmacologic therapy during one or more office visits. **Denominator:** All patients identified as smokers or other tobacco users **Inclusion(s):** None **Exclusion(s):** None	**4000F** **4001F**	Tobacco use cessation counseling Tobacco use cessation intervention, pharmacologic therapy

[1]Physician Consortium for Performance Improvement, www.ama-assn.org/go/quality
[2]National Committee on Quality Assurance (NCQA), Health Employer Data Information Set (HEDIS®), www.ncqa.org
[3]Joint Commission on Accreditation of Healthcare Organizations (JCAHO), ORYX Initiative Performance Measures, www.jcaho.org/pms

Brief Description of Performance Measure & Source	CPT Code(s)	Brief Code Descriptor
Drug Therapy for Lowering Cholesterol[1]—Percentage of patients who were prescribed a statin (based on current ACC/AHA guidelines) **Numerator:** Patients who were prescribed a statin **Denominator:** All patients with CAD **Inclusion(s):** None **Exclusion(s):** Documentation that a statin was not indicated; documentation of medical or patient reason(s) for not prescribing a statin	**4002F**	Statin therapy prescribed
Beta-Blocker Therapy- Prior Myocardial Infarction (MI)[1]—Percentage of CAD patients who also have prior MI who were prescribed beta-blocker therapy **Numerator:** Patients who were prescribed beta-blocker therapy **Denominator:** All patients with CAD **Inclusion(s):** Patients with prior MI **Exclusion(s):** Documentation that a beta-blocker was not indicated; documentation of medical or patient reason(s) for not prescribing a beta-blocker	~~**4003F**~~ **4006F***	Beta-blocker therapy prescribed
Angiotensin Converting Enzyme (ACE) Inhibitor Therapy[1]—Percentage of CAD patients who also have diabetes and/or left ventricular systolic dysfunction (LVSD) who were prescribed ACE inhibitor therapy **Numerator:** Patients who were prescribed ACE inhibitor therapy **Denominator:** All patients with CAD who also have diabetes and/or LVSD **Inclusion(s):** Patients with CAD who also have diabetes and/or LVSD, left ventricular ejection fraction (LVEF) < 40% or moderately or severely depressed left ventricular systolic function) **Exclusion(s):** Documentation that ACE inhibitor was not indicated (eg, patients on angiotensin receptor blockers; documentation of medical or patient reason(s) for not prescribing ACE inhibitor	~~**4004F**~~ **4009F***	Angiotensin Converting Enzyme (ACE) inhibitor prescribed
Antiplatelet Therapy[1]—Percentage of patients who were antiplatelet prescribed therapy **Numerator:** Patients who were prescribed antiplatelet therapy **Denominator:** All patients with CAD **Inclusion(s):** None **Exclusion(s):** Documentation that antiplatelet therapy was not indicated; documentation of medical or patient reason(s) for not prescribing a beta-blocker	~~**5005F**~~ **4011F***	Oral antiplatelet therapy prescribed

[1]Physician Consortium for Performance Improvement, www.ama-assn.org/go/quality
[2]National Committee on Quality Assurance (NCQA), Health Employer Data Information Set (HEDIS®), www.ncqa.org
[3]Joint Commission on Accreditation of Healthcare Organizations (JCAHO), ORYX Initiative Performance Measures, www.jcaho.org/pms
*The code listed under the stricken code reflects updates that have occurred in Appendix H of the 2006 CPT codebook since the publication of the codebook. The codes listed in the Category II section of the CPT codebook are correct as written. See the Category II section of the CPT Web site (www.ama-assn.org/go/CPT) for the most up-to-date information.

Brief Description of Performance Measure & Source	CPT Code(s)	Brief Code Descriptor
Hypertension (HTN)		
Blood Pressure Measurement[1]—Percentage of patient visits with blood pressure recorded for patients aged ≥ 18 years **Numerator:** Patient visits in the denominator with blood pressure measurement recorded **Denominator:** All patient visits for patients aged ≥ 18 years with hypertension **Inclusion(s):** None **Exclusion(s):** None	**2000F**	Blood pressure measured
Controlling High Blood Pressure[2]—Percentage of patients whose blood pressure is adequately controlled (BP ≤ 140/90) during the measurement year **Numerator:** Patients in the denominator whose blood pressure is adequately controlled (BP ≤ 140/90) during the measurement year **Denominator:** Patients aged 46 to 85 years with a diagnosis of hypertension and medical record review to confirm diagnosis and continuously enrolled for the measurement year **Inclusion(s):** None **Exclusion(s):** Exclude from eligible population all members diagnosed with end-stage renal disease anytime on or prior to December 31 of the measurement year	**3000F** **3002F**	Blood pressure ≤ 140/90 mm Hg Blood pressure > 140/90 mm Hg
Osteoarthritis (Adult)		
Composite Measure: Osteoarthritis Assessment— See individual measures listed below for: Osteoarthritis symptoms and functional status assessed (1006F), use of anti-inflammatory or over-the-counter (OTC) analgesic medications assessed (1007F), initial examination of the involved joint(s) (includes visual inspection, palpation, range of motion) (2004F)	**0005F**	Osteoarthritis assessed includes assessments 1006F, 1007F, 2004F
Symptom and Functional Assessment[1]—Percentage of osteoarthritis patient visits with assessment for current level of satisfaction with symptoms and functional status **Numerator:** Patient visits in the denominator with assessment for current level of satisfaction with symptoms and functional status **Denominator:** All patient visits for patients aged ≥ 21 years with osteoarthritis of the knee **Inclusion(s):** None **Exclusion(s):** None **Note:** Use when osteoarthritis is addressed during the patient encounter	**1006F**	Osteoarthritis symptoms and functional status assessed

[1]Physician Consortium for Performance Improvement, www.ama-assn.org/go/quality
[2]National Committee on Quality Assurance (NCQA), Health Employer Data Information Set (HEDIS®), www.ncqa.org
[3]Joint Commission on Accreditation of Healthcare Organizations (JCAHO), ORYX Initiative Performance Measures, www.jcaho.org/pms

Brief Description of Performance Measure & Source	CPT Code(s)	Brief Code Descriptor
Assessment for Use of Anti-inflammatory or Analgesic OTC medications[1] Percentage of osteoarthritis patient visits with assessment for use of anti-inflammatory or analgesic over-the-counter (OTC) medications **Numerator:** Patient visits in the denominator with assessment for use of anti-inflammatory or analgesic OTC medications **Denominator:** All patient visits for patients aged ≥ 21 years with osteoarthritis of the knee **Inclusion(s):** None **Exclusion(s):** None **Note:** Use when osteoarthritis is addressed during the patient encounter	**1007F**	Use of anti-inflammatory or analgesic over-the-counter (OTC) medications assessed
Non-steroidal Anti-inflammatory Drug (NSAID) Risk Assessment[1] Percentage of patients on prescribed or OTC NSAIDs who were assessed for gastrointestinal and renal risk factors **Numerator:** Patients who were assessed for all of the following risk factors: • GI bleed • History of peptic ulcer disease • Concomitant use of glucocorticoids or anticoagulants • Smoking • Significant alcohol use • Age > 65 years • Renal disease (Creatinine (Cr) > 2.0 mg/dl) • Hypertension • Heart failure • Concomitant use of diuretic or angiotensin converting enzyme (ACE) inhibitor **Denominator:** All patients aged ≥ 21 years with osteoarthritis **Inclusion(s):** None **Exclusion(s):** None	**1008F**	Gastrointestinal and renal risk factors assessed
Physical Examination of the Knee[1] Percentage of osteoarthritis patients for whom a physical examination of the knee was performed during the initial visit **Numerator:** Patients in the denominator for whom a physical examination of the knee was performed during the initial visit **Denominator:** All patients aged ≥ 21 years with osteoarthritis of the knee **Inclusion(s):** None **Exclusion(s):** None **Note:** Use only for initial osteoarthritis visit or for visits for new joint involvement	**2004F**	Initial examination of the involved joint(s)

[1]Physician Consortium for Performance Improvement, www.ama-assn.org/go/quality
[2]National Committee on Quality Assurance (NCQA), Health Employer Data Information Set (HEDIS®), www.ncqa.org
[3]Joint Commission on Accreditation of Healthcare Organizations (JCAHO), ORYX Initiative Performance Measures, www.jcaho.org/pms

Brief Description of Performance Measure & Source	CPT Code(s)	Brief Code Descriptor
Osteoarthritis (Adult), *continued*		
Anti-inflammatory/Analgesic Therapy[1] Percentage of patient visits during which an anti-inflammatory agent or analgesic was considered **Numerator:** Patient visits in the denominator during which an anti-inflammatory agent or analgesic was considered **Denominator:** All patient visits for patients aged ≥ 21 years with osteoarthritis of the knee **Inclusion(s) (Numerator):** Documentation that an anti-inflammatory agent or analgesic was not indicated; documentation of medical reason(s) for not prescribing an anti-inflammatory agent or analgesic (eg, allergy, drug interaction, contraindication); documentation of patient reasons(s) for not prescribing an anti-inflammatory agent or analgesic (eg, economic, social, religious); documentation that an anti-inflammatory agent or analgesic was prescribed **Exclusion(s):** None	**4016F**	Anti-inflammatory/analgesic agent prescribed
Gastrointestinal Prophylaxis[1] Percentage of patients visits during which GI prophylaxis was considered **Numerator:** Patient visits in the denominator during which GI prophylaxis was considered **Denominator:** All patient visits for patients aged ≥ 21 years with osteoarthritis on prescribed or OTC NSAIDs **Inclusion(s) (Numerator):** Documentation that GI prophylaxis was not indicated (eg, patients on COX-2 inhibitors); documentation of medical reason(s) for not prescribing GI prophylaxis (eg, allergy, drug interaction, contraindication); documentation of patient reason(s) for not prescribing GI prophylaxis (eg, economic, social, or religious); documentation that GI prophylaxis was prescribed **Exclusion(s):** None	**4017F**	Gastrointestinal prophylaxis for NSAID use prescribed
Therapeutic Exercise for the Knee[1] Percentage of patient visits during which therapeutic exercise for the involved joint(s) (therapeutic exercised instructed or physical therapy prescribed) was considered **Numerator:** Patient visits during which therapeutic exercise for the knee was considered **Denominator:** All patient visits for patients aged ≥ 21 years with OA of the knee **Inclusion(s) (Numerator):** Documentation that therapeutic exercise was not indicated; documentation of medical reason(s) for not instructing therapeutic exercise for the knee or prescribing physical therapy for the knee; documentation of patient reason(s) for not instructing therapeutic exercise for the knee or prescribing physical therapy for the knee (eg, economic, social, religious); documentation that therapeutic exercise for the knee was instructed; documentation that physical therapy for the knee was prescribed **Exclusion(s):** None	**4018F**	Therapeutic exercise for the involved joint(s) instructed or physical therapy prescribed

[1]Physician Consortium for Performance Improvement, www.ama-assn.org/go/quality
[2]National Committee on Quality Assurance (NCQA), Health Employer Data Information Set (HEDIS®), www.ncqa.org
[3]Joint Commission on Accreditation of Healthcare Organizations (JCAHO), ORYX Initiative Performance Measures, www.jcaho.org/pms

Brief Description of Performance Measure & Source	CPT Code(s)	Brief Code Descriptor
Prenatal-Postpartum Care		
Timeliness of Prenatal Care[2]—Percentage of patients in the denominator who received prenatal care **Numerator:** Number of women in the denominator who received a prenatal care visit as a member of the managed care organization (MCO) in the first trimester or within 42 days of enrollment in the MCO **Denominator:** Women who had live births between November 6th of the year prior to the measurement year and November 5th of the measurement year, who were continuously enrolled at least 43 days prior to delivery through 56 days after delivery **Inclusion(s):** None **Exclusion(s):** None	**0500F**	Initial prenatal care visit
Prenatal Flow Sheet[1]—Percentage of patients in the documenteddenominator with a prenatal flow sheet in use by the first physician visit **Numerator:** Percentage of patients in the denominator with a flow sheet in use by the date of the first physician visit, which contains at a minimum: blood pressure, weight, urine protein, uterine size, fetal heart tones, and estimated date of delivery **Denominator:** Pregnant women seen for prenatal care **Inclusion(s):** None **Exclusion(s):** Patients seen for consultation only, not for continuing care	**0501F**	Prenatal flow sheet
Frequency of Ongoing Prenatal Care[2]—Percentage of patients in the denominator with expected number of prenatal visits **Numerator:** Number of women in the denominator who had an unduplicated count of < 21%, 21%-40%, 41%-60%, 61%-80%, or ≥ 81% of the expected number of prenatal care visits, adjusted for the month of pregnancy at time of enrollment and gestational age **Denominator:** Women who had live births during the measurement year **Inclusion(s):** None **Exclusion(s):** MCOs must exclude members for whom a prenatal visit is not indicated	**0502F**	Subsequent prenatal care visit
Postpartum Care[2]—Percentage of patients in the denominator who had a postpartum visit between 21 and 56 days after delivery **Numerator:** Number of women in the denominator who had a postpartum visit on or between 21 days and 56 days after delivery **Denominator:** Women who had live births between November 6th of the year prior to the measurement year and November 5th of the measurement year, who were continuously enrolled at least 43 days prior to delivery through 56 days after delivery **Inclusion(s):** None **Exclusion(s):** None	**0503F**	Postpartum care visit

[1]Physician Consortium for Performance Improvement, www.ama-assn.org/go/quality
[2]National Committee on Quality Assurance (NCQA), Health Employer Data Information Set (HEDIS®), www.ncqa.org
[3]Joint Commission on Accreditation of Healthcare Organizations (JCAHO), ORYX Initiative Performance Measures, www.jcaho.org/pms

Appendix I

Rationale

The list of modifiers for genetic testing has been updated and revised to make the modifier system more accurate and easier to use by those providing the service.

Neoplasia (solid tumor, excluding sarcoma and lymphoma) includes 0N, 0O, 0P, and 0Z. *Neoplasia (sarcoma)* includes 1A, 1B, 1C, 1D, 1E, 1F, 1G, 1H, 1I, and 1J. *Neoplasia (lymphoid/hematopoietic)* includes 2L, 2M, 2N. 2O, 2T, 2Q, 2R, and 2S. *Non-neoplastic hematology/coagulation* includes 3K. *Histocompatibility/blood typing/identity/microsatellite* includes 4I, 4J, 4K, 4L, 4M, 4N, and 4O. *Muscular, non-neoplastic* includes 6E and 6F. *Metabolic, other* includes 7F. *Metabolic, transport* includes 8B. *Metabolic-pharmacogenetics* includes 9B, 9C, and 9D.

Genetic Testing Code Modifiers

This listing of modifiers is intended for reporting with molecular laboratory procedures related to genetic testing. Genetic testing modifiers should be used in conjunction with CPT and HCPCS codes to provide diagnostic granularity of service to enable providers to submit complete and precise genetic testing information without altering test descriptors. These modifiers are categorized by mutation. The first (numeric) digit indicates the disease category and the second (alpha) digit denotes gene type. Introductory guidelines in the molecular diagnostic and molecular cytogenetic code sections of CPT provide further guidance in interpretation and application of genetic testing modifiers.

Neoplasia (solid tumor, excluding sarcoma and lymphoma)

0A BRCA1 (Hereditary breast/Ovarian cancer)

0B BRCA2 (Hereditary breast cancer)

0C Neurofibromin (Neurofibromatosis, type 1)

0D Merlin (Neurofibromatosis, type 2)

0E c-RET (Multiple endocrine neoplasia, types 2A/B, familial medullary thyroid carcinoma)

0F VHL (Von Hippel Lindau disease, renal carcinoma)

0G SDHD (Hereditary paraganglioma)

0H SDHB (Hereditary paraganglioma)

0I ERRB2, commonly called Her-2/neu

0J MLH1 (HNPCC, mismatch repair genes)

0K MSH2, MSH6, or PMS2 (HNPCC, mismatch repair genes)

0L APC (Hereditary polyposis coli)

0M Rb (Retinoblastoma)

0N TP53, commonly called p53

0O PTEN (Cowden's syndrome)

0P KIT, also called CD117 (gastrointestinal stromal tumor)

0Z Solid tumor gene, not otherwise specified

Neoplasia (sarcoma)

1A WT1 or WT2 (Wilm's tumor)

1B PAX3, PAX7, or FOXO1A (Alveolar rhabdomyosarcoma)

1C FLI1, ERG, ETV1, or EWSR1 (Ewing's sarcoma, desmoplastic round cell)

1D DDIT3 or FUS (Myxoid liposarcoma)

1E NR4A3, RBF56, or TCF12 (Myxoid chondrosarcoma)

1F SSX1, SSX2, or SYT (Synovial sarcoma)

1G MYCN (Neuroblastoma)

1H COL1A1 or PDGFB (Dermatofibrosarcoma protuberans)

1I TFE3 or ASPSCR1 (Alveolar soft parts sarcoma)

1J JAZF1 or JJAZ1 (Endometrial stromal sarcoma)

1Z Sarcoma gene, not otherwise specified

Neoplasia (lymphoid/hematopoietic)

2A RUNX1 or CBFA2T1, commonly called AML1 or ETO, genes associated with t(8;21) AML1—also ETO (Acute myelogenous leukemia)

2B BCR or ABL1, genes associated with t(9;22) (Chronic myelogenous or acute leukemia) BCR—also ABL (Chronic myeloid, acute lymphoid leukemia)

2C PBX1 or TCF3, genes associated with t(1;19) (Acute lymphoblastic leukemia) CGF1

2D CBFB or MYH11, genes associated with inv 16 (Acute myelogenous leukemia) CBF beta (leukemia)

2E MLL (acute leukemia)

2F PML or RARA, genes associated with t(15;17) (Acute promyelocytic leukemia) PML/RAR alpha (Promyelocytic leukemia)

2G ETV6, commonly called TEL, gene associated with t(12;21) (acute leukemia) TEL (Leukemia)

2H BCL2 (B cell lymphoma, follicle center cell origin) bcl-2 (Lymphoma)

2I CCND1, commonly called BCL1, cyclin D1 (Mantle cell lymphoma, myeloma) bcl-1 (Lymphoma)

2J MYC (Burkitt lymphoma) c-myc (Lymphoma)

2K IgH (Lymphoma/leukemia)

2L IGK (Lymphoma/leukemia)

2M TRB, T cell receptor beta (Lymphoma/leukemia)

2N TRG, T cell receptor gamma (Lymphoma/leukemia)

2O SIL or TAL1 (T cell leukemia)

2T BCL6 (B cell lymphoma)

2Q API1 or MALT1 (MALT lymphoma)

2R NPM or ALK, genes associated with t(2;5) (Anaplastic large cell lymphoma)

2S FLT3 (Acute myelogenous leukemia)

2Z Lymphoid/hematopoietic neoplasia, not otherwise specified

Non-neoplastic hematology/coagulation

3A F5, commonly called Factor V (Leiden, others) (Hypercoagulable state)

3B FACC (Fanconi anemia)

3C FACD (Fanconi anemia)

3D HBB, beta globin (Thalassemia, Sickle cell anemia, other hemoglobinopathies)

3E HBA, commonly called alpha globin (Thalassemia)

3F MTHFR (Elevated homocystinemia)

3G F2, commonly called prothrombin (20210, others) (Hypercoagulable state) Prothrombin (Factor II, 20210A) (Hypercoagulable state)

3H F8, commonly called Factor VIII (Hemophilia A/VWF)

3I F9, commonly called Factor IX (Hemophilia B)

3K F13, commonly called Factor XIII (bleeding or hypercoagulable state) Beta globin

3Z Non-neoplastic hematology/coagulation, not otherwise specified

Histocompatibility/blood typing/identity/microsatellite

4A	HLA-A
4B	HLA-B
4C	HLA-C
4D	HLA-D
4E	HLA-DR
4F	HLA-DQ
4G	HLA-DP
4H	Kell
4I	Fingerprint for engraftment (post-allogeneic progenitor cell transplant)
4J	Fingerprint for donor allelotype (allogeneic transplant)
4K	Fingerprint for recipient allelotype (allogeneic transplant)
4L	Fingerprint for leukocyte chimerism (allogeneic solid organ transplant)
4M	Fingerprint for maternal versus fetal origin
4N	Microsatellite instability
4O	Microsatellite loss (loss of heterozygosity)
4Z	Histocompatiblity/blood typing, not otherwise specified

Neurologic, non-neoplastic

5A	ASPA, commonly called Aspartoacylase A (Canavan disease)
5B	FMR-1 (Fragile X, FRAXA, syndrome)
5C	FRDA, commonly called Frataxin (Freidreich ataxia)
5D	HD, commonly called Huntington (Huntington's disease)
5E	GABRA5, NIPA1, UBE3A, or ANCR GABRA (Prader Willi-Angelman syndrome)
5F	GJB2, commonly called Connexin-26 (Hereditary hearing loss) Connexin-32 (GJB2) (Hereditary deafness)
5G	GJB1, commonly called Connexin-32 (X-linked Charcot-Marie-Tooth disease)
5H	SNRPN (Prader Willi-Angelman syndrome)
5I	SCA1, commonly called Ataxin-1 (Spinocerebellar ataxia, type 1)
5J	SCA2, commonly called Ataxin-2 (Spinocerebellar ataxia, type 2)
5K	MJD, commonly called Ataxin-3 (Spinocerebellar ataxia, type 3, Machado-Joseph disease)

5L CACNA1A (Spinocerebellar ataxia, type 6)

5M ATXN7 Ataxin-7 (Spinocerebellar ataxia, type 7)

5N PMP-22 (Charcot-Marie-Tooth disease, type 1A)

5O MECP2 (Rett syndrome)

5Z Neurologic, non-neoplastic, not otherwise specified

Muscular, non-neoplastic

6A DMD, commonly called dystrophin (Duchenne/Becker muscular dystrophy)

6B DMPK (Myotonic dystrophy, type 1)

6C ZNF-9 (Myotonic dystrophy, type 2)

6D SMN1/SMN2 (Autosomal recessive spinal muscular atrophy)

6E MTTK, commonly called tRNAlys (myotonic epilepsy, MERRF)

6F MTTL1, commonly called tRNAleu (mitochondrial encephalomyopathy, MELAS)

6Z Muscular, not otherwise specified

Metabolic, other

7A APOE, commonly called apolipoprotein E (Cardiovascular disease or Alzheimer's disease)

7B NPC1 or NPC2, commonly called sphingomyelin phosphodiesterase (Nieman-Pick disease)

7C GBA, commonly called acid beta glucosidase (Gaucher disease)

7D HFE (Hemochromatosis)

7E HEXA, commonly called hexosaminidase A (Tay-Sachs disease)

7F ACADM (medium chain acyl CoA dehydrogenase deficiency)

7Z Metabolic, other, not otherwise specified

Metabolic, transport

8A CFTR (Cystic fibrosis)

8B PRSS1 (Hereditary pancreatitis)

8Z Metabolic, transport, not otherwise specified

Metabolic-pharmacogenetics

9A TPMT, commonly called (thiopurine methyltransferase) (patients on antimetabolite therapy)

9B CYP2 genes, commonly called cytochrome p450 (drug metabolism)

9C ABCB1, commonly called MDR1 or p-glycoprotein (drug transport)

9D NAT2 (drug metabolism)

9L Metabolic-pharmacogenetics, not otherwise specified

Dysmorphology

9M FGFR1 (Pfeiffer and Kallman syndromes)

9N FGFR2 (Crouzon, Jackson-Weiss, Apert, Saethre-Chotzen syndromes)

9O FGFR3 (Achondroplasia, Hypochondroplasia, Thanatophoric dysplasia, types I and II, Crouzon syndrome with acanthosis nigricans, Muencke syndromes)

9P TWIST (Saethre-Chotzen syndrome)

9Q DGCR, commonly called CATCH-22 (DiGeorge and 22q11 deletion syndromes)

9Z Dysmorphology, not otherwise specified

Appendix J

Rationale

Appendix J provides two coding references: a list of nerve families and a table of maximum number of studies.

The nerve families list provides nerve branches included within a nerve family and is intended to assist in appropriate assignment of codes for nerve conduction studies (95900, 95903, and 95904).

The maximum number of studies table summarizes the recommended maximum number of studies per diagnostic category necessary for a physician to arrive at a diagnosis in 90% of patients with that final diagnosis, when performing needle electromyography (EMG) tests (95860-95864 and 95867-95870); nerve conduction studies (95900, 95903, 95904); and other EMG studies (95934, 95936, 95937). The numbers in the table are to be used as a tool to detect outliers to assist in appropriate reporting. Each number in the table represents one study or unit. The maximum numbers are designed to apply to a diverse range of practice styles as well as practice types, including those at referral centers where more complex testing is frequently necessary. In simple, straightforward cases, fewer tests will be necessary. This is particularly true when results of the most critical tests are normal. In complex cases, the maximum numbers in the table will be insufficient for the physician to arrive at a complete diagnosis. In cases where there are borderline findings, additional tests may be required to determine if the findings are significant.

The appropriate number of studies to be performed should be left to the judgment of the physician performing the electrodiagnostic (EDX) evaluation; however, in the small number of cases that require testing in excess of the numbers listed in the table, the physician should be able to provide supplementary documentation to justify the additional testing. Such documentation should explain what other differential diagnostic problems needed to be ruled out in that particular situation. In some patients, multiple diagnoses will be established by EDX testing, and the recommendations listed in the table for a single diagnostic category will not apply. It should be noted that in some situations it is necessary to test an asymptomatic contralateral limb to establish normative values for an individual patient. Normal values based on the general population alone are less sensitive than this approach; therefore, restrictions on contralateral asymptomatic limb testing will reduce the sensitivity of electrodiagnostic tests.

Electrodiagnostic Medicine Listing of Sensory, Motor, and Mixed Nerves

This summary assigns each sensory, motor, and mixed nerve with its appropriate nerve conduction study code in order to enhance accurate reporting of 95900, 95903, and 95904. Each nerve constitutes one unit of service.

Codes 95900 and 95903 involve the following motor nerves:

I. Upper extremity/cervical plexus/brachial plexus motor nerves
   A. Axillary motor nerve to the deltoid
   B. Long thoracic motor nerve to the serratus anterior
   C. Median nerve
      1. Median motor nerve to the abductor pollicis brevis
      2. Median motor nerve, anterior interosseous branch, to the flexor pollicis longus
      3. Median motor nerve, anterior interosseous branch, to the pronator quadratus
      4. Median motor nerve to the first lumbrical
      5. Median motor nerve to the second lumbrical
   D. Musculocutaneous motor nerve to the biceps brachii
   E. Radial nerve
      1. Radial motor nerve to the extensor carpi ulnaris
      2. Radial motor nerve to the extensor digitorum communis
      3. Radial motor nerve to the extensor indicis proprius
      4. Radial motor nerve to the brachioradialis
   F. Suprascapular nerve
      1. Suprascapular motor nerve to the supraspinatus
      2. Suprascapular motor nerve to the infraspinatus
   G. Thoracodorsal motor nerve to the latissimus dorsi
   H. Ulnar nerve
      1. Ulnar motor nerve to the abductor digiti minimi
      2. Ulnar motor nerve to the palmar interosseous
      3. Ulnar motor nerve to the first dorsal interosseous
      4. Ulnar motor nerve to the flexor carpi ulnaris
   I. Other

II. Lower extremity motor nerves
   A. Femoral motor nerve to the quadriceps
      1. Femoral motor nerve to vastus medialis
      2. Femoral motor nerve to vastus lateralis
      3. Femoral motor nerve to vastus intermedialis
      4. Femoral motor nerve to rectus femoris
   B. Ilioinguinal motor nerve
   C. Peroneal (fibular) nerve
      1. Peroneal motor nerve to the extensor digitorum brevis
      2. Peroneal motor nerve to the peroneus brevis
      3. Peroneal motor nerve to the peroneus longus
      4. Peroneal motor nerve to the tibialis anterior

- D. Plantar motor nerve
- E. Sciatic nerve
- F. Tibial nerve
    1. Tibial motor nerve, inferior calcaneal branch, to the abductor digiti minimi
    2. Tibial motor nerve, medial plantar branch, to the abductor hallucis
    3. Tibial motor nerve, lateral plantar branch, to the flexor digiti minimi brevis
- G. Other

III. Cranial nerves and trunk

- A. Cranial nerve VII (facial motor nerve)
    1. Facial nerve to the frontalis
    2. Facial nerve to the nasalis
    3. Facial nerve to the orbicularis oculi
    4. Facial nerve to the orbicularis oris
- B. Cranial nerve XI (spinal accessory motor nerve)
- C. Cranial nerve XII (hypoglossal motor nerve)
- D. Intercostal motor nerve
- E. Phrenic motor nerve to the diaphragm
- F. Recurrent laryngeal nerve
- G. Other

IV. Nerve roots

- A. Cervical nerve root stimulation
    1. Cervical level 5 (CT)
    2. Cervical level 6 (C6)
    3. Cervical level 7 (C7)
    4. Cervical level 8 (C8)
- B. Thoracic nerve root stimulation
    1. Thoracic level 1 (T1)
    2. Thoracic level 2 (T2)
    3. Thoracic level 3 (T3)
    4. Thoracic level 4 (T4)
    5. Thoracic level 5 (T5)
    6. Thoracic level 6 (T6)
    7. Thoracic level 7 (T7)
    8. Thoracic level 8 (T8)
    9. Thoracic level 9 (T9)
    10. Thoracic level 10 (T10)
    11. Thoracic level 11 (T11)
    12. Thoracic level 12 (T12)
- C. Lumbar nerve root stimulation
    1. Lumbar level 1 (L1)
    2. Lumbar level 2 (L2)
    3. Lumbar level 3 (L3)
    4. Lumbar level 4 (L4)
    5. Lumbar level 5 (L5)
- D. Sacral nerve root stimulation
    1. Sacral level 1 (S1)
    2. Sacral level 2 (S2)

3. Sacral level 3 (S3)
4. Sacral level 4 (S4)

Code 95904 involves the following sensory and mixed nerves:

I. Upper extremity sensory and mixed nerves
   A. Lateral antebrachial cutaneous sensory nerve
   B. Medial antebrachial cutaneous sensory nerve
   C. Medial brachial cutaneous sensory nerve
   D. Median nerve
      1. Median sensory nerve to the first digit
      2. Median sensory nerve to the second digit
      3. Median sensory nerve to the third digit
      4. Median sensory nerve to the fourth digit
      5. Median palmar cutaneous sensory nerve
      6. Median palmar mixed nerve
   E. Posterior antebrachial cutaneous sensory nerve
   F. Radial sensory nerve
      1. Radial sensory nerve to the base of the thumb
      2. Radial sensory nerve to digit 1
   G. Ulnar nerve
      1. Ulnar dorsal cutaneous sensory nerve
      2. Ulnar sensory nerve to the fourth digit
      3. Ulnar sensory nerve to the fifth digit
      4. Ulnar palmar mixed nerve
   H. Intercostal sensory nerve
   I. Other
II. Lower extremity sensory and mixed nerves
   A. Lateral femoral cutaneous sensory nerve
   B. Medial calcaneal sensory nerve
   C. Medial femoral cutaneous sensory nerve
   D. Peroneal nerve
      1. Deep peroneal sensory nerve
      2. Superficial peroneal sensory nerve, medial dorsal cutaneous branch
      3. Superficial peroneal sensory nerve, intermediate dorsal cutaneous branch
   E. Posterior femoral cutaneous sensory nerve
   F. Saphenous nerve
      1. Saphenous sensory nerve (distal technique)
      2. Saphenous sensory nerve (proximal technique)
   G. Sural nerve
      1. Sural sensory nerve, lateral dorsal cutaneous branch
      2. Sural sensory nerve
   H. Tibial sensory nerve (digital nerve to toe 1)
   I. Tibial sensory nerve (medial plantar nerve)
   J. Tibial sensory nerve (lateral plantar nerve)
   K. Other

III. Head and trunk sensory nerves
   A. Dorsal nerve of the penis
   B. Greater auricular nerve
   C. Ophthalmic branch of the trigeminal nerve
   D. Pudendal sensory nerve
   E. Suprascapular sensory nerves
   F. Other

The following table provides a reasonable maximum number of studies performed per diagnostic category necessary for a physician to arrive at a diagnosis in 90% of patients with that final diagnosis. The numbers in each column represent the number of studies recommended. The appropriate number of studies to be performed is based upon the physician's discretion.

	Type of Study/Maximum Number of Studies				
		Nerve Conduction Studies (95900, 95903, 95904)		Other EMG Studies (95934, 95936, 95937)	
Indication	**Needle EMG (95860-95864 95867-95870)**	**Motor NCS With and/or Without F Wave**	**Sensory NCS**	**H-Reflex**	**Neuromuscular Junction Testing (Repetitive Stimulation)**
Carpal tunnel (unilateral)	1	3	4		
Carpal tunnel (bilateral)	2	4	6		
Radiculopathy	2	3	2	2	
Mononeuropathy	1	3	3	2	
Polyneuropathy/mononeuropathy multiplex	3	4	4	2	
Myopathy	2	2	2		2
Motor neuronopathy (eg, ALS)	4	4	2		2
Plexopathy	2	4	6	2	
Neuromuscular junction	2	2	2		3
Tarsal tunnel syndrome (unilateral)	1	4	4		
Tarsal tunnel syndrome (bilateral)	2	5	6		
Weakness, fatigue, cramps, or twitching (focal)	2	3	4		2
Weakness, fatigue, cramps, or twitching (general)	4	4	4		2
Pain, numbness, or tingling (unilateral)	1	3	4	2	
Pain, numbness, or tingling (bilateral)	2	4	6	2	

Appendix K

Product Pending FDA Approval

Some vaccine products have been assigned a CPT Category I code in anticipation of future approval from the Food and Drug Administration (FDA). Following is a list of the vaccine product codes pending FDA approval status that are identified in the CPT codebook with the ✗ symbol. Upon revision of the approval status by the FDA, notation of this revision will be provided via the AMA CPT "Category I Vaccine Codes" Internet listings (www.ama-assn.org/ama/pub/category/10902.html) and in subsequent publications of the CPT codebook.

90649

90680

90698

90710

90715

90736

Appendix L

✍ Rationale

The vascular families table in Appendix L identifies the applicable vessels within a vascular family. This appendix is provided as a resource to assist in the assignment of procedure codes based upon the vascular family and the order of the vessel within the family from the point of origin.

Vascular Families

Note: Assignment of branches to first, second, and third order in this table makes the assumption that the starting point is catheterization of the aorta. This categorization would not be accurate, for instance, if a femoral or carotid artery were catheterized directly in an antegrade direction. Arteries highlighted in bold are those more commonly reported during arteriographic procedures.

First Order	Second Order Branch	Third Order Branch	Beyond Third Order Branches
Innominate	**R. common carotid**	**R. internal carotid**	R. ophthalmic R. p. communicating R. middle cerebral R. a. cerebral
		R. external carotid	R. superior thyroid R. ascending pharyngeal R. facial R. lingual R. occipital R. p. auricular R. superficial temporal R. internal maxillary R. middle meningeal
	R. subclavian & axillary	**R. vertebral**	Basilar
		R. internal thoracic (internal mammary)	
		R. thyrocervical trunk	R. inferior thyroid R. suprascapular R. transverse cervical
		R. costocervical trunk	R. highest intercostal R. deep cervical
		R. lateral thoracic R. thoracoacromial R. humeral circumflex (A/P)	
		R. subscapular	R. circumflex scapular
		R. brachial	
		R. deep brachial	R. ulnar R. radial R. interosseous R. deep palmar arch R. superficial palmar arch R. metacarpals and digitals
L. common carotid	**L. internal carotid**	L. ophthalmic L. p. communicating L. middle cerebral L. a. cerebral	
	L. external carotid	L. superior thyroid L. ascending pharyngeal L. facial L. lingual L. occipital L. p. auricular L. superficial temporal	
		L. internal maxillary	L. middle meningeal

R = right, L = left, A = anterior, P = posterior

First Order	Second Order Branch	Third Order Branch	Beyond Third Order Branches
L. subclavian & axillary	**L. vertebral**		
	L. internal thoracic (internal mammary)		
	L. thyrocervical trunk	L. inferior thyroid	
		L. suprascapular	
		L. transverse cervical	
	L. costocervical trunk	L. highest intercostal	
		L. deep cervical	
	L. lateral thoracic		
	L. thoracoacromial		
	L. humeral circumflex (A/P)		
	L. subscapular	L. circumflex scapular	
	L. brachial		
	L. deep brachial	L. ulnar	
		L. radial	
		L. interosseous	L. deep palmar arch
			L. superficial palmar arch
			L. metacarpals and digitals
Intercostals			
Bronchials			
Recurrent esophageal			
Inferior phrenic	Superior suprarenal		
Celiac trunk	L. gastric	Esophageal branch	
	Splenic	Dorsal pancreatic	Inferior transverse pancreatic
		Great pancreatic	
		Caudal pancreatic	
		Gastroepiploic	
		Short gastrics	
	Common hepatic	Gastroduodenal	P. superior pancreaticoduodenal
			A. superior pancreaticoduodenal
		Proper hepatic	L. hepatic
			R. hepatic
			Cystic
			Gastroepiploic
			Supraduodenal
			Intermediate hepatic

R = right, L = left, A = anterior, P = posterior

First Order	Second Order Branch	Third Order Branch	Beyond Third Order Branches
Middle suprarenal			
Superior mesenteric	Middle colic		
	Inferior pancreaticoduodenal	P. inferior pancreaticoduodenal A. inferior pancreaticoduodenal	
	Jejunal		
	Ileocolic		
	Appendicular		
	P. cecal		
	A. cecal		
	Marginal		
	R. colic		
Renal	Inferior suprarenal		
Testicular / Ovarian			
Lumbar			
Inferior mesenteric	L. colic		
	Sigmoid	Rectosigmoid Superior rectal	

R = right, L = left, A = anterior, P = posterior

First Order	Second Order Branch	Third Order Branch	Beyond Third Order Branches
Middle sacral			
Common iliac	**Internal iliac**	Iliolumbar	
		Lateral sacral	
		Superior gluteal	
		Umbilical	
		Superior vesical	
		Obturator	
		Inferior vesical	
		Middle rectal	
		Inferior rectal	
		Internal pudendal	
		Inferior gluteal	
	External iliac	Inferior epigastric	Cremasteric
			Pubic
		Deep circumflex iliac	Ascending deep circumflex iliac
	Common femoral	**Profunda femoris**	Medial descending
			Perforating branches
			Lateral descending
			Lateral circumflex
		Deep external pudendal	
		Superficial external pudendal	
		Ascending lateral circumflex femoral	
		Descending lateral circumflex femoral	
		Transverse lateral circumflex femoral	
		Superficial femoral	Geniculate
			Popliteal
			A. tibial
			Peroneal
			P. tibial
R. & L. main pulmonary arteries (venous selective)			

Reference: Kadir S. *Atlas of Normal and Variant Angiographic Anatomy.* Philadephia, Pa: WB Saunders Co; 1991.

R = right, L = left, A = anterior, P = posterior

The Tabular Review of the Changes

The Tabular Review of the Changes

KEY: **Add** = Added
Del = Deleted
Rev = Revised
GR = Grammar revision
Cross = Cross-reference

Section/Code	Add	Del	Rev	GR	Cross
Anesthesia					
Obstetric					
01964		x			x
01965		x			
01966		x			
Other Procedures					
01995					x
Surgery					
Integumentary System					
Skin, Subcutaneous and Accessory Structures					
Excision Debridement					
11008					x
Repair (Closure)					
12001				x	
Skin Replacement Surgery and Skin Substitutes					
Surgical Preparation					
15000			x		x
15001				x	x
Grafts					
Autograft/Tissue Cultured Autograft					
15040	x				
15100			x		

Section/Code	Add	Del	Rev	GR	Cross
Autograft/Tissue Cultured Autograft—continued					
15110	x				
15111	x				x
15115	x				
15116	x				x
15120			x		
15130	x				
15131	x				x
15135	x				
15136	x				x
15150	x				
15151	x				x
15152	x				x
15155	x				
15156	x				x
15157	x				x
Acellular Dermal Replacement					
15170	x				
15171	x				x
15175	x				
15176	x				x
Allograft/Tissue Cultured Allogeneic Skin Substitute					
15300	x				
15301	x				x
15320	x				
15321	x				x
15330	x				
15331	x				x
15335	x				
15336	x				x

Section/Code	Add	Del	Rev	GR	Cross
15340	x				
15341	x				x
15342		x			x
15343		x			x
15350		x			x
15351		x			x
15360	x				
15361	x				x
15365	x				
15366	x				x
Xenograft					
15400			x		
15401			x		
15420	x				
15421	x				x
15430	x				
15431	x				x
Other Procedures					
15810		x			
15811		x			x
Burns, Local Treatment					
16010		x			
16015		x			x
16020			x		
16025			x		
16030			x		
16036					x
Breast					
Excision					
19272					x

Section/Code	Add	Del	Rev	GR	Cross
Musculoskeletal System					
20000				X	
Head					
21010				X	
Fracture and/or Dislocation					
21493		X			
21494		X			X
21495					X
Neck (Soft Tissues) and Thorax					
Incision					
21501					X
Spine (Vertebral Column)					
21935				X	
Incision					
22010	X				
22015	X				X
Vertebral Body, Embolization or Injection					
22523	X				
22524	X				
22525	X				X
Forearm and Wrist					
25000				X	
Foot and Toes					
Repair, Revision, and/or Reconstruction					
28297				X	
Other Procedures					
28890	X				X
Application of Casts and Strapping					
29000					X

Section/Code	Add	Del	Rev	GR	Cross
Endoscopy/Arthroscopy					
29866					x
29867					x
29868					x

Respiratory System

Section/Code	Add	Del	Rev	GR	Cross
Nose					
Excision					
30130			x		x
30140			x		x
Destruction					
30801			x		x
30802					x
Other Procedures					
30930			x		x
Larynx					
Endoscopy					
31526			x		
31531			x		
31536			x		
31541			x		
31561			x		
31571			x		
Repair					
31585		x			
31586		x			x
Trachea and Bronchi					
Endoscopy					
31620					x

Section/Code	Add	Del	Rev	GR	Cross
Lungs and Pleura					
Incision					
32002					X
32020					X
32100					X
32160					X
Excision					
32445					X
32500					X
32503	X				
32504	X				X
32520		X			
32522		X			
32525		X			X
Surgical Collapse Therapy; Thoracoplasty					
32900					X
Cardiovascular System					
Heart and Pericardium					
Wounds of the Heart and Great Vessels					
33315				X	
Cardiac Valves					
Pulmonary Valve					
33478					X
Coronary Artery Anomalies					
33502			X		
33507	X				
Arterial Grafting for Coronary Artery Bypass					
33548	X				X
Single Ventricle and Other Complex Cardiac Anomalies					
33608					X

Section/Code	Add	Del	Rev	GR	Cross
33617					X
Shunting Procedures					
33768	X				X
Endovascular Repair of Descending Thoracic Aorta					
33880	X				X
33881	X				X
33883	X				X
33884	X				X
33886	X				X
33889	X				X
33891	X				X
Pulmonary Artery					
33918		X			
33919		X			X
33924					X
33925	X				
33926	X				X
Arteries and Veins					
Endovascular Repair of Abdominal Aortic Aneurysm					
34833			X		
34834			X		
Direct Repair of Aneurysm or Excision (Partial or Total) and Graft Insertion for Aneurysm, Pseudoaneurysm, Ruptured Aneurysm, and Associated Occlusive Disease					
35001					X
Bypass Graft					
Other Than Vein					
35606					X
Arterial Transposition					
35694					X
Venous					
36400				X	

Section/Code	Add	Del	Rev	GR	Cross
Central Venous Access Procedures					
Other Central Venous Access Procedures					
36598	x				x
Transcatheter Procedures					
Arterial Mechanical Thrombectomy					
37184	x				x
37185	x				x
37186	x				x
Venous Mechanical Thrombectomy					
37187	x				x
37188	x				x
Other Procedures					
37205					x
37209			x		
Ligation					
37700					x
37718	x				x
37720		x			x
37722	x				x
37730		x			x
37735					x

Digestive System

Salivary Gland and Ducts

Section/Code	Add	Del	Rev	GR	Cross
Incision					
42325		x			
42326		x			x

Esophagus

Section/Code	Add	Del	Rev	GR	Cross
Endoscopy					
43239					x

Section/Code	Add	Del	Rev	GR	Cross
Stomach					
Excision					
43638		x			
43639		x			x
Bariatric Surgery					
Laparoscopy					
43770	x				x
43771	x				
43772	x				
43773	x				x
43774	x				x
Other Procedures					
43848			x		x
43886	x				
43887	x				
43888	x				x
Intestines (Except Rectum)					
Incision					
44005					x
Laparoscopy					
Incision					
44180	x				
Enterostomy—External Fistulization of Intestines					
44186	x				
44187	x				x
44188	x				x
44200		x			x
44201		x			x
Excision					
44202			x		

Section/Code	Add	Del	Rev	GR	Cross
Excision—*continued*					
44213	x				x
Repair					
44227	x				x
Other Procedures					
44239		x			x
Enterostomy—External Fistulization of Intestines					
44310			x		x
44320			x		x
Repair					
44626					x
Rectum					
Excision					
45110					x
45119			x		x
Laparoscopy					
Excision					
45395	x				x
45397	x				x
Repair					
45400	x				x
45402	x				x
45499	x				
Repair					
45540			x		x
45550			x		x
Other Procedures					
45990	x				x
45999					x

Section/Code	Add	Del	Rev	GR	Cross
Anus					
Introduction					
46505	x				x
Repair					
46710	x				
46712	x				
Abdomen, Peritoneum, and Omentum					
Excision, Destruction					
49201					x

Urinary System

Section/Code	Add	Del	Rev	GR	Cross
Kidney					
Excision					
50250	x				x
Introduction					
Renal Pelvis Catheter Procedures					
Internally Dwelling					
50382	x				x
50384	x				x
Externally Accessible					
50387	x				x
50389	x				x
Laparoscopy					
50542					x
Other Procedures					
50592	x				x
Ureter					
Introduction					
50688			x		

Section/Code	Add	Del	Rev	GR	Cross
Bladder					
Laparoscopy					
51999	X				
Vesical Neck and Prostate					
52647			X		
52648			X		
Male Genital System					
Prostate					
Incision					
55700					X
Female Genital System					
Vagina					
Repair					
57295	X				
Endoscopy					
57421			X		X
Cervix Uteri					
Endoscopy					
57461					X
Corpus Uteri					
Excision					
58100					X
58110	X				X
Maternity Care and Delivery					
Cesarean Delivery					
59510				X	
59515				X	
59525				X	

Section/Code	Add	Del	Rev	GR	Cross
Nervous System					
Skull, Meninges, and Brain					
Endovascular Therapy					
61630	x				
61635	x				x
61640	x				
61641	x				
61642	x				x
Extracranial Nerves, Peripheral Nerves, and Autonomic Nervous System					
Destruction by Neurolytic Agent (eg, Chemical, Thermal, Electrical or Radiofrequency)					
Somatic Nerves					
64613			x		
64614					x
Sympathetic Nerves					
64650	x				
64653	x				x
Eye and Ocular Adnexa					
Anterior Segment					
Anterior Sclera					
Excision					
66172					x
Ocular Adnexa					
Eyelids					
Repair (Brow Ptosis, Blepharoptosis, Lid Retraction, Ectropion, Entropion)					
67901			x		
67902			x		
Auditory System					
Middle Ear					
Introduction					
69410		x			x

Radiology

Diagnostic Radiology (Diagnostic Imaging)

Section/Code	Add	Del	Rev	GR	Cross
Head and Neck					
70470					x
70482					x
70488					x
70492					x
Chest					
71270					x
Spine and Pelvis					
72133					x
72194					x
Upper Extremities					
73202					x
Lower Extremities					
73702					x
Abdomen					
74170					x
Vascular Procedures					
Veins and Lymphatics					
75801				x	
Transcatheter Procedures					
75900			x		
75956	x				x
75957	x				x
75958	x				x
75959	x				x
Other Procedures					
76012			x		
76013					x

Section/Code	Add	Del	Rev	GR	Cross
76362					X
76375		X			X
76376	X				X
76377	X				X
76394					X

Diagnostic Ultrasound

Ultrasonic Guidance Procedures

76940					X

Radiation Oncology

Radiation Treatment Delivery

77412			X		
77421	X				X

Neutron Beam Treatment Delivery

77422	X				
77423	X				

Hyperthermia

77600				X	

Nuclear Medicine

Diagnostic

Hematopoietic, Reticuloendothelial and Lymphatic System

78160		X			
78162		X			
78170		X			
78172		X			X

Cardiovascular System

78455		X			X
78472					X

Other Procedures

78810					X

Section/Code	Add	Del	Rev	GR	Cross

Pathology and Laboratory

Therapeutic Drug Assays

80195	X				

Consultations (Clinical Pathology)

80502				X	

Chemistry

82180				X	
82270			X		
82271	X				
82272	X				
82273		X			
82274					X
82726					X
83036			X		
83037	X				
83090				X	
83630			X		
83631	X				
83695	X				
83700	X				
83701	X				
83704	X				
83715		X			
83716		X			X
83721					X
83890					X
83898			X		
83900	X				
83901			X		X

Section/Code	Add	Del	Rev	GR	Cross
83907	X				
83908	X				X
83909	X				
83914	X				
84238			X		

Immunology

86000					X
86064		X			X
86200	X				
86355	X				
86357	X				
86367	X				X
86379		X			X
86480	X				
86580					X
86585		X			X
86587		X			X

Transfusion Medicine

86923	X				X
86960	X				

Microbiology

87177					X
87209	X				
87900	X				
87901					X
87904			X		

Cytopathology

88173					X
88175			X		

Section/Code	Add	Del	Rev	GR	Cross

Surgical Pathology

88333	x				
88334	x				x
88384	x				
88385	x				
88386	x				x

Other Procedures

89049	x				

Reproductive Medicine Procedures

89320				x	

Medicine

Immunization Administration for Vaccines/Toxoids

90465					x

Vaccines, Toxoids

90649	x				
90680			x		
90713			x		
90714	x				
90715			x		
90736	x				

Hydration, Therapeutic, Prophylactic, and Diagnostic Injections and Infusions (Excludes Chemotherapy)

90749					x
Hydration					
90760	x				x
90761	x				x
Therapeutic, Prophylactic, and Diagnostic Injections and Infusions					
90765	x				

Section/Code	Add	Del	Rev	GR	Cross
90766	x				x
90767	x				x
90768	x				x
90772	x				x
90773	x				
90774	x				x
90775	x				x
90779	x				x
Therapeutic or Diagnostic Infusions (Excludes Chemotherapy)					
90780		x			
90781		x			
Therapeutic, Prophylactic or Diagnostic Injections					
90782		x			
90783		x			
90784		x			
90788		x			
90799		x			
Psychiatry					
90801				x	
Psychiatric Therapeutic Procedures					
Other Psychiatric Services or Procedures					
90862					x
90870			x		
90871		x			x
Dialysis					
Hemodialysis					
90939		x			x
90940			x		

Section/Code	Add	Del	Rev	GR	Cross
Gastroenterology					
91022	X				X
91065				X	
Ophthalmology					
Ocular Prosthetics, Artificial Eye					
92330		X			
92335		X			
92340					X
Spectacle Services (Including Prosthesis for Aphakia)					
92371					X
Supply of Materials					
92390		X			
92391		X			
92392		X			
92393		X			
92395		X			
92396		X			
Special Otorhinolaryngologic Services					
92506			X		
92507			X		
92510		X			X
92520			X		X
Audiologic Function Tests With Medical Diagnostic Evaluation					
92568			X		
92569			X		
Evaluative and Therapeutic Services					
92602					X
92626	X				
92627	X				X

Section/Code	Add	Del	Rev	GR	Cross
92630	X				
92633	X				
Cardiovascular					
Cardiography					
93018					X
Intracardiac Electrophysiological Procedures/Studies					
93662					X
Non-Invasive Vascular Diagnostic Studies					
Cerebrovascular Arterial Studies					
93882					X
Allergy and Clinical Immunology					
Allergy Testing					
95078					X
Endocrinology					
95250			X		
95251	X				X
Neurology and Neuromuscular Procedures					
Muscle and Range of Motion Testing					
95858		X			
95860					X
Electromyography and Nerve Conduction Tests					
95865	X				X
95866	X				
95873	X				
95874	X				X
95875					X
Intraoperative Neurophysiology					
95920				X	

Section/Code	Add	Del	Rev	GR	Cross
Central Nervous System Assessments/Tests (eg, Neuro-Cognitive, Mental Status, Speech Testing)					
96100		X			
96101	X				X
96102	X				
96103	X				
96115		X			X
96116	X				
96117		X			X
96118	X				
96119	X				
96120	X				
Chemotherapy Administration					
96400		X			
96401	X				X
Injection and Intravenous Infusion Chemotherapy					
96402	X				
96405			X		
96406			X		X
96408		X			
96409	X				
96410		X			
96411	X				X
96412		X			
96413	X				X
96414		X			
96415	X				X
96416	X				X
96417	X				X

Section/Code	Add	Del	Rev	GR	Cross
Intra-Arterial Chemotherapy					
96423			X		X
96425					X
Other Chemotherapy					
96520		X			
96521	X				X
96522	X				X
96523	X				X
96530		X			
96542					X
96545		X			
96549					X

Special Dermatological Procedures

96900				X	

Physical Medicine and Rehabilitation

Modalities					
Supervised					
97020		X			X
97024			X		
Therapeutic Procedures					
97504		X			X
97520		X			
97530					X
97542			X		
Tests and Measurements					
97703		X			X
Orthotic Management and Prosthetic Management					
97760	X				X
97761	X				
97762	X				

Section/Code	Add	Del	Rev	GR	Cross
Other Procedures					
97770					X
Acupuncture					
97810					X
97811			X		X
97813			X		X
97814			X		X
Education and Training for Patient Self-Management					
98960	X				X
98961	X				
98962	X				
Special Services, Procedures and Reports					
Miscellaneous Services					
99050			X		
99051	X				
99052		X			X
99053	X				
99054		X			X
99056			X		
99058			X		
99060	X				
99070					X
Sedation With or Without Analgesia (Conscious Sedation)					
99141		X			
99142		X			
Moderate (Conscious) Sedation					
99143	X				X
99144	X				
99145	X				X

Section/Code	Add	Del	Rev	GR	Cross
99148	X				
99149	X				
99150	X				X

Other Services and Procedures

99170					X

Evaluation and Management

Office or Other Outpatient Services

New Patient

99201				X	
99204				X	
99205				X	

Hospital Observation Services

99217				X	

Hospital Inpatient Services

Initial Hospital Care

New or Established Patient

99221				X	

Subsequent Hospital Care

99231				X	

Consultations

Initial Inpatient Consultations

New or Established Patient

99254				X	

Follow-Up Inpatient Consultations

Established Patient

99261		X			
99262		X			
99263		X			

Section/Code	Add	Del	Rev	GR	Cross
Confirmatory Consultations					
New or Established Patient					
99271		X			
99272		X			
99273		X			
99274		X			
99275		X			
99281					X

Continuing Intensive Care Services

99300	X				

Nursing Facility Services

Initial Nursing Facility Care					
New or Established Patient					
99301		X			
99302		X			
99303		X			X
99304	X				
99305	X				
99306	X				
Subsequent Nursing Facility Care					
New or Established Patient					
99307	X				
99308	X				
99309	X				
99310	X				
99311		X			
99312		X			
99313		X			X
Other Nursing Facility Services					
99318	X				X

Section/Code	Add	Del	Rev	GR	Cross
Domiciliary, Rest Home (eg, Boarding Home), or Custodial Care Services					
99321		X			X
New Patient					
99322		X			
99323		X			X
99324	X				
99325	X				
99326	X				
99327	X				
99328	X				
Established Patient					
99331		X			
99332		X			
99333		X			X
99334	X				
99335	X				
99336	X				
99337	X				
Domiciliary, Rest Home (eg, Assisted Living Facility), or Home Care Plan Oversight Services					
99339	X				X
99340	X				X
Prolonged Services					
Prolonged Physician Service With Direct (Face-To-Face) Patient Contact					
99354				X	
99356					X
Care Plan Oversight Services					
99374					X

Section/Code	Add	Del	Rev	GR	Cross

Category II Codes

0001F	X				X

Composite Measures

0005F	X				X

Patient History

1003F	X				
1004F	X				
1005F	X				
1006F	X				
1007F	X				
1008F	X				

Physical Examination

2000F				X	
2001F	X				
2002F	X				
2003F	X				
2004F	X				

Diagnostic/Screening Processes or Results

3000F	X				
3002F	X				

Therapeutic, Preventive or Other Interventions

4003F	X				
4011F				X	
4012F	X				
4014F	X				
4015F	X				X
4016F	X				
4017F	X				
4018F	X				

Section/Code	Add	Del	Rev	GR	Cross

Category III Codes

Section/Code	Add	Del	Rev	GR	Cross
0010T		X			X
0019T			X		X
0020T		X			X
0023T		X			X
0033T		X			X
0034T		X			X
0035T		X			X
0036T		X			X
0037T		X			X
0038T		X			X
0039T		X			X
0040T		X			X
0067T				X	

Online Medical Evaluation

Section/Code	Add	Del	Rev	GR	Cross
0078T			X		
0089T	X				
0090T	X				
0091T	X				
0092T	X				X
0093T	X				
0094T	X				
0095T	X				X
0096T	X				X
0097T	X				X
0098T	X				X
0099T	X				
0100T	X				
0101T	X				X
0102T	X				X

Section/Code	Add	Del	Rev	GR	Cross
Online Medical Evaluation—*continued*					
0103T	x				
0104T	x				
0105T	x				
0106T	x				
0107T	x				
0108T	x				
0109T	x				
0110T	x				
0111T	x				x
Medication Therapy Management					
0115T	x				
0116T	x				
0117T	x				x
0120T	x				x
0123T	x				
0124T	x				
0126T	x				
0130T	x				
0133T	x				
0135T	x				
0137T	x				x
0140T	x				

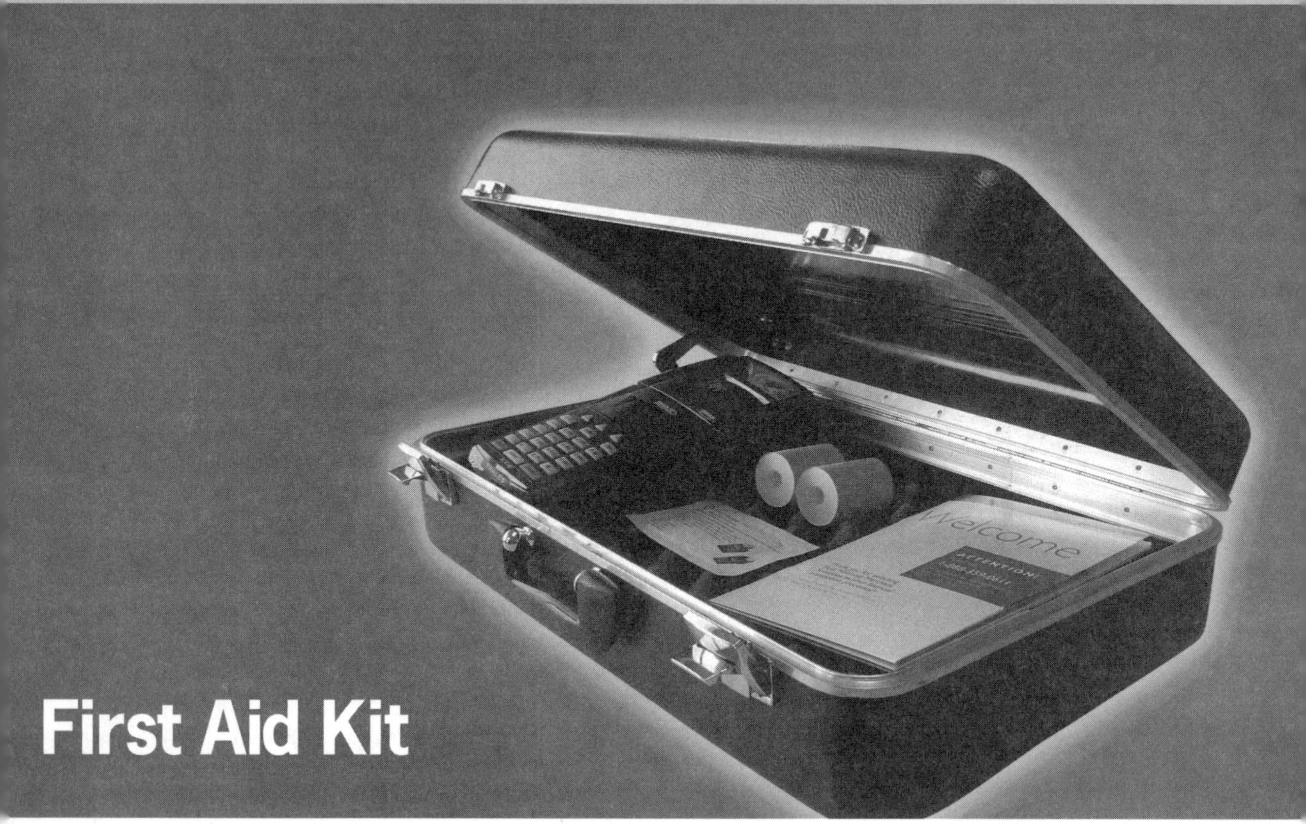
First Aid Kit